IM... GY
A SEL... OACH

IMMUNOLOGY
A SELF-INSTRUCTIONAL APPROACH

CATHERINE E. ROESEL
Professor of Cell and Molecular Biology
School of Medicine and School of Graduate Studies
Medical College of Georgia

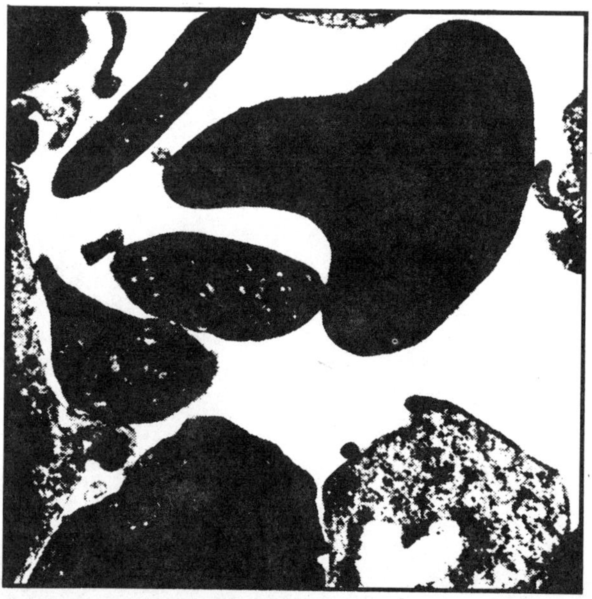

McGRAW-HILL BOOK COMPANY

New York St. Louis San Francisco Auckland Bogotá
Düsseldorf Johannesburg London Madrid Mexico
Montreal New Delhi Panama Paris São Paulo Singapore
Sydney Tokyo Toronto

Library of Congress Cataloging in Publication Data

Roesel, Catherine E.
Immunology: a self-instructional approach.

Bibliography: p.
Includes index.
1. Immunology. I. Title. [DNLM: 1. Immunology—Programmed texts. QW18 R718i]
QR181.R55 616.07'9 78-9319
ISBN 0-07-053411-X

IMMUNOLOGY: A SELF-INSTRUCTIONAL APPROACH

1 2 3 4 5 6 7 8 9 0 WHWH 7 8 3 2 1 0 9 8

This book was set in Press Roman by The Whitlock Press, Inc. The editor was Stuart D. Boynton; the copy editor was Elizabeth Richardson; the production supervisor was Milton J. Heiberg. The Whitlock Press, Inc., was printer and binder.

To the memory of

Dr. J. J. Bronfenbrenner

Pioneer in the field of immunology, former Chairman, Department of Microbiology and Immunology, Washington University School of Medicine, St. Louis, Missouri

Preface

Immunology has applications in all fields of medicine. The objective of this self-instructional book is to help students in the health sciences obtain a functional knowledge and working vocabulary of fundamental immunology.

In 1971 I attended a workshop in the preparation of self-instructional material, where the participants were required to prepare a short self-instructional package. Later I used this material with students; since the feedback was generally very favorable, I continued to prepare other packages, which were also well received. The self-instructional material was revised many times and with the encouragement of the publisher developed into this book.

I wish to thank Dr. Lloyd A. Lewis, Chairman of the Committee for the Development of Self-instructional Material, Medical College of Georgia, and the members of this committee for their interest and help. The illustrations were produced by the Section of Medical Illustration, Medical College of Georgia. Artwork was by Karen L. Waldo, Leslie A. Dessauer and Mickey Sentarik; photography was by Peter Ide. Special recognition is due Margaret R. Stafford and Marian T. Gregory for their assistance in preparation of the manuscript.

I wish to acknowledge the support of my Department Chairman, Dr. Titus H. J. Huisman, and the assistance of my colleagues, J. Fred Denton, Fred A. Garver, John C. Howard, William S. Harms, Beth Kenimer, David F. Lapp, Fred H. Leibach, Thomas F. McDonald, Betty P. Barton, Linda L. Smith and George H. Brownell.

Catherine E. Roesel

Introduction

The basic principles of immunology are presented in a stepwise manner. Since the subdivisions of immunology are highly interrelated, the most effective use of this self-instructional material is to start with Chap. 1 and proceed in order through Chap. 11; however, each chapter is written as an independent unit to cover the material outlined at the beginning of the chapter. Occasionally references are made to material in other chapters for more complete coverage. Instead of dividing the material into basic principles and clinical applications, the two are presented together. Learning appears easier for students when they are able to appreciate some of the practical applications of the material being studied.

Questions (with answers) are distributed throughout a chapter, and not placed at the end, so that students can check their comprehension of the material as they go. Sections of the book are numbered to facilitate cross-references. Specific references to the literature will be found at the end of each chapter. For a general review of the basic principles of immunology and their clinical applications Review Questions are included at the end of the book.

Chapter 2 is on B and T lymphocytes and their role in immune responses. Since B and T cells are now under intensive investigation, the information in Chap. 2 will probably be more subject to change during the next few years than that in other chapters. At present there are many areas of dispute, but controversial subjects have been avoided as much as possible. Not many years ago the function of lymphocytes was not known, but now an understanding of their role holds great promise, especially in such areas as organ transplantation and cancer therapy.

Chapter 11, included as an appendix, is on serologic tests used to help diagnose syphilis. Since *Treponema pallidum,* the causative agent of syphilis, has never been propagated in vitro in sufficient quantities for use as antigen in serologic tests, many of the common tests for syphilis employ a nonspecific antigen. It is very important for health science students to be aware of the limitations of these tests. *T. pallidum* propagated in vivo is available for a limited number of specific tests, the significance of which is discussed. The development of microtechniques in immunology has facilitated testing where reagents like *T. pallidum* antigen cannot be produced on a large scale.

Contents

IMMUNOLOGY
A SELF-INSTRUCTIONAL APPROACH

Recommended reading for students studying Human Biology (A.E.B. 642.). The sections listed below and marked with a pencil cross in the text are relevant to this syllabus. Sections 2.18-2.21 may be ommitted if the concepts are found too difficult or confusing.

Chapter 1: 1-1,-2,-3,-4,-5,-6,-7,-8,-9,-10,-11,-12,-13,-14,
-15,-16,-17,-18,-19,-20,-21,-22,-23,-24,-25
-26,-27,-28,-29,-30,-31.

Chapter 2: 2-1, -4, -6, -8,-9,-10, -12,-13,-14, -17,
(-18,-19,-20,-21,) -26,-27,-28, -34,-35,-36.

Chapter 3: 3-2,-3,-4,-5,-6, -9,-10, -12, Table 3-2,
-26, -28, -30.

Chapter 4: 4-1, -12.

Chapter 5: 5-1,-2, -5, -10, -16,-17,-18, -20,-21,-22,
-33,-34, table 5-4, -36, -40,-41, -47, -50.

Chapter 8: 8-6.

Chapter9: 9-1,-2, -4, -7,-8.

Do attempt those questions set on the sections read.

M.G.Y.

1

Resistance Mechanisms of the Host before and after Immunization

HOST AND PARASITE INTERACTIONS

1-1 The human host and parasitism by microorganisms will be considered. *Pathogenic microorganisms* are those which are able to cause disease. An infection occurs when microorganisms invade the tissues of the host and multiply there. Not all infections result in disease. A *subclinical infection* is one which is aborted and does not give rise to recognizable clinical infection or disease. A few pathogenic microorganisms are saprophytes rather than parasites in that they are unable to multiply on or in living tissue; e.g., *Corynebacterium diphtheriae*, the causative agent of diphtheria, multiplies in the throat on dead tissue and excretes a very powerful toxin called an *exotoxin*; thus it is the exotoxin which enters the bloodstream, is transported to all areas of the body, and causes a highly fatal disease if untreated. A similar situation exists with tetanus, which is caused by the production of an exotoxin excreted by *Clostridium tetani*, also a saprophyte. In a later discussion of specific resistance, we shall see that in both diphtheria and tetanus we must immunize against the exotoxin, not the microorganism. A substance called *toxoid* is used for active immunization against the effects of exotoxin. Toxoid is exotoxin which has been suitably detoxified. Of course, diphtheria toxoid must be used for diphtheria and tetanus toxoid must be used for tetanus.

1-2 Pathogenic microorganisms are relatively few in number compared with the numbers of microorganisms existing around us everywhere. Nonpathogenic bacteria carry out many essential activities. If it were not for bacteria, dead plants and animals would not undergo decay with the return of simple chemical substances to the environment. Most of these bacteria are harmless to human beings because they are unable to overcome the natural or innate barriers of the human host to infection. We speak of these natural barriers as being *nonspecific* because they serve as barriers to many different species of microorganisms in our environment. Sometimes when the natural defense mechanisms are lowered, e.g., by trauma or certain drugs, bacteria which usually are not pathogenic will invade the tissues and cause reactions leading to disease. Such microorganisms are termed *opportunists*.

1-3 Microorganisms like bacteria and viruses contain chemical substances called *antigens*. An antigen or antigenic substance has a structure which stimulates an immune response in the host. Usually in order to be antigenic, a substance must appear foreign to the host. One type of immune response is the production of *antibody*. Antibody is a globulin and is found in serum. An outstanding characteristic of antibodies is that they react very specifically with the antigens which stimulated their production. For example, antibody elicited in response to infection with poliomyelitis virus reacts with that virus and not with viruses like influenza. Naturally occurring antigens are usually proteins of high molecular weight although certain high-molecular-weight polysaccharides, e.g., those making up the capsules of pneumococci, are antigenic in human beings and in some other animal species but not all. *Specific resistance* refers to resistance to a particular microorganism through previous exposure to an antigen of that microorganism.

1-4 To prevent or control an infectious disease it is often necessary to know how the causative (or *etiologic*) agent enters and leaves the body. These pathways are commonly referred to as *portals of entry* and *portals of exit*. Portals of entry are listed in Table 1-1 with some familiar examples.

Some of the ways by which microorganisms leave the body are as follows:

Exudate from skin lesion

Droplet nuclei from respiratory tract; discharges from the mouth and nose

Blood removed by biting insects or by needles and syringes

Feces

Urine

Exudate from lesion on the genitalia

Exudate from eye

1-5 The *incubation period* is the interval between the time of exposure and the appearance of symptoms of disease. Whether or not infection occurs after exposure depends mainly on the virulence of the microorganism, the number of organisms to which the host is exposed, and the

Table 1-1 Portals of Entry

Portal of entry	Examples of microorganisms entering at portal
Skin	Staphylococcus by wounds Rabies virus by bite of rabid dog Malaria parasite by bite of mosquito Hepatitis viruses by injection of infected blood or serum; use of virus-contaminated instruments
Respiratory tract	Meningococcus, german measles virus
Alimentary tract	Typhoid bacillus, poliomyelitis virus, hepatitis viruses
Genitourinary tract	Gonococcus, spirochete of syphilis
Eye	Trachoma agent
Placenta	Spirochete of syphilis, german measles virus

resistance of the host. If the portal of entry is one by which the microorganism normally invades, the above three-factors can be combined into the following equation:

$$\text{Infection} = \frac{\text{virulence} \times \text{number (microorganism)}}{\text{resistance (host)}}$$

Questions for Secs. 1-1 to 1-5

1. What is a pathogenic microorganism?
2. What is a parasite?
3. What is a saprophyte?
4. (*a*) Can saprophytes be pathogenic? (*b*) If your answer is yes, give an example.
5. What is a subclinical infection?
6. What is meant by an opportunist or opportunistic microorganism?
7. What is an antigen or antigenic substance?
8. What is antibody?
9. What is the difference between nonspecific and specific resistance of the host to infection?

*The section of the text in which the material was presented is given in parentheses at the end of each answer. Occasionally details not found in the text are included in an answer.

10. Name five portals of entry whereby microorganisms can invade the host.
11. What is the incubation period of an infectious disease?
12. Name three factors which may determine whether or not an infection will occur after exposure to a microorganism.

Answers*

1. A pathogenic microorganism is one capable of causing disease in the host. (Sec. 1-1.)
2. A parasite is an organism capable of multiplying on or in living tissue. (Sec. 1-1.)
3. A saprophyte is an organism incapable of multiplying on or in living tissue; it grows on dead tissue. (Sec. 1-1.)
4. (*a*) Yes, some saprophytes are pathogens. (*b*) The bacteria which cause diphtheria and tetanus multiply on damaged tissue in a localized area of the body but are pathogens because they excrete a very harmful exotoxin which must be neutralized in order to save a patient's life. (Sec. 1-1.)
5. A subclinical infection is an infection which is cleared up by the body shortly after the infection begins, so that clinical symptoms of the disease do not appear. (Sec. 1-1.)
6. Opportunists, or opportunistic microorganisms, especially bacteria and fungi, are microorganisms which are not usually considered pathogens but which may cause disease if the resistance of the host is decreased. (Sec. 1-2.)
7. An antigen or antigenic substance is one which is capable of stimulating an immune response such as the production of antibody; antigens are usually (but not always) foreign proteins of high molecular weight. (Sec. 1-3.)
8. Antibody is a globulin which reacts very specifically with the antigen which elicited it. (Sec. 1-3.)
9. Nonspecific resistance refers to the general defense mechanisms of the host against a wide variety of microorganisms; specific resistance is due to an immune response which is effective against a particular microorganism. (Sec. 1-3.)
10. Portals of entry of the host for microorganisms are the skin, respiratory tract, alimentary tract, genitourinary tract, eye, and placenta. (Sec. 1-4.)
11. The incubation period of an infectious disease is the time between exposure to the microorganism and the development of clinical symptoms of disease. (Sec. 1-5.)

12. Three factors which are important in the initiation of an infection are the virulence and number of microorganisms to which the host is exposed and the resistance of the host. (Sec. 1-5.)

NONSPECIFIC (INNATE) RESISTANCE OF THE HOST TO INFECTION

1-6 *Nonspecific resistance* of the host refers to mechanisms of resistance which are present at the time of birth or which develop naturally due to maturation of the host. Nonspecific resistance mechanisms may be due to the following:

1. Factors such as age, race, species, nutrition, and hormones
2. Physical barriers at the portal of entry
3. Chemical barriers, e.g., the high acidity of gastric contents and the bactericidal action of fatty acids of the skin for some bacteria
4. Biochemical tissue constituents, e.g., interferon
5. Normal flora and antagonism of the normal flora for other microorganisms
6. Alternate complement pathway
7. Phagocytosis
   a. Reticuloendothelial or macrophage system (mononuclear phagocytes)
   b. Neutrophils (polymorphonuclear leukocytes) of the blood
8. Inflammatory response

1-7 Not all aspects of nonspecific resistance will be discussed here; emphasis will be placed on specific resistance and on the basic principles of immunology. Nonspecific resistance is just as important to the host as specific resistance, and possibly even more important, because it is effective against many different microorganisms; when nonspecific resistance breaks down, specific resistance often does also. For example, the antibody *opsonin* reacts with microorganisms like pneumococci so that the pneumococci are more easily phagocytized and destroyed. Pneumococcus has a capsule which repels phagocytes, but when antibody (opsonin) reacts with the capsular polysaccharide, this organism is easily phagocytized. Phagocytosis is a process in which host cells, such as macrophages, take up or engulf foreign particles, such as microorganisms. When phagocytosis occurs after reaction of the microorganism with opsonin, the process is called *opsonization.* Opsonization is an example of a specific resistance of the host (opsonin) that is dependent on a nonspecific resistance mechanism (phagocytosis).

1-8 Opsonization is increased by the presence of *complement*, a heat-labile protein which has several components and is present in normal serum. The term *heat-labile opsonin* has been used to refer to complement in opsonization. The complement system is described in Chap. 3. Heat-stable opsonin is an antibody. Most antibodies are considered to be heat-stable in that they are not inactivated at 56°C for 30 min. Complement is inactivated in this way. In addition to its role in opsonization, complement is associated with many other reactions in the host, both specific and nonspecific. Complement is also used with in vitro serologic tests (Sec. 4-37). The alternate complement pathway (Sec. 3-34) is considered a nonspecific resistance mechanism since it does not require an antigen-antibody reaction for activation.

Reticuloendothelial System Phagocytosis

Mononuclear Phagocytes or Macrophages and the Reticuloendothelial System

1-9 The reticuloendothelial system (RES) is also known as the macrophage system or the mononuclear phagocyte system (MPS). Figure 2-1 shows a transmission electron micrograph of rat spleen. One of the cells shown is a macrophage which contains fragments of red blood cells and leukocytes. Macrophages remove from the circulation old or damaged cellular material of the host and foreign material such as microorganisms which gain entrance to the host's tissues. Ingested material is broken down by a variety of hydrolytic enzymes, which are contained in cytoplasmic granules known as *lysosomes*; however, not all microorganisms are destroyed after being phagocytized by macrophages. In addition to playing an important role in nonspecific resistance, macrophages participate in immune reactions, which will be considered later.

1-10 Macrophages constitute a separate cell line which originates in the bone marrow as promonocytes. The promonocytes undergo division to form monocytes, which go to the bloodstream and after a brief period of circulation move on to the tissues to form macrophages. Macrophages are usually larger and more phagocytic than monocytes. Blood monocytes range from about 12 to 18 μm, while tissue macrophages range from 25 to 50 μm. Stages in the development of macrophages or mononuclear phagocytes are outlined in Table 1-2. Macrophages are often referred to by different names according to tissue locations (Table 1-3).

1-11 In 1882 Metchnikoff first observed ingestion of foreign material by phagocytes and recognized phagocytosis as a mechanism of resistance. By derivation phagocyte means "eating cell." Metchnikoff used the term macrophages (*macro-* means "large") to refer to tissue histiocytes and microphages (*micro-* means "small") for polymorphonuclear leukocytes of the blood. He observed that macrophages are capable of ingesting large particles, e.g., damaged red blood cells, but that microphages ingest smaller particles, e.g., bacteria. In 1924 Aschoff viewed the macrophages of the host as belonging to a functional system which he called the *reticuloendothelial system.* In other words, the total body pool of macrophages constitutes the reticuloendothelial system. It was shown that if vital dyes or carbon particles are injected intravenously into an experimental animal, the dye or particles will be taken up by the macrophages. This technique makes it easy to trace where the macrophages are localized throughout the body. The name reticuloendothelial came from Aschoff's observation that organs where macrophages localize, e.g., the spleen, are composed of a network of supporting reticular cells which may become phagocytic; endothelial cells which line the sinusoids in these organs appeared to Aschoff to differ from the endothelial cells which line ordinary blood capillaries in seeming to be much more phagocytic. These observations were made with a light microscope. More recent studies with the electron microscope indicate that the sinusoids of bone marrow and spleen are

Table 1-2 Origin and Development of Mononuclear Phagocytes

Bone Marrow	Blood	Tissues
Promonocyte		
(cell division)		
monocyte ↙ ↘ monocyte →	→ monocyte (reduced capacity to divide) →	→ macrophage (may divide under certain stimuli)
↓ macrophage		

Table 1-3 Names for Macrophages According to Tissue Locations

Location	Name	Location	Name
Connective tissue	Histiocyte	Serous cavity	Peritoneal macrophage
Liver	Kupffer cell	Bone tissue	Osteoclast
Lung	Alveolar macrophage or "dust" cell	Nervous system	Microglial cell
Spleen		Spleen	Sinusoidal lining cell

lined with endothelial cells which are probably no more phagocytic than ordinary endothelium; the endothelial cells of sinusoids are associated very closely with macrophages which are just outside their walls or project between them.

Neutrophilic Polymorphonuclear Leukocytes

1-12 *Neutrophilic polymorphonuclear leukocytes* (or *neutrophils*) are actively phagocytic cells which are important in maintaining host resistance. Neutrophils have a markedly lobulated nucleus, and it is because of the many shapes the nucleus can assume that the neutrophils have been described as polymorphonuclear or polymorphs. Neutrophils are about 10 to 12 μm. They are present in the blood in large numbers, which increase with a slight infection. Neutrophils do not multiply, but a reserve pool of mature neutrophils is stored in bone marrow. Neutrophils may migrate out of blood vessels into tissues where infection has been initiated. They can function effectively under both aerobic and anaerobic conditions. Neutrophils or polymorphonuclear neutrophils (PMN) are also called granulocytes because they characteristically have granules in their cytoplasm. These granules, known as *lysosomes,* contain enzymes which are released on contact with phagocytized material and act to degrade it. It was pointed out earlier that encapsulation of microorganisms often prevents phagocytosis; however, phagocytosis may take place even in the absence of opsonins if the phagocytes are able to trap encapsulated microorganisms in some manner, e.g., against tissue surfaces, between other leukocytes, or in the mesh of fibrin clots. Destruction occurs after ingestion with the exception of a few microorganisms which are able to survive and even to multiply within the phagocyte. When opsonins are present, they provide a means for attachment of microorganisms to the surface of phagocytes so that phagocytes do not have to trap microorganisms against a surface in order to phagocytize them. Figure 1-1 shows the major events which occur during phagocytosis of a pneumococcus after reaction with opsonins. When antibody is involved, resistance becomes specific. The attraction of a phagocyte to an object is known as *chemotaxis.* Ordinarily neutrophils move in a zigzag pattern, but under the influence of chemotactic substances, e.g., certain complement components, the neutrophils move in a straight line. Phagocytosis should not be confused with pinocytosis, which means "cell drinking." It proceeds at the surface of the cell by the cell's taking in water globules within vacuoles by invagination of the plasma membrane in a manner similar to phagocytosis of particulate matter. Pinocytosis and phagocytosis are both examples of endocytosis.

Blood Leukocytes

1-13 In addition to neutrophils, there are two other kinds of blood granulocytes based on the staining characteristics of their cytoplasmic granules, namely *eosinophils* and *basophils.* Blood leukocytes may be classified as granular and nongranular leukocytes, as shown in Table 1-4, which also gives the mean percentage of each type of leukocyte in blood. Mature granulocytes are end cells, incapable of further differentiation or of mitotic division. After 8 to 12 h in the blood, they leave the circulation at random times and go to the tissues, where they survive for only a few days. In mature granulocytes, the granules of eosinophils and basophils, stained by Wright's blood stain, are more prominent than those of neutrophils. Eosinophils and basophils are similar in size to neutrophils. Eosinophils contain acidophilic granules, which are lysosomes. Eosinophils become more numerous in blood during parasitic infestations and allergic diseases (Chap. 5). They are reported to be phagocytic with a preference for antigen-antibody complexes. Eosinophils also have been reported to play a role in removing toxic substances such as histamine. The phagocytic ability of basophils does not appear to be great. Basophils are very similar to tissue mast cells, and their granules, like those of tissue mast cells, contain heparin and histamine; the release of histamine from tissue mast cells and basophils is responsible for some immediate-type allergic reactions (Chap. 5). Lymphocytes known as B and T lymphocytes, described in Chap. 2, are the main cells responsible for immune responses of the host. Stem cells under the influence of a lymphoid structure, the bursa of Fabricius of chickens and an equivalent lymphoid structure in human beings, develop into B lymphocytes. On contact with antigen B lymphocytes differentiate into plasma cells, which

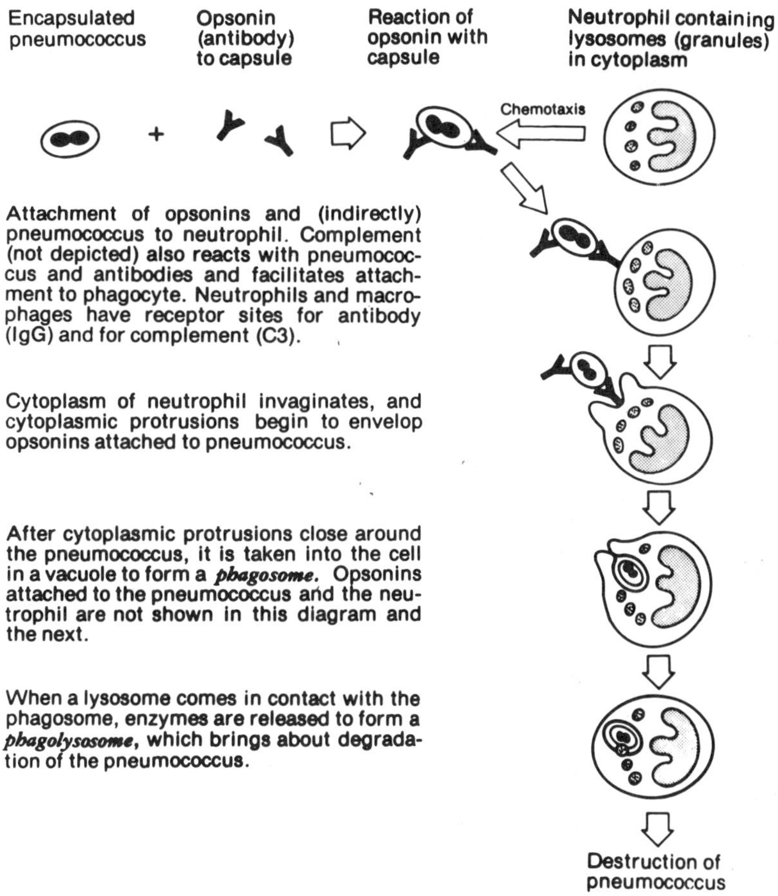

Figure 1-1 Phagocytosis of a pneumococcus by a polymorphonuclear neutrophil after reaction of the pneumococcus with opsonins.

secrete antibodies. Stem cells under the influence of another lymphoid organ, the thymus, differentiate into T lymphocytes. On contact with antigen T lymphocytes become activated to carry out cell-mediated immune reactions. Figure 1-2 shows the derivation of lymphocytes, other cells discussed in this chapter, and platelets. *Platelets* (also called *thrombocytes*) are nonnucleated cells formed from the cytoplasm of megakaryocytes. In human beings megakaryocytes are found only in bone marrow and along the walls of vascular sinuses, into which their pseudopodia extend, giving rise to platelets. Platelets are essential for blood clotting. Platelets are also involved in some reactions which are not favorable to the host, e.g., hypersensitivity (Sec. 5-32), and in autoimmune reactions to platelets, e.g., thrombocytopenic purpura (Sec. 6-7). Platelets have a life-span of about 10 days.

Table 1-4 White Blood Cells (Leukocytes) and Mean Percentage of Each Type in Blood*

Granular	%	Nongranular	%
Neutrophils	59.0	Monocytes	4.0
Eosinophils	2.7	Lymphocytes	34.0
Basophils	0.3		

*Normal white blood cell count is 5 to 9 × 10^9 per liter.

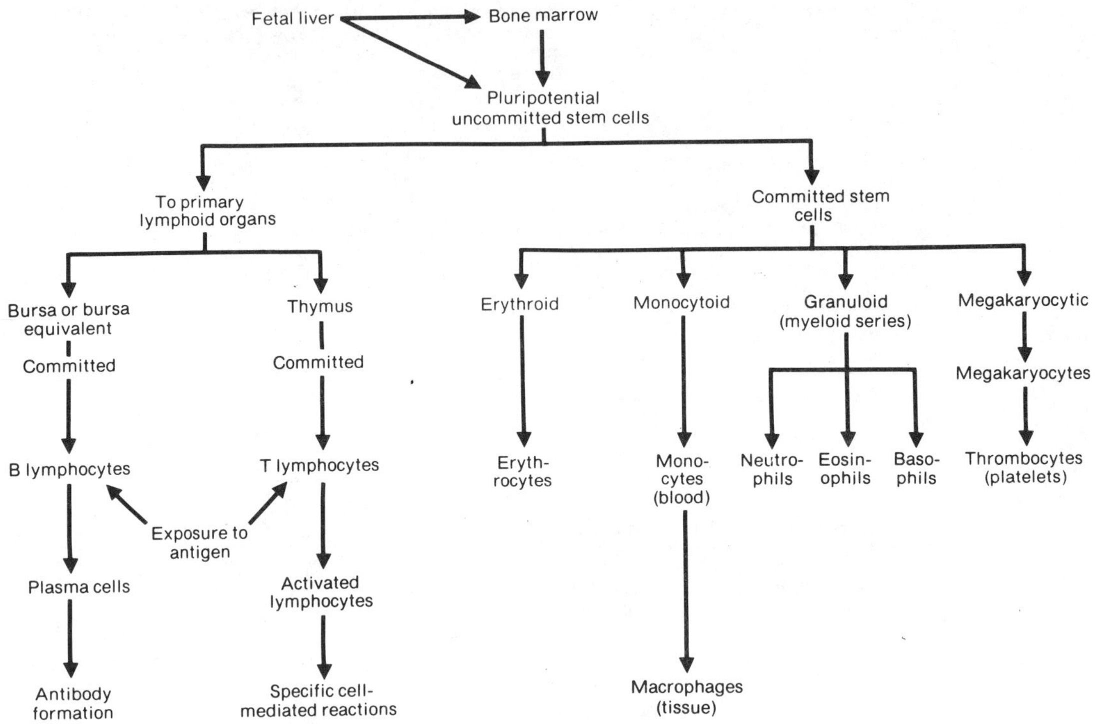

Figure 1-2 Summary of the possible interrelationships in the development of B and T lymphocytes and other hematopoietic cells.

Inflammation

1-14 Inflammation is considered one of the nonspecific resistance mechanisms of the host for localizing an infection, and clearing it up, but the inflammatory response of the host is not always beneficial. It may be harmful, with considerable damage to tissue, e.g., the inflammatory response in certain allergic disorders (Chap. 5). The reactions which take place in inflammation initiated by infection are as follows.

Permeability changes in blood vessels with exudation of plasma and the formation of fibrin Blood vessels supplying the affected area become dilated, so that the blood supply is increased. Because of an increase in permeability, plasma passes through the blood-vessel walls into the surrounding area. A network of fibrin is formed, which may serve to trap bacteria, occlude lymphatic channels, and thus limit spread of bacteria from the site of invasion. The flow of plasma into the area brings in bactericidal substances and complement.

Migration of polymorphonuclear leukocytes through blood-vessel walls to area of infection with subsequent phagocytosis of bacteria Because of chemotaxis, circulating polymorphonuclear leukocytes stick to blood-vessel walls at the site of infection and then migrate by diapedesis through the endothelium and its basement membrane. As soon as neutrophils reach the area of infection, they phagocytize bacteria and begin to destroy them by the many enzymes and bactericidal substances released from lysosomes. The pH of the inflamed area becomes more acid. Not all bacteria which are phagocytized are destroyed by neutrophils; instead the neutrophils lyse and release their intracellular contents. Neutrophils which are present in large numbers die after a short time as a result of the events of phagocytosis, the change in environmental pH, their limited life-span, and the inability to multiply. When there are large numbers of dead and dying leukocytes, the accumulation of cells appears creamy in color and consistency and is known as *pus.*

Infiltration of macrophages into area and resolution of infection Macrophages phagocytize leukocytic debris and any microorganisms not destroyed by neutrophils. Local tissue macrophages participate in cleaning up the area, but most of the macrophages in an inflamed area are derived from circulating monocytes, which leave the blood vessels by diapedesis and, as they move to the site of inflammation, change into macrophages (review scheme in Sec. 1-10). Other leukocytes, e.g., lymphocytes and eosinophils, may also be observed in an inflammed area. Unlike neutrophils, macrophages can multiply under certain stimuli; they have a fairly long life-span and can persist in tissue for weeks. In some cases, e.g., infection with tubercle bacilli and certain fungi, the macrophages may not be able to destroy the microorganisms but accumulate around them and fuse to form *multinucleated giant cells.* The accumulation of giant cells often serves to wall off the infection. In chronic inflammation, the accumulation of macrophages may be so great that nodules, called *granulomata,* are formed. Tuberculosis is often referred to as a granulomatous disease.

Production of Interferon

1-15 Interferon was first recognized by Isaacs and Lindenmann (1957).* The ability to produce interferon is one of the most important nonspecific resistance mechanisms of the host against viral infection. Interferon is a soluble protein substance (or family of substances) produced by virus-infected cells which acts as a nonspecific inhibitor of viral replication to protect uninfected cells exposed to virus. The action of interferon is not on the virus particle (virion) but on the cell, so that intracellular multiplication of viruses cannot occur. Interferon is not virus-specific because interferon produced by cells infected with a certain virus can act on other cells to protect them against a wide variety of unrelated viruses. With regard to animal species, the action of interferon is specific in that interferon produced in such laboratory animals as chickens and mice is not effective in protecting human cells from virus infection. Interferon is produced not only by cells of an intact living animal but also by tissue cells in culture. It has recently been reported that macrophages and activated T lymphocytes produce interferon. Preformed interferon may be present in leukocytes before virus invasion or may be produced de novo after infection. Interferon can be induced not only by viruses (living or inactivated) but also by other intracellular microorganisms, e.g., rickettsiae, and by certain chemical substances. Many agents which are potent inducers of interferon contain double-stranded ribonucleic acid (RNA). In view of the fact that antibiotics are not effective in controlling virus diseases, it was hoped when interferon was discovered that it could be used as a therapeutic agent. This hope has not yet materialized. It is apparent, however, that recovery from many virus infections is due to the production of interferon. Within 12 to 48 h after virus titers reach a maximum, interferon in the infected animal is produced in large quantities and virus production rapidly decreases. Interferon levels subside in a few days. The production of cell-mediated immunity helps more than antibody-mediated immunity to terminate a viral infection. Interferon is one of the substances produced by activated T lymphocytes, which are prominent cells in specific cell-mediated reactions (Chap. 2). Antibodies are produced after interferon; the role of antibodies in recovery from viral infections is not clear. Antiviral antibodies probably have little effect on an established intracellular viral infection, but they are effective in preventing viral infections.

Questions for Secs. 1-6 to 1-15

A number of mechanisms of resistance and the cells which take part have been considered. Since these mechanisms or their components occur throughout basic immunology, it is essential that you understand what has been covered. Check yourself by answering the following questions.

13. Give two other names by which the reticuloendothelial system is known.

14. (*a*) Name two mononuclear phagocytes. (*b*) What is the origin of each, and where is each mainly found? (*c*) Which has the greatest phagocytic power?

15. What macrophages would you expect to ingest and destroy microorganisms entering the body (*a*) by invasion of the bloodstream, (*b*) by inhalation, and (*c*) by injection into connective tissue?

*A date in parentheses signifies that a citation is listed in the References at the end of the chapter.

16. Place a check mark in the spaces below for any cells which fit the characteristics listed in the column on the left.

Characteristic	Macro-phage	Mono-cyte	Lympho-cyte	Neutro-phil	Eosin-ophil	Baso-phil
Arise from bone-marrow stem cells						
Mononuclear						
Polymorphonuclear						
Also known as granulocyte						
Main cells of reticuloendothelial system						
Phagocytic						
Main cell in immune response						
Capable of multiplication with appropriate stimulus						
Similar to tissue mast cells						
Predominant leukocyte in blood						
Main cell in first line of defense in inflammatory response to infection						
Main cell in second line of defense in inflammatory response to infection						

17. (*a*) About what percentage of leukocytes in the blood are lymphocytes? (*b*) Where else in the body besides blood are lymphocytes found? (*c*) Give the name of the cells which produce antibodies; what are these cells derived from?

18. What are opsonins?

19. What is complement?

20. (*a*) Can phagocytosis of bacteria take place in the absence of opsonins? (*b*) Explain.

21. How are bacteria destroyed by the phagocyte after ingestion?

22. (*a*) What are the main reactions which take place during the inflammatory response to a bacterial infection? (*b*) Is inflammation always beneficial to the host?

23. (*a*) What is interferon? (*b*) What agents besides viruses can be used to induce interferon?

24. Compare the properties of interferons induced by viruses with those of antibodies induced by viruses by filling in the spaces in the table with yes or no. See page 11.

Answers

13. The reticuloendothelial system is also known as the macrophage system or the mononuclear phagocyte system (MPS). (Sec. 1-9.)

14. (*a*) Two mononuclear phagocytes are the monocyte and the macrophage. (*b*) Both monocytes and macrophages are derived from bone marrow from the same cell line. Mono-

Property	Interferon	Antiviral antibodies
Protein structure		
Produced by many kinds of tissue cells		
Action on cells		
Action directly on virus		
Virus specific		
Specific for animal species		

cytes are found in the blood for a few days; then they enter various tissues and change into macrophages. (*c*) Tissue macrophages are much more phagocytic than blood monocytes. (Sec. 1-10.)

15. (*a*) Microorganisms which enter the body by the bloodstream are taken up by Kupffer cells (macrophages) of the liver and macrophages of the spleen. (*b*) Microorganisms which enter the lungs are taken up by alveolar macrophages. (*c*) Microorganisms which enter by injection into connective tissue are taken up by macrophages called histiocytes. (Sec. 1-10.)

16. See Table 1-5. (Secs. 1-9, 1-10, and 1-12 to 1-14.)

Table 1-5 Characteristics of Blood Leukocytes and Tissue Macrophages

Characteristic	Macrophage	Monocyte	Lymphocyte	Neutrophil	Eosinophil	Basophil
Arise from bone-marrow stem cells	√	√	√	√	√	√
Mononuclear	√	√	√			
Polymorphonuclear*				√	√	√
Also known as granulocyte				√	√	√
Main cells of reticuloendothelial system	√	√				
Phagocytic	√	√		√	√	?
Main cell in immune response			√			
Capable of multiplication with appropriate stimulus	√	√	√			
Similar to tissue mast cells						√
Predominant leukocyte in blood				√		
Main cell in first line of defense in inflammatory response to infection				√		
Main cell in second line of defense in inflammatory response to infection	√					

* The term *polymorphs* is often used to refer to neutrophils.

17. (*a*) About 30 percent of leukocytes in the blood are lymphocytes. (*b*) Lymphocytes are found not only in blood but also in such lymphoid tissue as lymph nodes, spleen, etc. (*c*) Plasma cells derived from B lymphocytes produce antibodies. (Sec. 1-13.)

18. Heat-stable opsonins are antibodies which combine with microorganisms in such a way that they are more easily phagocytized by such phagocytes as neutrophils and macrophages. Certain complement components (sometimes called heat-labile opsonins) enhance phagocytosis. (Secs. 1-7 and 1-8.)

19. Complement is a complex set of interacting proteins present in normal serum of mammals; complement is heat-labile and can be inactivated by heating at 56°C for 30 min; complement has chemotactic properties; complement enters into many host reactions, including immune reactions. (Sec. 1-8.)

20. (*a*) Yes. (*b*) Phagocytosis of bacteria can take place in the absence of opsonins if the phagocyte can trap the bacteria against the surface of tissue, between leukocytes, in the interstices of a fibrin clot, or in some other manner. (Sec. 1-12.)

21. After being phagocytized by macrophages or neutrophils, bacteria come in contact with granules in the cytoplasm which are known as lysosomes and which contain a number of bactericidal substances and enzymes capable of killing and degrading bacteria. (Sec. 1-12.)

22. (*a*) The main reactions which take place during the inflammatory response to a bacterial infection are (1) permeability changes in blood vessels with exudation of plasma and the formation of a fibrin network which may serve to trap some bacteria; (2) migration of leukocytes through blood-vessel walls to the area of infection with phagocytosis of bacteria by neutrophils; (3) migration of macrophages into the area with phagocytosis by macrophages of dead or dying neutrophils, leukocytic debris, and remaining bacteria. (*b*) No, inflammation is not always beneficial to the host because it can involve considerable injury to tissue. (Sec. 1-14.)

23. (*a*) Interferon is a soluble nonviral protein (or family of proteins) produced by virus-infected cells which confers antiviral resistance on normally virus-susceptible animal cells of the same species. (*b*) Interferon production may be induced by viruses and other intracellular microorganisms and also by certain chemical substances. (Sec. 1-15.)

24. See Table 1-6 for a comparison of the properties of interferons and antiviral antibodies. (Sec. 1-15.)

SPECIFIC RESISTANCE OR IMMUNITY OF THE HOST

1-16 Specific resistance or immunity depends on an immune response. In contrast to nonspecific or innate resistance mechanisms of the host, which are active against many different kinds of microorganisms, specific resistance is active against, or specific for, a particular microorganism. For example, antibody to rabies virus will neutralize rabies virus but no other virus. It has already been pointed out that microorganisms contain antigens which stimulate the production of antibodies. Antigens are usually foreign to the host (a different species) and are protein in nature or made up of

Table 1-6 Comparison of Interferons and Antiviral Antibodies

Property	Interferons	Antiviral antibodies
Protein structure	Yes	Yes
Produced by many kinds of tissue cells	Yes	No
Action on cells	Yes	No
Action directly on virus	No	Yes
Virus-specific	No	Yes
Specific for animal species	Yes	No

chemical substances bound to proteins. A single species of bacteria usually contains many different antigens. Because of their structure and small size viruses have a limited number of antigens. Some antigens of microorganisms and the antibodies specific for them are necessary for the establishment of immunity; some are not. It was observed many years ago that a person who had had a certain disease was immune to subsequent attacks of it. In 1798 Edward Jenner was the first person to immunize against a disease. He immunized against smallpox using material from cowpox lesions. Jenner had noted that milkmaids developed lesions on their hands from milking cows with cowpox but that during epidemics of smallpox they did not develop that disease. Although Jenner showed that material taken from lesions of cowpox, a mild disease, was protective against smallpox, a severe or highly fatal disease, his work was not readily accepted by the medical profession. It did not seem reasonable that material taken from a cow could protect against smallpox. Many years later other investigators showed that smallpox and cowpox are caused by viruses and that the two viruses are very similar antigenically although quite different with respect to severity of infection produced in the human host. Vaccinia virus is now used for immunization against smallpox. Vaccinia virus does not occur in nature but is a mutant strain of virus which arose in the laboratory during research with smallpox and cowpox viruses. The term *vaccine*, derived from the Latin *vacca*, meaning "cow," was coined many years later by Pasteur to honor and recognize the work of Jenner. Specific resistance or immunity can be acquired as outlined below:

1. Active immunity
   a. Naturally acquired
   b. Artificially acquired
2. Passive immunity
   a. Naturally acquired
   b. Artificially acquired

With regard to antibody production, active immunity refers to that type of immunity in which a person has a very active part in development of his own immunity because antibody is produced in significant amounts by his own cells about 7 to 14 days after exposure to antigen. In contrast, passive immunity is immunity conferred by the injection of antibodies produced in another person or animal in order to provide a nonimmune person with immediate protection.

Active Immunity

Naturally Acquired

1-17 Active immunity may be naturally acquired either by having a subclinical infection with a particular microorganism or by actually having the disease. Some diseases, e.g., poliomyelitis, appear to produce a much more lasting type of immunity than others, e.g., influenza. The poliomyelitis virus enters through the alimentary tract, multiplies in the intestinal tract, and enters the bloodstream before it reaches the central nervous system, where symptoms of poliomyelitis are produced. If specific antibodies are in the blood, the virus is neutralized before reaching the central nervous system and a typical case of poliomyelitis does not occur. In this disease, the portal of entry (alimentary tract) is not the attack organ (central nervous system), and during passage of virus from one to the other, virus can be neutralized if specific antibodies are in the blood. In a previously exposed individual, there may be a rapid rise in serum antibodies (anamnestic response, Sec. 1-22) before virus reaches the attack organ. In contrast, influenza virus enters the respiratory tract, and the infection causing the disease takes place in the respiratory tract. In other words, the portal of entry (respiratory tract) is also the attack organ (respiratory tract). In order to prevent influenza, neutralization of virus must occur in the respiratory tract at the time of invasion by influenza virus. The antibody secretory IgA is usually responsible for neutralization of viruses in the respiratory tract; IgA is also in blood. The different kinds of immunoglobulins (IgA, IgG, IgM, IgE, and IgD) are described in Chap. 3.

Table 1-7 Types of Vaccines

Composition	Example
Bacterial vaccine, killed	Whooping cough (pertussis)
Attenuated (living)	Tuberculosis, designated BCG (bacille Calmette-Guérin); not used in United States
Virus vaccine, killed	Salk vaccine for poliomyelitis
Attenuated (living)	Sabin vaccine for poliomyelitis
Toxoid	Tetanus and diphtheria toxoids for immunization against exotoxin
Structural components of infectious agents	Polysaccharide of pneumococcus capsule
	Subviral antigens of influenza vaccine

Artificially Acquired

1-18 Active immunity is artificially acquired through the use of vaccines. Some of the many types of vaccines in use today are given in Table 1-7. An attenuated strain of a microorganism is one which is still living although virulence has been decreased. In order for a living microorganism to be used in a vaccine, it must be attenuated to the extent that it is no longer capable of causing disease, but it must be unchanged antigenically. A vaccine composed of living attenuated organisms is preferred to a killed vaccine because it is a more effective immunizing agent; i.e., immunity induced by this type of vaccine persists longer. Toxoid is soluble exotoxin treated so that its toxic properties are destroyed without affecting it antigenically. One way toxoid can be prepared is by treatment with formalin under mild conditions. Antibodies to toxoid will neutralize the specific exotoxin. In contrast, neither toxoid nor effective neutralizing antibodies can be produced with bacterial endotoxins. There are two kinds of influenza vaccines, *whole-virus* and *split-virus*, for use in the United States; the latter type, produced by disrupting the virus, causes fewer side effects, especially in children.

1-19 The antigenic composition of most microorganisms is fairly stable. Influenza virus, especially type A, is a notable exception and presents problems for preparation of effective influenza vaccines. Influenza virus vaccine has a protective effect only when the viruses incorporated into the vaccine are antigenically similar to those causing the epidemic or outbreak of influenza. Influenza virus demonstrates *antigenic drift* or *shift.* At least 18 different antigenic components have been determined in type A strains of influenza virus. There may be a finite number of antigens even though they vary in proportion from one influenza strain and epidemic to the next; they may exert their influence as major or minor antigenic components. It has been observed that in childhood the activity of influenza antibodies produced is narrow but becomes progressively broader with age due to exposure to a number of influenza virus strains varying in antigenic composition. The apparent short period of immunity to influenza virus following infection could be due to antigenic drift and not to the lack of persistence of protective antibody.

1-20 It has been suggested that influenza virus vaccine could be given by instillation into the respiratory tract in order to increase IgA production and local immunity at the site of viral invasion. Most vaccines are given by injection but not all. The Sabin poliomyelitis vaccine is administered orally by the alimentary tract because it is a vaccine composed of living attenuated viruses and this is the route by which poliomyelitis viruses usually invade. As the result of a transient mild type of infection caused by the attenuated virus, local immunity with secretory IgA is produced in the intestinal tract. Neutralizing antibodies are also produced in the blood (IgM, IgG, IgA). Three antigenic types of poliomyelitis viruses, designated 1, 2, and 3, are in the vaccine. Whenever there is more than one antigenic type of a microorganism, all types which are known to be responsible for an outbreak of the disease should be included in the vaccine. The vaccine DTP, routinely given to children by injection, is composed of diphtheria toxoid, tetanus toxoid, and a killed suspension of *Bordetella pertussis*, the causative agent of whooping cough. Whenever several antigens are mixed together, it must be determined that there is no competition between the different antigens and that the combination of antigens does not decrease the immune response which would have been produced to a single antigen. Since DTP is given to children, the combination of antigens allows immunization with fewer injections. Also an *adjuvant* may be used to increase the immune response to antigen so that fewer injections are required. For immunization of children, antigens are often precipitated with alum. When alum is mixed with sodium hydroxide in the presence of antigen, a white insoluble precipitate of aluminum hydroxide is formed with antigen adsorbed to it. There are a number of different kinds of adjuvants which act in different ways. An adjuvant used for human vaccines should not be antigenic. Since alum-precipitated antigens are held in the tissue longer, the antigenic stimulus is prolonged.

Passive Immunity

Naturally Acquired

1-21 Passive immunity occurs when antibodies produced in one individual are transferred to another individual. Passive immunization confers protection immediately. An example of naturally acquired passive immunity is transfer of the mother's antibodies across the placenta to the fetus. The immunoglobulin (antibody) designated IgG has characteristics which enable it to pass the placental barrier. Other immunoglobulins have not been reported to pass the placenta. The baby is born with the mother's antibodies of the IgG type. These antibodies persist for about 2 to 4 months and protect the child. Meanwhile, the child begins to produce its own antibodies when exposed to various microorganisms in the environment. In some animal species, e.g., the dog, the mother's antibodies do not pass the placenta but for a short time after delivery of the offspring are present in colostrum, the first milk after parturition. Colostrum contains secretory IgA, IgM, and IgG. Since the digestive system of the newborn is poorly developed, antibodies of colostrum may be absorbed from the intestinal tract. It has been reported that when transplacental passage of antibodies is relatively inefficient, intestinal adsorption of antibodies in colostrum is more efficient. These two forms of passive immunization, which are acquired naturally, may complement each other.

Artificially Acquired

1-22 Passive immunity may be used therapeutically or prophylactically. If a sick child is diagnosed as having diphtheria, passive immunization must be given immediately in order to neutralize diphtheria exotoxin. Antibiotics, which are lifesaving in other diseases, will not neutralize diphtheria exotoxin. Some antibiotics are inhibitory for *C. diphtheriae* and would prevent continued growth and excretion of exotoxin but would not neutralize exotoxin already formed. The administration of diphtheria antitoxin to a child who is showing symptoms of diphtheria is mandatory and is an example of therapeutic passive immunity. The longer the delay in treatment after the appearance of symptoms, the larger the amount of antitoxin which must be given to save a life. Special precautions must be taken to prevent immediate-type hypersensitivity reactions to a foreign protein if the antitoxin which is used was prepared in an animal such as the horse (Chap. 5). A person not previously actively immunized against tetanus who is exposed to tetanus should receive a small amount of tetanus antitoxin to prevent tetanus from occuring. This is an example of prophylactic passive immunity in which protection is conferred immediately after injection. Human tetanus antitoxin is now available commercially. If the person had been actively immunized in the past, a booster injection with tetanus toxoid would cause a fairly rapid production of antibody. The booster injection is based on the reaction known as *immunologic memory* or the *anamnestic response.* Primary active immunization requires about 10 to 14 days for the patient to develop a fairly high level of antibodies. After primary immunization has been carried out, the booster injection given at a later date elicits in 1 to 3 days sufficient antibody for protection against tetanus as a result of immunologic memory. If a person develops tetanus, tetanus antitoxin may be given, but its value in affecting the course of the disease is questionable. Tetanus exotoxin appears to combine rapidly and firmly with neural tissue, so that antitoxin may not have any effect.

× **1-23** Since antibodies are mainly in the gamma-globulin fraction of serum, gamma globulin is usually separated from antiserum. This procedure concentrates the antibodies and eliminates unwanted proteins. In human serum, which could contain hepatitis viruses, the procedure for separation of gamma globulins removes hepatitis virus if it happens to be present. Sometimes a blood donor has one of the hepatitis viruses in the blood before showing symptoms of disease and becoming aware of infection. Passive immunization may be used for prevention of viral infections after exposure but before symptoms of disease develop. After symptoms of a virus disease occur, passive immunization appears to have little or no effect because viruses multiply within cells and are inaccessible to antibodies. Human gamma globulin prepared from normal adult serum or immune serum has been used for the prevention of a number of virus diseases. If the incidence of a disease is fairly high, gamma globulin prepared from normal adult sera has a sufficient amount of antibody to be used for passive immunization for the disease. For example, about 90 percent of the adult population in this country has been exposed to measles, and normal adult serum has a fairly high concentration of antibodies to measles virus. For diseases in which the incidence is lower, e.g., mumps, gamma globulin for passive immunization should be prepared from convalescent serum or the serum of recently immunized persons. In contrast to active immunization, which may persist for years, passive immunization lasts only a few weeks.

Questions for Secs. 1-16 to 1-23

25. Outline four ways specific immunity can be acquired and give an example of each.

26. What is the difference between active and passive immunization?

27. (*a*) Are vaccines composed of antigens? (*b*) Are vaccines used for active or passive immunization?

28. (*a*) Is an attenuated microorganism dead? (*b*) Is an attenuated microorganism more or less virulent than the parent strain?

29. (*a*) What is the difference between toxin and toxoid? (*b*) Are toxoids used for active or passive immunization?

30. (*a*) Why is Sabin vaccine administered orally? (*b*) If Sabin vaccine has not been stored properly, and the virus is dead will immunization to poliomyelitis take place? (*c*) Explain.

31. If local immunization occurs in the intestinal tract, what differences would you expect to observe with regard to excretion of virus by two children exposed during an epidemic of poliomyelitis if one had previously been immunized with Sabin vaccine and the other with Salk vaccine?

32. (*a*) What is an adjuvant? (*b*) Is it permissible to mix several antigens for the preparation of a vaccine?

33. Fill out the chart by checking the type(s) of immunity related to the cause.

34. How long do the antibodies from the mother transferred in utero serve to protect the child after birth?

Cause of immunity	Naturally acquired	Artifically acquired	Active	Passive
(1) Mumps (exposure to a case)				
(2) Influenza vaccine				
(3) Diphtheria toxoid				
(4) Newborn infant has immunity acquired from mother				

35. (*a*) Do you think that horse antibodies (from an injection of horse antiserum) would persist in the human host as long as antibodies of human origin? (*b*) Explain. (*c*) Compare the duration of immunity after active and passive immunization.

36. (*a*) What is colostrum? (*b*) Are proteins usually absorbed without alteration from the intestinal tract?

37. (*a*) With regard to passive immunization, what are the differences between antiserum, immune serum, hyperimmune serum, and gamma globulin? (*b*) Why is whole human serum not used for passive immunization?

38. (*a*) Why is gamma globulin prepared from normal adult serum satisfactory for prevention of measles in an exposed nonimmunized child? (*b*) Why is gamma globulin prepared from mumps immune serum (serum of person recently immunized against mumps or convalescing from mumps) used for prevention of mumps instead of gamma globulin prepared from normal adult serum?

Answers

25. Specific immunity can be acquired: (1) Naturally by having a disease or subclinical infection; the result is active immunization by natural means. (2) Naturally by placental passage of mother's antibodies to child before birth; the result is passive immunization by natural means. (3) Artificially by injection of antigens contained in vaccines; the result is active immunization by artificial means. (4) Artificially by injection of gamma globulin containing antibodies; the result is passive immunization by artificial means. (Secs. 1-16 to 1-18, 1-21, and 1-22.)

26. In active immunization the cells of a person exposed to antigens or vaccines produce antibodies; in passive immunization in order to obtain immediate protection a person receives antibodies formed in another person or animal. (Sec. 1-16.)

27. (*a*) Yes, vaccines are composed of antigens. (*b*) Vaccines are used for active immunization. (Sec. 1-18.)

28. (*a*) No, an attenuated microorganism is living. (*b*) An attenuated microorganism is less virulent than the parent strain. (Sec. 1-18.)

29. (*a*) Toxin may be exotoxin or endotoxin. Exotoxin is a soluble protein which is excreted by certain bacteria, which is active in very small amounts, and which, unless neutralized, combines irreversibly with host tissue and may even lead to death. Toxoid is exotoxin detoxified but unchanged antigenically. (*b*) Toxoids are used for active immunization and cause the production of antitoxin, which neutralizes exotoxin. (Sec. 1-18.)

30. (*a*) The Sabin vaccine is given orally because it is composed of living attenuated viruses which usually invade the body by the oral route and then multiply in the intestinal tract. (*b*) If the virus is dead because of improper storage, immunity will not result. (*c*) Immunization depends on multiplication of the virus in the intestinal tract. (Sec. 1-20.)

31. The child who was immunized with the Sabin vaccine should have local immunity in the intestinal tract and should neutralize any virus there to which he was exposed during the epidemic; therefore, wild-type virus (virulent) of the epidemic should not be excreted. If virus should happen to reach the bloodstream, it would also be neutralized there. The child immunized with Salk vaccine has antibody in the blood to neutralize the virus if he is exposed but does not have local immunity in the intestinal tract and would excrete virulent virus of the epidemic. (Sec. 1-20.)

32. (*a*) An adjuvant is a substance like alum which is mixed with the antigens of a vaccine in order to increase the immune response of the host. (*b*) Several antigens may be included in a vaccine and injected at the same time provided tests are made to be sure that there is no competition between the antigens or that they do not interfere with the antigenicity of each other. (Sec. 1-20.)

33. (1) naturally acquired, active; (2) artificially acquired, active; (3) artificially acquired, active; (4) naturally acquired, passive. (Secs. 1-17, 1-18, and 1-21.)

34. The mother's antibodies acquired in utero by placental passage usually protect a child for about 2 to 4 months after birth. (Sec. 1-21.)

35. (*a*) Human antibodies persist in the human host longer than horse antibodies. (*b*) Horse antibodies are foreign, are treated as a foreign substance, and are more rapidly degraded. (*c*) Active immunity lasts for several months to years; passive immunity lasts only about 2 weeks if antibodies of a different species are injected, while antibodies of the same species persist a little longer. (Sec. 1-23.)

36. (*a*) Colostrum contains antibodies and is the first milk after parturition. (*b*) Unlike most proteins, colostrum antibodies are absorbed without alterations in some animal species for a short time after birth. (Sec. 1-21.)

37. (*a*) Antiserum, immune serum, hyperimmune serum, and preparations of gamma globulin all contain antibodies and are used for passive immunization; immune serum implies that it comes from an immunized animal; hyperimmune serum comes from an animal which has been intensively immunized or has received so many injections that there is a high level of antibodies; since gamma globulin is the fraction of serum which contains most antibodies, separation of the gamma-globulin fraction is a means of concentrating the antibodies and getting rid of unwanted serum proteins. (*b*) Whole human serum is not used because of the danger of transferring hepatitis viruses; also a patient does not have to receive as large an injection of gamma globulin as of whole serum in order to obtain the same level of antibodies. (Secs. 1-22 and 1-23.)

38. (*a*) A pool of normal adult serum or plasma has a high level of antibodies to measles virus because until the recent introduction of the measles vaccine there was a high incidence of the disease in the general population; measles is a highly communicable disease. (*b*) Whenever there is not a high incidence of a disease in the general population, gamma globulin for passive immunization should be prepared either from convalescent sera or the sera of recently immunized persons. (Sec. 1-23.)

Comparison of Active and Passive Immunization

1-24 No attempt has been made to include schedules for immunization or the amounts of vaccine or gamma globulin to be given. The principles on which active and passive immunization are based have been presented with examples. The characteristics of active and passive immunization are summarized in Table 1-8.

Combined Active and Passive Immunization

1-25 Active immunization is almost always used for prevention of a disease before exposure occurs because for most diseases the incubation period is too short to permit primary active immunization after exposure. An exception to this rule is rabies. The average incubation period in rabies is about 4 weeks, and this should allow time to actively immunize a patient before rabies virus reaches the central nervous system. Except for one or two questionable cases which have been reported, rabies is fatal after symptoms of the disease occur. Duck-embryo rabies vaccine containing inactivated virus is most frequently used for active immunization. When a patient has been bitten on the face, neck, or hands, the incubation period is much shorter than when the bite is elsewhere on the body. It is also shorter when there has been severe exposure, e.g., with wolf bites. If a shortened incubation period is expected, the patient should receive passive immunization followed by active immunization. Hyperimmune serum to rabies virus is injected immediately in order to protect the patient passively with antibodies to the virus until the patient can build up his own antibodies. Also, after thoroughly cleansing the wound, the wound should be infiltrated with hyperimmune serum in order to try to neutralize rabies virus at the site of entry. Since the quantity of antibodies used for passive immunization against rabies virus may be great enough to interfere with active immunization, precautions must be taken to ensure active immunity. Booster injections of rabies vaccine are given 10 and 20 days after the last dose in the series of daily injections for rabies immunization. The World Health

Table 1-8 Comparison of Active and Passive Immunization

Characteristic	Active immunization	Passive immunization
Role of host	Active	Passive
Method of induction	Exposure to antigens of infectious agents or vaccines	Injection of antibodies (preformed in another human being or animal)
Kinds of immunity involved	Antibody-mediated or cell-mediated	Antibody-mediated only*
Acquired immunity:		
Naturally	Subclinical infection or clinical disease	IgG by way of placenta Ingestion of colostrum
Artificially	Immunization with vaccines including toxoid	Injection of antibodies: Antitoxin for prophylaxis and therapy Antiviral antibodies for prophylaxis only
Time for development	7 to 14 days	Immediately after injection of antibodies
Effectiveness	Good	Fair to good depending on disease
Duration of immunity	Months to years	A few weeks
Booster of immunity by additional injection	Anamnestic (recall) response in 1 to 3 days by single small injection of antigen	Reinforcement only by amount of antibody injected
Precautions	Be aware of contraindications; in general, do not give live attenuated virus vaccine to: Those receiving immunosuppressive drugs Those with immunodeficiency diseases Pregnant women	Test for possible hypersensitivity reactions caused by sensitization to protein of different species

*Adoptive immunization or injection of sensitized lymphocytes from another host in order to transfer cell-mediated immunity is dangerous and can even be fatal.

Organization (WHO) has made recommendations to follow after exposure to rabies.* With regard to measles, if a nonimmunized child is exposed to measles, gamma globulin containing antibodies to measles virus is given to prevent or modify the disease; for future protection, active immunization with living attenuated virus is delayed several weeks until the remaining amount of passively transferred antibodies to measles virus is no longer considered great enough to neutralize the virus of the vaccine. It has been observed that in some cases of passive transfer of maternal antibodies in utero, antibody formation by the infant may be temporarily depressed until there is a significant drop in maternal antibodies. In contrast, standard procedure allows the combination of both passive and active immunization of a patient exposed to tetanus who has not been previously immunized. A small amount of tetanus toxoid is given as the first in a series of injections for active immunization. Toxoid is strongly antigenic or immunogenic, so that active immunization of the patient in this case is barely affected by passive immunization.

*Expert Committee Report on Rabies, *6th Rep. WHO Tech. Rep. Ser.* 523, World Health Organization, Geneva, 1973.

Preparation and Use of Vaccines

1-26 Diphtheria, tetanus, whooping cough, poliomyelitis, and measles (rubeola) are serious diseases and vaccines are available for routine immunization of children against them. Children are also actively immunized against German measles (rubella) although it is not a serious disease in children. Active immunization with the recently developed living attenuated rubella vaccine is carried out in an attempt to prevent another epidemic like the one in the United States in 1964. Many thousands of children were born with malformations as a result of exposure of pregnant women to rubella followed by infection and transplacental passage of rubella virus and infection in utero. At that time there was no vaccine, and passive immunization proved unreliable. In some cases of passively immunized pregnant women, the women did not develop the characteristic rash of rubella, but their babies were born deformed. A nonimmune female adult has less chance of being exposed to rubella virus in a population of immunized children. The vaccine also has the advantage that female children who are immunized should not be susceptible when they reach the childbearing age. A nonimmune female adult should not be immunized unless pregnancy is prevented during the period of immunization. Another vaccine is the one for mumps. Mumps is not a very serious virus disease except for certain sequelae, e.g., involvement of the central nervous system, deafness, and sterility, which may follow infection. About 5 percent of males who have mumps during or after adolescence develop bilateral orchitis and may become sterile. Measles, rubella, and mumps vaccines may be combined for immunization of children.

1-27 A number of vaccines are not used for the entire population but only for certain groups of people, e.g., those planning foreign travel, those located in certain geographical areas, and those in the army or in institutions. The following diseases either do not occur in the United States or occur so infrequently that immunization is not warranted unless someone is planning to travel outside the country:*

Cholera

Plague

Smallpox

Typhoid fever

Typhus fever

Yellow fever

Some diseases, e.g., Rocky Mountain spotted fever, are usually confined to certain sections of the United States, and vaccines are given only in the areas where the disease occurs. A number of vaccines have been designed for use by the army or in institutions or places where many people come together from different areas, so that conditions favor an outbreak of disease. For example, outbreaks of meningococcal meningitis or mycoplasma pneumonia are frequent in the army, especially in new recruits. The pneumococcal polysaccharide vaccine is especially recommended for the elderly, such as residents of nursing homes. Although a frequent infection in institutions is that with hepatitis viruses, no vaccine for hepatitis is yet available.

1-28 Another problem concerned with preparation of vaccines is attenuation of a microorganism if it is to be used in the living state. In 1880 Pasteur showed that cultures of bacteria which cause fowl cholera lose their virulence if they are allowed to age and the time interval between transfers is increased. Pasteur showed that immunity could be induced by injection with bacterial cultures which had been rendered avirulent by laboratory manipulation. He also showed that rabies virus in saliva from rabid dogs found on the streets of France (known as *street virus*) became less virulent for dogs

*Requirements and recommendations for foreign travel can be found in Health Information for International Travel 1977, supplement to U.S. Department of Health, Education and Welfare, Public Health Service, Center for Disease Control, *Morb. Mortal. Wkly. Rep.*, vol. 26, August 1977.

after serial passage intracranially in rabbits. With continued passage of the virus intracranially in rabbits, neurotropism of the virus was enhanced and the incubation period for rabbits became progressively shorter, until additional rabbit passage caused no further reduction in the incubation period. This virus was called *fixed rabies virus.* Fixed rabies virus was less virulent for dogs by subcutaneous injection than street virus; however, fixed virus was still too virulent to be used for immunization of human beings without inactivation, which was carried out by drying over potassium hydroxide. For his first injections Pasteur used neural tissue (spinal cord) which had been dried for a long time and therefore probably contained only inactivated fixed virus. Later injections were made with tissue which had been dried for shorter times so that some fixed virus was probably still viable in the injections given at the end of the series. The Flury vaccine for rabies was attenuated by passage in embryonated eggs. The strain known as LEP (low egg passage) is used for immunization of dogs; the HEP (high egg passage) strain is used for immunization of cats and cattle, especially where bat rabies is prevalent. To bring about attenuation, microorganisms are often grown under conditions other than those considered optimum with regard to temperature, tissue affinity, etc. Many viruses have been attenuated for preparation of vaccines by serial passage in tissue culture. Whenever an attenuated strain is used in a vaccine, there is always the possibility of a back mutation to virulence. During World War II, American troops were immunized against yellow fever virus with the attenuated mutant strain of yellow fever virus known as 17D. When many soldiers who had been immunized with virus developed jaundice, which is one of the symptoms of yellow fever, it was feared that back mutation to virulence had occurred in the 17D strain. Yellow fever has a short incubation period, but a long time had elasped between injection of vaccine and the development of jaundice. It was noted that soldiers who developed jaundice were immunized with a vaccine lot number stabilized by the same pool of human plasma. The jaundice was not caused by 17D yellow fever virus but by a hepatitis virus present in human plasma which up to that time was unrecognized.

x **1-29** Autogenous vaccines are seldom used now although they were frequently employed many years ago with staphylococcal infections. The derivation of the word autogenous (*auto-* means "self") indicates that the vaccine is composed of material derived from the patient such as the strain of *Staphylococcus aureus* causing the infection. These vaccines, if used, are often prepared in a local hospital laboratory; care must be taken to be sure that the antigenicity of the autogenous vaccine is in no way altered by the method for inactivation of the organism, i.e., chemical treatment or heat. Inactivation by heat should not exceed 60°C for 60 min. Antibodies would be formed to altered antigens in the vaccine, but these antibodies would not combine effectively with those of the microorganism as it occurs in the patient or in nature.

Precautions for Immunization

x **1-30** Whenever a vaccine is to be used for immunization, the person administering it should be fully aware of any dangers associated with it and precautions which should be exercised. Some reactions which follow immunization are unpredictable and occur regardless of precautions taken. The Guillain-Barrē syndrome (Chap. 6) very infrequently follows immunization. Its occurrence in a few persons during the 1976 national swine influenza immunization program had an adverse effect on the program. One of the most dread conditions is *subacute sclerosing panencephalitis* (SSPE), which is caused by a slow virus infection of the brain. The virus is usually described as being measleslike. SSPE has been estimated to follow immunization with live measles vaccine at a rate of 0.5 to 1.1 cases per million doses of measles vaccine distributed. SSPE follows measles infection in children at a rate of approximately 5 to 10 cases for every million children who develop measles; therefore, the risk of SSPE following a case of measles appears to be significantly greater than that following immunization for measles. Some of the complications which have been observed to occur with vaccines are outlined below.

Pertussis vaccine Children with a history of convulsions or disease of the central nervous system should not be given pertussis vaccine unless it is given in small divided doses separately from other immunizations and after 1 year of age. This vaccine contains a suspension of *Bordetella pertussis*, a gram-negative bacillus which contains an endotoxin with properties of an adjuvant. The bacteria are killed, but the properties of the endotoxin are not destroyed. Babies need immunization against pertussis because antibodies of the mother to *B. pertussis* appear not to pass the placenta.

Typhoid, cholera, and plague vaccines The bacteria in these vaccines are gram-negative bacilli which have an endotoxin. Injection of these vaccines separately is often associated with local and systemic side effects. If these vaccines are given simultaneously (at separate sites) for foreign travel, the side effects may be accentuated.

Poliomyelitis vaccine The Sabin poliomyelitis vaccine, which contains live virus, appears to be better attenuated for children and young adults than for the middle age group. For this reason, it has been recommended that oral poliomyelitis vaccine not be given to adults who live in an area free of endemic or epidemic poliomyelitis. The Sabin vaccine is still the one recommended for immunization of children in spite of the recent controversy over the use of the Sabin versus the Salk vaccine, which is inactivated. There are a few cases in which attenuated strains of the Sabin vaccine have been reported to cause poliomyelitis.

Rickettsial and viral vaccines containing egg protein If microorganisms like rickettsiae and viruses are propagated in chicken embryos for preparation of vaccines, sensitivity reactions to egg protein can occur unless the vaccine is highly purified. Influenza virus propagated in embryonated eggs is separated from egg protein by zonal ultracentrifugation.

Living attenuated virus vaccines If these vaccines are administered by parenteral injection, they should not be given to pregnant women because of the chance of transplacental passage of live virus and harm to the fetus. Nor should living attenuated virus vaccines be given to anyone receiving immunosuppressive drugs or suffering from immunodeficiency disorders, especially those affecting cell-mediated immunity.

Smallpox vaccine In recent years, extremely adverse reactions following smallpox immunization and the fact that smallpox no longer occurs in the United States have warranted dropping the requirement for immunization against smallpox in this country. A condition known as *vaccinia necrosum* or *vaccinia gangrenosum* may be observed in individuals lacking the capacity to produce cell-mediated immunity; in these people the smallpox inoculation does not begin to clear up within 14 days but continues to spread, involving the entire arm and shoulder, sometimes necessitating amputation. Smallpox immunization should not be given to children with skin problems such as eczema because of the danger of the development of generalized vaccinia. Parents should be cautioned not to allow these children to go near children or adults recently vaccinated against smallpox because vaccinia virus multiplies at the inoculation site unless the person is already immune. If there is an outbreak of smallpox, children for whom active immunization would be dangerous can be passively protected by vaccinia immune globulin prepared from the serum of recently immunized individuals such as those in military service. Smallpox is an extremely serious and disfiguring disease with a high case fatality rate.

Rabies vaccine Active immunization for rabies after the bite of a rabid animal is dangerous because encephalitis occurs as a result of immunization in about 1 to 500 to 25,000 persons immunized (statistics vary). Three vaccines currently used for immunization are (1) the duck-embryo vaccine (DEV) and P-DEV (P = purified), inactivated with β-propiolactone; (2) the Semple vaccine, which is similar to Pasteur's vaccine for rabies but contains phenol-inactivated fixed rabies virus propagated in brain tissue; and (3) the human diploid rabies vaccine, a new vaccine available from the Center for Disease Control (CDC). There appears to be greater chance of encephalomyelitis following immunization with vaccine containing brain tissue, possibly because of an organ-specific antigen and an allergic reaction to brain tissue. Encephalomyelitis occurs more often in persons who receive a second series of injections because of another exposure to rabies. This vaccine appears to be more immunogenic than duck-embryo vaccine, but the latter is preferred because it is less likely to cause neuroparalytic reactions. Since rabies has a case fatality rate of almost 100 percent, serum of an immunized person should be tested for protective antibodies (Sec. 4-44). Human diploid rabies vaccine has been provided by the CDC when immunization with duck-embryo vaccine produced antibody titers below those assumed to be protective. Duck-embryo vaccine is considered sufficiently safe for preexposure immunization of persons in high-risk groups such as veterinarians. P-DEV is less likely to cause allergic reactions to duck protein.

1-31 In passive immunization, gamma globulin containing concentrated antibodies should be given by intramuscular and not by intravenous injections because the preparation may contain small amounts of aggregated gamma globulin which could cause severe or even fatal systemic reactions. As pointed out previously, whole human serum should not be used for passive immunization because of the possibility of transferring one of the hepatitis viruses. If antiserum from a different species such as horse serum is the only serum available for passive immunization and has to be used, the patient must be tested for hypersensitivity to protein of the foreign species. Failure to do so can result in anaphylactic shock and death. If the patient is hypersensitive, desensitization is carried out before administering heterologous antiserum from the foreign species (Chap. 5). Human immune globulin is available for almost all types of passive immunization.

Licensing of Vaccines and Immune Serum Globulin

1-32 Inactivated measles virus (rubeola) vaccine was licensed for use in addition to the attenuated vaccine. Later it was recommended that the inactivated measles vaccine be withdrawn when it was realized that on exposure to the disease many children immunized with this vaccine developed atypical measles with pneumonia and other serious reactions. Also it was observed that children immunized with inactivated respiratory syncytial (RS) virus developed a more severe illness than unimmunized children on infection with virulent RS virus. The basis for this type of reaction after immunization with inactivated measles and RS virus was not understood; it was thought to be caused by the lack of sufficient stimulation of secretory IgA in the respiratory tract to neutralize virus but the development of hypersensitivity to virus so that immune complexes were formed in the lung (Sec. 5-32). A vaccine with living attenuated RS virus should prove effective, like the living attenuated measles virus vaccine. A vaccine and immune serum against *Pseudomonas aeruginosa* have been prepared and are being evaluated. *P. aeruginosa*, a gram-negative bacillus, is an opportunist which is resistant to most antibiotics and creates life-threatening situations in burn cases and other hospital patients with lowered resistance. *P. aeruginosa* is composed of at least seven major immunological types, so that a polyvalent vaccine and polyvalent immune serum are necessary. Another vaccine which is being tested for future use is one composed of capsular polysaccharide, type b, of *Hemophilus influenzae*. *H. influenzae* is a gram-negative bacillus which causes a highly fatal type of meningitis in young children, usually between 2 months and 3 years old. During the first few months, babies seem to be protected by maternal antibodies; by 3 years of age they have developed their own resistance, which evidently is acquired through exposure. Meningitis is associated with type b. This vaccine has not proved very effective. A vaccine against viral hepatitis, types A and B, has been sought for many years without success, partly because of the difficulty experienced in isolating and propagating these viruses. There are no vaccines against venereal diseases. The type of immunity which exists in syphilis, sometimes called *infection immunity*, is not understood. An infected person shows resistance to superinfection, but after suitable treatment this person is again susceptible to reinfection. Research on a vaccine for syphilis has been hampered by failures to culture the spirochete of syphilis in vitro (Chap. 11). The high incidence of gonorrhea in the United States is a public health problem which might be helped by active immunization if an effective vaccine could be prepared. The causative agent can be grown in vitro, but vaccines prepared with suspensions of the organism appear to confer immunity only against the serotype(s) or strain(s) present in the vaccine. When structural appendages of the gonococcus known as *pili* and their role in attachment to tissue surfaces were recognized, it was thought that vaccines composed of pili might be effective, but results to date have not been conclusive. Also a vaccine composed of ribosomes of gonococci has been used experimentally to immunize against gonococcal infection in an animal model. The use of ribosomes of other microorganisms to immunize against the respective infections caused by these microorganisms is now being investigated. The use of ribosomes separated from bacterial cells either as immunizing agents or as skin-test antigens is a relatively new experimental procedure.

Questions for Secs. 1-24 to 1-32

39. (*a*) Why must active immunization be given before exposure to a disease? (*b*) Why is rabies an exception? (*c*) Under what circumstances are both active and passive immunization used for protection against rabies?

40. (*a*) Give two ways in which microorganisms have been attenuated for use in vaccines. (*b*) What general precautions should be taken when living attenuated vaccines are injected parenterally? (*c*) What general precautions should be exercised when passive immunization is given?

41. (*a*) Are attenuated microorganisms nonpathogenic for all individuals regardless of the status of their capacity to produce an immune response? (*b*) Why is immunization with living, attenuated, supposedly nonvirulent viruses considered potentially fatal in children with cell-mediated immunodeficiency?

42. Why do you think that the Sabin vaccine would be considered safe for young pregnant women if they require immunization against poliomyelitis?

43. (*a*) What is the difference between homologous and heterologous antiserum? (*b*) What is meant by polyvalent vaccine and polyvalent antiserum?

In questions 44 to 56 review the situations and state in the first column whether vaccine, toxoid, antitoxin, or immune serum globulin (ISG) would be used for immunization. (Toxoid is a vaccine which specifically contains detoxified exotoxin.) In the second column state whether the type of immunization is active or passive.

44. Nonimmunized person exposed to tetanus	________	________
45. Routine immunization of child for diphtheria	________	________
46. Routine immunization of child for tetanus	________	________
47. Routine immunization of child for whooping cough (pertussis)	________	________
48. Person needs immunization against smallpox for foreign travel	________	________
49. 3-year-old sickly child not previously immunized against measles is exposed	________	________
50. Booster for tetanus	________	________
51. Child suspected of having diphtheria	________	________
52. 14-year-old boy without previous history of mumps or immunization for mumps is exposed	________	________
53. Husband ate same food at church supper as wife, who has just developed symptoms of botulism (exotoxin food poisoning produced by more than one type of toxin)	________	________
54. Young man bitten on leg by rabid dog	________	________
55. Child bitten on face by suspected rabid dog	________	________
56. Person bitten on leg by untraced dog;	________	________
not known whether it is rabid or nonrabid	________	________

Answers

39. (*a*) Active immunization must be given before exposure to a disease because it takes at least 7 to 14 days to build up an effective level of immunity. The incubation period of many diseases is less than 14 days, so that an effective level of immunity may not be attained if the vaccine is given after exposure. (*b*) Rabies is an exception because since there is usually a fairly long incubation period of about 4 weeks, an effective level of immunity can be achieved after exposure before rabies develops. (*c*) If a person is bitten on the face or on the upper extremities by a rabid animal, the incubation period is known to be shorter; therefore, passive immunization is used for immediate protection and active immunization is carried out for additional and more lasting protection since the incubation period in rabies is quite variable, sometimes being as long as 6 months, during which time passive immunity would no longer be effective. (Sec. 1-25.)

40. (*a*) Microorganisms can be attenuated by serially passaging them in an animal or environment other than that in which they usually grow, e.g., serial passage in embryonated eggs or tissue culture. Microorganisms can also be attenuated by aging and growth at temperatures other than optimum. (*b*) Living attenuated vaccines should not be given to persons who have immunodeficiency diseases or who are receiving immunosuppressive drugs. Living attenuated viruses should not be injected parenterally into pregnant women because of the danger of transplacental passage to the fetus. (*c*) For passive immunization, gamma globulin should not be injected intravenously. If serum or gamma globulin is from an animal of a different species, the patient should first be skin-tested to rule out allergy to the foreign protein. (Secs. 1-28 and 1-30.)

41. (*a*) Attenuated microorganisms which are used in vaccines are considered nonpathogenic for normal individuals but may be pathogenic for those suffering from immunodeficiency disorders or for those taking immunosuppressive drugs. (*b*) If specific antibodies are at the site of invasion by a virus, the virus is neutralized and viral infection does not occur. After viral infection occurs, antibodies are ineffective and only cell-mediated immunity is believed to be responsible for termination of a viral infection. If a child is lacking in cell-mediated immunity, even an attenuated virus may cause progressive and even fatal viral infection. (Sec. 1-30.)

42. Sabin vaccine is considered safe for immunization of young pregnant women because the virus is given by mouth and causes a mild infection of the intestinal tract. Since it is not injected parenterally, there should be less chance of transplacental passage of the virus to the fetus. (Sec. 1-30.)

43. (*a*) Homologous serum is serum from an animal of the same species; heterologous serum is from an animal of a different, or foreign, species. (*b*) Polyvalent vaccine contains antigens from more than one immunological type; polyvalent antiserum contains antibodies to more than one immunological type. (Secs. 1-31 and 1-32.)

44. Antitoxin;* passive

45. Toxoid; active

46. Toxoid; active

47. Vaccine; active

48. Vaccine; active

49. ISG; passive

50. Toxoid; active

51. Antitoxin; passive

52. ISG; passive

53. Antitoxin;† passive

54. Vaccine; active

55. ISG; passive; vaccine; active

56. Vaccine;‡ active

(Secs. 1-18, 1-22, 1-23, and 1-25.)

REFERENCES

Ammann, A. J., J. Addiego, D. W. Wara, B. Lubia, W: B. Smith and W. C. Mentzner (1977): Pneumococcal Immunization in Sickle-Cell Anemia and Asplenia, *N. Engl. J. Med.*, **297**:897–900.

Berg, J. M. (1958): Neurologic Complications of Pertussis Immunization, *Br. Med. J.*, 2:24–27.

Briody, B. A., and R. E. Gillis (1974): "Microbiology and Infectious Disease," McGraw-Hill, New York.

Brock, T. D. (1961): "Milestones in Microbiology," American Society for Microbiology, Washington, D.C.

*The first injection of toxoid for active immunization may also be given.

†Since there is more than one immunological type of exotoxin secreted by strains of *Clostridium botulinum*, a polyvalent antitoxin must be used.

‡Before immunization, consult local health official for presence of rabies in region.

Cunningham-Rundles, U. F. (1976): The Reticuloendothelial System, pp. 289-303 in F. H. Bach and R. A. Good (eds.), "Clinical Immunobiology," vol. 2, Academic, New York.
Davidson, I., and D. A. Nelson (1974): The Blood, pp. 100-310 in I. Davidson and J. B. Henry (eds.), "Todd-Sanford Clinical Diagnosis by Laboratory Methods," 15th ed., Saunders, Philadelphia.
Davis, B. D., R. Dulbecco, H. N. Eisen, H. S. Ginsberg, W. B. Wood, and M. McCarty (1973): "Microbiology," 2d ed., Harper & Row, Hagerstown, Md.
Douglas, R. G., Jr. (1975): Respiratory Virus Vaccines: Recent Advances, pp. 409-415 in D. Schlessinger (ed.), "Microbiology: 1975" American Society for Microbiology, Washington, D.C.
Eickhoff, T. C. (1971): Committee on Immunization against Influenza: Rationale and Recommendations, *J. Infect. Dis.*, **123**:446-453.
Enders, J. F., S. Katz, M. V. Milovanie, and S. Holloway (1960): Studies of an Attenuated Measles Vaccine, I: Development and Preparation of the Vaccine, *N. Engl. J. Med.* **263**:153-159.
Finter, N. B. (ed.) (1973): "Interferons and Interferon Inducers," American Elsevier, New York.
Fisher, M. W. (1975): Polyvalent Vaccine and Human Globulin for Controlling *Pseudomonas aerugenosa* Infections, p. 416 in D. Schlessinger (ed.), "Microbiology: 1975" American Society for Microbiology, Washington, D.C.
Freedman, S. O. and P. Gold (eds.) (1976): "Clinical Immunology," 2d ed. Harper & Row, Hagerstown, Md.
Fulginiti, V. A. (1971): Abnormalities in Vaccine Responsiveness, pp. 245-261 in B. M. Kagan and E. R. Stiehm (eds.), "Immunologic Incompetence" Year Book, Chicago.
———J. J. Eller, A. W. Downie, and C. H. Kempe (1967): Altered Reactivity to Measles Virus: Atypical Measles in Children Previously Immunized with Inactivated (Killed) Measles Vaccines, *JAMA*, **202**:1075-1080.
Gellis, S. S., A. C. McGuinnes, and M. Peters (1945): A Study on the Prevention of Mumps Orchitis by Gamma Globulin, *Am. J. Med. Sci.*, **210**:661-664.
Glezen, W. P., and F. W. Denner (1973): Epidemiology of Acute Lower Respiratory Disease in Children, *N. Engl. J. Med.*, **288**:498-505.
Goerke, L. S., P. Roberts, and J. M. Chapman (1958): Neo-natal Responses to D. T. P. Vaccines, *Public Health Rep.*, **73**:511-518.
Goldstein, A. L., G. B. Thurman, C. H. Cohen, and J. A. Hooper (1975): The role of Thymosin and the Endocrine Thymus on the Ontogenesis and Function of T-cells, pp. 243-265 in E. E. Smith and D. W. Ribbons (eds.), Molecular Approaches to Immunology, *Miami Winter Sym.* vol. 9, Academic, New York.
Greep, R. O., and L. Weiss (1973): "Histology," 3d ed., McGraw-Hill, New York.
Ham, A. W. (1974): "Histology," 7th ed., Lippincott, Philadelphia.
Hilleman, M. R., E. B. Bunyak, R. E. Weibel, and J. Stokes (1968): Live Attenuated Mumps-Virus Vaccine, *N. Engl. J. Med.*, **278**:227-232.
Horstmann, D. M. (1971): Rubella: The Challenge of Its Control, *J. Infect. Dis.*, **123**:640-654.
Isaacs, A., and J. Lindenmann (1957): Virus Interference, I: The Interferon, *Proc. R. Soc.*, **147**:258-267.
Kempe, C. H. (1971): To Vaccinate or Not? pp. 274-279 in R. A. Good and D. W. Fisher (eds.), "Immunobiology," Sinauer, Stamford, Conn.
Krugman, S., J. P. Giles, and J. Hammond (1971): Viral Hepatitis, Type B (MS-2 Strain): Studies on Active Immunization, *JAMA*, **217**:41-45.
Larson, H. E., P. D. Parkman, W. J. Davis, H. E. Hopps, and H. M. Meyer (1971): Inadvertant Rubella Virus Vaccination during Pregnancy, *N. Engl. J. Med.*, **284**:870-873.
Modlin, J. F., J. T. Jabbour, J. J. Witte, and N. A. Halsey (1977): Epidemiologic Studies of Measles, Measles Vaccine, and Subacute Sclerosing Panencephalitis, *Pediactrics*, **59**:505-512.
Nelson, D. S. (ed.) (1976): "Immunobiology of the Macrophage," Academic, New York.
Nelson, K. E., V. Vithayasai, S. Makornkawkayoon, M. D. Batt, K. Panas-Amporn, and J. T. Anderson (1977): Purified Duck Embryo Rabies Vaccine: An Accelerated Schedule for Pre-exposure Immunization against Rabies, *JAMA*, **238**:218-220.
Nightingale, E. O. (1977): Recommendations for a National Policy on Poliomyelitis Vaccination, *N. Engl. J. Med.*, **297**:249-253.
North, R. J. (1974): Cell-mediated Immunity and the Response to Infection, pp. 185-219 in R. T. McClusky and S. Cohen (eds.), "Mechanisms of Cell-mediated Immunity," Wiley, New York.
Nowell, P. C., and D. B. Wilson (1971): Lymphocytes and Hemic Stem Cells, *Am. J. Pathol.*, **65**:641-652.
Pumper, R. W., and H. M. Yamashiroga (1975): "Essentials of Medical Virology," Saunders, Philadelphia.

Report (1942): Jaundice Following Yellow Fever Vaccination, *JAMA*, **119**:1110.
Report (1942): Outbreak of Jaundice in the Army, *JAMA*, **120**:51-53.
Robbins, J. R. (1975): Acquisition of "Natural" and Immunization Induced Immunity to *Haemophilus influenzae* Type b Diseases, pp. 400-405 in D. Schlessinger (ed.), "Microbiology: 1975," American Society for Microbiology, Washington, D.C.
Sabin, A. B. (1963): Is there an Exceedingly Small Risk Associated with Oral Poliovirus Vaccine? *JAMA*, **183**:268-271.
——R. H. Michaels, S. Krugman, M. E. Eigen, P. H. Berman, and J. Warren (1963): Effect of Oral Poliovaccine in Newborn Children, 1: Excretion of Virus after Injection of Large Doses of Type 1 or of Mixtures of All Three Types in Relation to the Level of Placentally Transmitted Antibody, *Pediatrics*, **31**:623-640.
——P. Ziring, S. Krugman, and J. Warren (1963): Effect of Oral Poliovaccine in Newborn Children, 2: Intestinal Resistance and Antibody Response at 6 Months in Children Fed Type 1 Vaccine at Birth, *Pediatrics*, **31**:641-650.
Salk, J., and D. Salk (1977): Control of Influenza and Poliomyelitis with Killed Virus Vaccines, *Science*, **195**:834-847.
Scribner, D. J., and D. Fahrney (1976): Neutrophil Receptors for IgG and Complement: Their Roles in the Attachment and Ingestion Phases of Phagocytosis, *J. Immunol.*, **116**:892-897.
Sever, J. L., K. B. Nelson, and M. R. Gilkeson (1965): Rubella Epidemic 1964: Effect on 6000 Pregnancies, *Am. J. Dis. Child.*, **110**:395-407.
Shvartzman, Ya. S., and M. P. Zykov (1976): Secretory Anti-influenza Immunity, *Adv. Immunol.*, **22**:291-330.
Stiehm, E. R., and V. A. Fulginiti (1973): "Immunologic Disorders in Infants and Children," Saunders, Philadelphia.
Strom, J. (1960): Is Universal Vaccination against Pertussis Always Justified?, *Br. Med. J.*, **2**:1184-1186.
Terry, L. (1962): The Association of Cases of Poliomyelitis with the Use of Type 3 Oral Poliomyelitis Vaccines: A Technical Report, U.S. Department of Health, Education and Welfare, Sept. 20, 1962.
Waldman, R. H., S. H. Wood, E. J. Torres, and P. A. Small (1970): Influenza Antibody Response Following Aerosol Administration of Inactivated Virus, *Am. J. Epidemiol.*, **91**:575-584.
Weihl, C. (1963): Extracted Pertussis Antigen: A Clinical Appraisal, *Am. J. Dis. Child.*, **106**:210-215.
Wintrobe, M. W., G. R. Lee, D. R. Boggs, T. C. Bithell, J. W. Athens, and J. Forrester (1974): "Clinical Hematology," 7th ed., Lea & Febiger, Philadelphia.
Wong, K. H., R. J. Arko, L. C. Logan, and J. C. Bullar (1976): Immunological and Serological Diversity of *Neisseria gonorrhoeae*: Gonococcal Serotypes and Their Relationship with Immunotypes, *Infect. Immun.*, **14**:1297-1301.

2
The Action of B and T Lymphocytes in Humoral and Cell-mediated Immune Responses

IMMUNE RESPONSES OF THE HOST TO ANTIGEN

2-1 Specific immunological reactions of the host to antigens may include four distinct responses:

1. The production of antibody
2. The development of specific cell-mediated reactions
3. The production of immunological memory
4. The production of specific immunological unresponsiveness

The production of antibody Antibody production may be either beneficial or harmful to the human host. Examples of the protective action of antibodies are elimination of pathogenic bacteria from tissues of the host after reaction with antibodies, neutralization of exotoxins, and neutralization of viruses. Examples of the harmful action of antibodies are immediate-type hypersensitivity reactions, e.g., anaphylactic shock and atopy. Immediate-type hypersensitivity reactions can be caused by the production of antibodies to antigens like those found in horse serum, bee venom, and plant pollens. The body produces antibodies to any foreign substance which enters it provided the foreign substance has the properties of an antigen (or immunogen).

The development of specific cell-mediated reactions Cell-mediated reactions of the host to antigen result in cell-mediated immunity or in delayed-type hypersensitivity. Examples associated with protection are resistance of the host to tuberculosis and destruction of host cells when they are transformed into cancer cells. An example of delayed-type hypersensitivity is contact dermatitis to chemicals, e.g., those found in poison ivy. Rejection of skin and organ grafts is also associated with delayed-type hypersensitivity.

The production of immunological memory Immunological memory is initiated during the primary response but becomes manifest during the secondary response and usually any time thereafter when the host is exposed to the specific antigen. Immune responses, including both antibody production and cell-mediated reactions, take place more rapidly and to a greater extent when reexposure to an antigen occurs after primary immunization. Immunological memory is the basis of the booster injection of a vaccine and is also known as the anamnestic response.

The production of specific immunological unresponsiveness If an animal is exposed to an antigen in utero and expósure to the antigen occurs again after birth, the antigen is not recognized as being foreign. Both production of antibody and cell-mediated immunity may be affected. Only certain kinds of antigens produce immunological unresponsiveness, also called immunologic tolerance. Tolerance may be produced experimentally by injection of appropriate antigens immediately after birth. Tolerance is more readily produced to soluble antigens such as serum albumin than to particulate antigens, i.e., those contained in particulate structures like bacteria. When in utero infection occurs with certain microorganisms, e.g., the spirochete of syphilis, tolerance is not produced.

Phylogeny of the Immune System

2-2 The ability to produce the immune responses cited above is limited to vertebrate animals. The immune responses described are viewed as adaptations of higher vertebrates for maintaining the integrity of the body even though some immune reactions turn out to be unfavorable to the host. Lower vertebrates have a simple immune system; some produce only IgM antibodies, which are considered to be the most primitive type of immunoglobulins. In human beings, IgM antibodies are produced in utero by the fetus in response to transplacental infection and are the first type to be produced after birth in response to an antigen. We shall see later (Chaps. 4 and 11) that in utero production of IgM is made use of in diagnosing congenital infections. The study of the immune system beginning with phyla of lower vertebrates such as fish and continuing up the phlogenetic scale of complexity to that of higher vertebrates such as mammals and human beings is often referred to as the *phylogeny of immunity*. Ontogeny is a biological term used to refer to the development of the individual organism. We shall study the development of the immune system in human beings and in other animals insofar as a study of the latter helps us understand the human immune system.

Questions for Secs. 2-1 and 2-2

1. List four basically distinct immunologic responses which could occur in the human host after exposure to an antigen (or immunogen) depending on the biologic state of the host and the nature of the antigen.

2. (*a*) Is the production of antibody always a favorable response for the host? (*b*) Give examples to illustrate your answer.

3. (*a*) Is the production of specific cell-mediated reactions always favorable to the host? (*b*) Give examples to illustrate your answer.

4. (*a*) What is meant by immunological memory? (*b*) Does the production of immunologic memory on reexposure to an antigen apply to both antibody production and cell-mediated reactions? (*c*) What is another name for immunologic memory?

5. What is the difference between immunologic tolerance and the type of unresponsiveness which is achieved by giving drugs to suppress immune responses in general?

6. The production of specific immunologic unresponsiveness is easy to achieve in experimental animals but not in the human host. Can you think of a case where specific immunologic unresponsiveness or tolerance would be very desirable in human beings?

7. (*a*) What is considered to be the main function of the immune system? (*b*) Do invertebrates form immunoglobulins (antibodies)? (*c*) Which immunoglobulin is considered to be the most primitive type produced by vertebrates? (*d*) What immunoglobulin may be produced in utero in response to infection during development of the human fetus?

8. (*a*) What is meant by phylogeny of immunity? (*b*) What is meant by ontogeny of immunity?

Answers

1. Four basically distinct immunologic reactions are (1) production of antibody, (2) production of cell-mediated reactions, (3) production of immunologic memory, and (4) production of specific immunologic unresponsiveness or tolerance. (Sec. 2-1.)

2. (*a*) Antibody production is not always favorable to the host. (*b*) Antibody to a microorganism may afford protection. In contrast, antibody to a foreign protein like that in bee venom can cause immediate-type hypersensitivity reactions and even death if a sensitized person (one containing this antibody) is stung by a bee. (Sec. 2-1.)

3. (*a*) Specific cell-mediated reactions are not always favorable. (*b*) Cell-mediated reactions are associated with resistance to tuberculosis and cancer. Cell-mediated reactions are the basis of delayed-type hypersensitivity, e.g., contact dermatitis and rejection of skin grafts. (Sec. 2-1).

4. (*a*) Immunological memory refers to the more rapid immune response of the host on reexposure to an antigen than after first exposure. (*b*) Immunological memory occurs with both antibody production and cell-mediated reactions. (*c*) The anamnestic response by derivation means "to recall to memory." (Sec. 2-1.)

5. Suppression of immune responses by giving drugs is nonspecific in that immune responses to a wide variety of antigens including bacteria, viruses, tumor cells, etc., may be suppressed; immunologic tolerance is specific for a particular antigen. (Sec. 2-1.)

6. For organ grafts, e.g., heart transplantation, it would be desirable to produce specific unresponsiveness or tolerance to the foreign heart tissue in order to prevent rejection without affecting the patient's resistance to microorganisms and tumor cells. (Sec. 2-1.)

7. (*a*) Maintenance of the body's integrity is considered to be the main function of the immune system. (*b*) No, invertebrates do not form immunoglobulins (antibodies). (*c*) IgM is the most primitive type of immunoglobulin. (*d*) IgM may be produced in utero by human fetus in response to infection. (Sec. 2-2.)

8. (*a*) Phylogeny of immunity refers to the study of the immune system starting with the phyla of lower vertebrates and ending with the phyla of vertebrates, showing the greatest degree of development, e.g., that of human beings. (*b*) Ontogeny of immunity refers to the development of the immune system of an individual, e.g., a human child from conception to adult life. (Sec. 2-2.)

THE DEVELOPMENT OF HUMORAL AND CELL-MEDIATED IMMUNITY

Early Distinction between Humoral and Cell-mediated Immunity

2-3 It was recognized by von Behring in 1890 that antibodies are responsible for neutralization of diphtheria exotoxin and protection against many bacterial diseases such as pneumococcal pneumonia. Protection associated with antibodies was known as *humoral immunity*. It was also recognized that antibodies could be harmful and even cause fatal allergic reactions such as anaphylactic shock. Because of the short time which elapsed between injection of the antigen and the appearance of allergic symptons, this type of allergy associated with antibodies became known as *immediate hypersensitivity*. Both humoral immunity and immediate hypersensitivity could be passively transferred with antiserum containing antibodies. Protection could be conferred immediately, but transfer of sensitivity could be demonstrated only after several hours. It was postulated then that time was required for antibodies to be fixed to tissue; that this is true for IgE has been recognized.

2-4 In contrast to the findings just cited, it was observed that antibodies did not confer any protection against diseases like tuberculosis. It was also noted that when material called *tuberculin* prepared from cultures of tubercle bacilli was injected intradermally into the skin of a patient with tuberculosis, a reaction did not appear at once at the injection site but was delayed for several hours. This type of allergic reaction could not be passively transferred with serum antibodies but could be transferred to other animals by injection of a suspension of cells (leukocytes). Resistance to tuberculosis and allergy in this disease became known as *cell-mediated* or *delayed hypersensitivity*. Cellular transfer of delayed hypersensitivity was demonstrated by Landsteiner and Chase (1942) with experiments on contact hypersensitivity to picryl chloride in guinea pigs. They used peritoneal exudate cells from hypersensitive animals. Chase extended these studies on cell transfer of allergy to other cases of delayed hypersensitivity, e.g., the tuberculin reaction. It was not shown until much later that the cells responsible for transfer of delayed hypersensitivity are lymphocytes which are now known as *sensitized* or *activated T lymphocytes*. These cells are considered immunologically competent cells because on contact with antigen they are capable of immune responses. Transfer of immunity or sensitivity with cells is known as *adoptive immunization*. This procedure can lead to a very serious reaction, the graft-versus-host reaction, especially when these cells are injected into a person with an immunologic deficiency disorder. Each individual has individual specific tissue antigens, designated *HLA antigens*, which are foreign to a graft unless it comes from an identical twin. HLA antigens are also known as *histocompatibility* or *transplantation antigens*. Since lymphocytes have high concentrations of HLA antigens, a suspension of lymphocytes is used for tissue typing before transplantation (Chap. 9). If a graft-versus-host reaction occurs in an immunologic-deficient individual, instead of rejection of the graft by the host, the graft rejects the host to cause disease and sometimes even death of the host.

2-5 Lawrence (1954) reported that a cell-free extract of human leukocytes from peripheral blood is capable of transferring cell-mediated immunity in human beings. He called his extract *transfer factor*. Transfer factor is now being investigated extensively for treatment of individuals showing cell-mediated deficiency disorders. Transfer factor is not associated with the graft-versus-host reaction and appears safe for injection, but the mechanism of its action is not known. Transfer factor has been shown to have the following properties: it is effective only in human beings and not in any of the lower animal species tested; it is a low-molecular-weight (less than 10,000) nonimmunogenic heat-labile dialyzable substance of polypeptide-polynucleotide composition. For a further discussion of transfer factor and its use, see Chap. 7.

Ontogeny of the Immune System

2-6 For many years little was known about the basis for development of humoral and cell-mediated types of immune responses. Glick, Chang, and Jaap (1956) reported that removal of a lymphoid structure in chickens shortly after hatching destroys their ability to develop humoral immunity; the ability to produce cell-mediated immunity was not affected. The lymphoid structure was the bursa of Fabricius, which is located in the cloacal region. This important discovery seems to have been a fortunate accident because the bursa had been removed to study its effect on sexual development. The chickens which were normal except for bursectomy were later used in a class experiment to demonstrate antibody production, but antibody production did not occur. This was one of the findings which led to the extensive study by many other investigators of the effect of primary lymphoid organs on the development of the immune system. Mammals have no bursa of Fabricius; lymphoid tissue in the gut, e.g., Peyer's patches and the appendix, has been studied to determine whether its role is the same as that of the bursa. Lymphoid tissue in the gut is referred to as *gut-associated lymphoid tissue* (GALT). So far the human equivalent of the bursa has not been definitely determined, but it appears to be the bone marrow.

2-7 The importance of the thymus in the maturation of the immune system was reported by Miller (1961), who showed that neonatal thymectomy of mice causes a severe depletion of lymphocytes and a marked deficiency in reactions associated with cell-mediated immunity or delayed-type hypersensitivity. The results of many investigators indicated that interference with development of the bursa affects antibody production primarily, while interference with thymus development affects cell-mediated reactions. (Review Fig. 1-2.) The critical period in the development of the immune system is when lymphoid tissue is forming; both the bursa and the thymus exert their influence on immunologic development during early life. The weight of the human thymus is maximal at puberty, after which its size and function decrease. A thymus hormone may influence development of the immune system. It has been shown experimentally with neonatally thymectomized mice that thymus tissue implanted in these mice but enclosed in porous chambers largely corrects the known thymus deficiency. A thymus hormonal effect is indicated because the pores of the chamber were too small to allow passage of cells but large enough to allow passage of a hormone.

2-8 The cells directly concerned with humoral and cell-mediated reactions eventually reside in peripheral or secondary lymphoid tissues, e.g., lymph nodes and spleen. Cells responsible for antibody production are called *B lymphocytes* because they become committed to antibody production under the influence of the bursa in chickens or equivalent bursa structure in other animals. As stated above, it was earlier believed that gut-associated lymphod tissue (GALT) in man might be the bursa equivalent; more recent evidence indicates bone marrow. Lymphocytes committed to cell-mediated reactions are under the influence of the thymus and are called T lymphocytes or thymus-dependent lymphocytes. On contact with antigen, B cells are stimulated to form antibody-producing plasma cells; after reaction with antigen, T lymphocytes are called *activated T lymphocytes, sensitized T lymphocytes*, or *effector cells of cell-mediated reactions.* When it was realized that it was not the time differences between immediate and delayed hypersensitivity reactions which were important but the basic underlying mechanisms, it was recommended that the terms immediate-type and delayed-type be used to differentiate hypersensitivity. The mechanisms concerned with cell-mediated immunity are essentially the same as those for delayed-type hypersensitivity.

2-9 Additional information about the development of humoral and cell-mediated immunity can be gathered by studying children with immunodeficiency diseases concerned with antibody production or cell-mediated reactions or both. Bruton (1952) described the first case of congenital sex-linked agammaglobulinemia. Children with Bruton's agammaglobulinemia have B-cell deficiencies, so that they produce very little antibody; cell-mediated immunity is not affected. Actually, the term hypogammaglobulinemia (*hypo*- means "decreased") better describes the condition than agammaglobulinemia (*a*- means "without") since there is a severe deficiency but not a complete absence of gamma globulin. These children recover from viral infections as if they had a normal immune mechanism but must be given antibiotics and gamma globulin to protect them from bacterial infections. DiGeorge (1965) described the syndrome named after him, which is not a genetic disease but is caused by failure during embryogenesis of the third and fourth pharyngeal pouches, from which the thymus is derived. It can be shown at autopsy that these children lack a thymus. Children with this syndrome have very few circulating lymphocytes, which in normal children are mainly T cells. They have B cells and produce antibody, but T-cell deficiency means that they cannot produce cell-mediated immunity and are very susceptible to viral and fungal infections. Recently a few children with the DiGeorge syndrome have been reconstituted immunologically with a thymus graft from aborted human fetuses. As pointed out previously, the injection of immunocompetent cells into a patient with an immunologic deficiency disorder is dangerous and can cause a graft-versus-host reaction. At present there are several immunologic deficiency disorders in which both B- and T-cell deficiences have been recognized. These include the Wiskott-Aldrich syndrome and Swiss-type agammaglobulinemia. Transfer factor has been used successfully in the treatment of some children with these two conditions. Transfer factor is not curative; it has to be given again when relapses occur.

Questions for Secs. 2-3 to 2-9

9. (*a*) Answer in the space whether you would use serum or cells for the transfer of the types of immune reactions shown.

________(1) Humoral immunity
________(2) Immediate-type hypersensitivity
________(3) Cell-mediated immunity
________(4) Delayed-type hypersensitivity

(*b*) What in the serum is responsible for transfer of humoral immunity or immediate-type hypersensitivity? (*c*) What kind of cells are capable of transferring cell-mediated immunity or delayed-type hypersensitivity? (*d*) What is adoptive immunization? (*e*) Is adoptive immunization considered safe? (*f*) If your answer to part (e) is no, explain.

10. (*a*) What are immunocompetent cells? (*b*) What are HLA antigens? (*c*) What are two general terms which are used to refer to HLA antigens? (*d*) Why is a suspension of lymphocytes used for tissue typing for transplantation?

11. (*a*) What are the source and nature of transfer factor? (*b*) What type of reactivity is transferred with transfer factor? (*c*) Is transfer factor effective only in human beings? (*d*) Can transfer factor be used for therapeutic purposes? (*e*) What is the mechanism of action of transfer factor?

12. (*a*) What primary lymphoid organ is necessary for the development of that part of the immune system responsible for antibody production? (*b*) What is the effect of the removal of this organ from adult animals? (*c*) What is the effect of the removal of this organ from newborn animals?

13. (*a*) In what animal is the bursa of Fabricius found? (*b*) Where is the bursa located? (*c*) What type of structure is it? (*d*) What is the bursa equivalent in human beings?

14. (*a*) What primary lymphoid organ is necessary for the development of that part of the immune system responsible for cell-mediated immunity and delayed-type hypersensitivity? (*b*) What is the effect of the removal of this organ from adult animals? (*c*) What is the effect of the removal of this organ from newborn animals?

15. (*a*) Does the thymus produce a hormone which influences the development of cell-mediated immunity (or delayed-type hypersensitivity)? (*b*) Explain.

16. (*a*) What are B and T lymphocytes? (*b*) With reference to lymphocytes, what is the origin of the letters B and T?

17. Use the letters A and C to denote whether the conditions listed are antibody-mediated (A) or mainly cell-mediated (C).

_____ (*a*) Resistance to tuberculosis
_____ (*b*) Termination of viral infections
_____ (*c*) Neutralization of viruses
_____ (*d*) Resistance to fungal infections
_____ (*e*) Immediate-type hypersensitivity
_____ (*f*) Anaphylactic shock and atopy
_____ (*g*) Delayed-type hypersensitivity
_____ (*h*) Contact dermatitis (hypersensitivity)
_____ (*i*) Graft-versus-host reaction
_____ (*j*) Graft rejection by host
_____ (*k*) Neutralization of diphtheria exotoxin
_____ (*l*) Immune surveillance or destruction of cancer cells

18. In the chart, check whether the immunodeficiency disorders listed in first column were due to B or T lymphocytes and which part of the immune system was affected.

Immunodeficiency disorder	Population of lymphocytes affected		Immune response(s) affected	
	B cells	T cells	Antibody production	Cell-mediated
Bruton's agammaglobulinemia				
DiGeorge syndrome				
Swiss-type agammaglobulinemia				
Wiskott-Aldrich syndrome				

9. (*a*) (1) Serum, (2) serum, (3) cells, (4) cells. (*b*) Antibodies in the serum. (*c*) Activated T lymphocytes can transfer cell-mediated immunity or delayed-type hypersensitivity to another animal. (*d*) Adoptive immunization is transfer of immunity or hypersensitivity with cells, e.g., a suspension of blood leukocytes which has a fairly high concentration of T lymphocytes. (*e*) No. (*f*) The immunologically competent transferred cells can act against the cells of the host, especially in a person with an immunodeficiency disorder, so that a graft-versus-host reaction takes place. (Secs. 2-3 and 2-4.)

10. (*a*) Immunocompetent cells are cells capable of immune responses. This does not mean that the cells have to be actively engaged at the time in an immune response. (*b*) HLA antigens are individual specific antigens found in human tissue and in high concentration on lymphocytes; HLA antigens are responsible for graft rejection. (*c*) HLA antigens are referred to as histocompatibility antigens and transplantation antigens. (*d*) A suspension of lymphocytes is used for tissue typing or matching before transplantation because they have a high concentration of HLA antigens. (Sec. 2-4.)

11. (*a*) Transfer factor is prepared from an extract of blood leukocytes, the main cells being the T lymphocytes; transfer factor is a heat-labile, nonantigenic low-molecular-weight dialyzable substance of polypeptide-polynucleotide composition. (*b*) Cell-mediated immunity or delayed-type hypersensitivity. (*c*) Yes, transfer factor is effective in human beings but not in any of the lower animal species tested. (*d*) Transfer factor can be used for therapeutic purposes provided the individual(s) from whose cells it was prepared had the desired resistance. It has been used for treating T-cell deficiencies. Where there is a combined B- and T-cell deficiency, the B-cell deficiency is treated with antibiotics and gamma globulin. (*c*) The mechanism of action of transfer factor is not understood. (Sec. 2-5.)

12. (*a*) The bursa of Fabricius in chickens or the bursa equivalent in other animals. (*b*) Usually little or no effect on immune responses. (*c*) These animals do not develop the capacity to produce antibodies. (Secs. 2-6 and 2-7.)

13. (*a*) The bursa of Fabricius is found in chickens. (*b*) The bursa is in the cloacal region of chickens. (*c*) The bursa is a primary lymphoid organ. (*d*) The bursa equivalent in human beings has not been definitely established but is believed to be bone marrow; at one time, gut-associated lymphoid tissue (GALT) was thought to be the bursa equivalent. (Sec. 2-6.)

14. (*a*) Thymus. (*b*) Usually little or no effect on immune responses. (*c*) These animals do not develop the capacity to produce cell-mediated immunity or delayed type-hypersensitivity. (Sec. 2-7.)

15. (*a*) Yes, there is some evidence that the thymus produces a hormone which brings about differientiation of precursor lymphocytes into T cells. (*b*) Thymus tissue implanted into neonatally thymectomized mice helps correct the T-cell deficiency when thymus is implanted in a chamber with pores of such a size that intact cells cannot pass but a hormone can. (Sec. 2-7.)

16. (*a*) B and T lymphocytes are immunocompetent cells responsible for antibody production and specific cell-mediated reactions, respectively. (*b*) The letter B comes from bursa and T from thymus since B cells were originally observed to develop under the influence of the bursa in chickens and T cells under the influence of the thymus; B at the present time is also used to denote bone marrow since there is some evidence that bone marrow is the bursa equivalent for human beings. (Sec. 2-8.)

17.

(*a*) C	(*b*) C	(*c*) A	(*d*) C
(*e*) A	(*f*) A	(*g*) C	(*h*) C
(*i*) C	(*j*) C	(*k*) A	(*l*) C

(Secs. 2-1, 2-4, and 2-9.)

18.

Immunodeficiency disorder	Population of lymphocytes affected		Immune response(s) affected	
	B cells	T cells	Antibody production	Cell-mediated
Bruton's agammaglobulinemia	√		√	
DiGeorge syndrome		√		√
Swiss-type agammaglobulinemia	√	√	√	√
Wiskott-Aldrich syndrome	√	√	√	√

(Sec. 2-9.)

THE FUNCTIONING OF B AND T LYMPHOCYTES IN IMMUNE RESPONSES

Physical Properties of B and T Cells

2-10 B and T cells are lymphocytes and are found mainly in blood, lymph, lymphoid tissue, and connective tissue. Lymphocytes have a large nucleus, which almost completely fills the cytoplasm. A cluster of lymphocytes can be observed in the electron micrograph in Fig. 2-1. Lymphocytes are

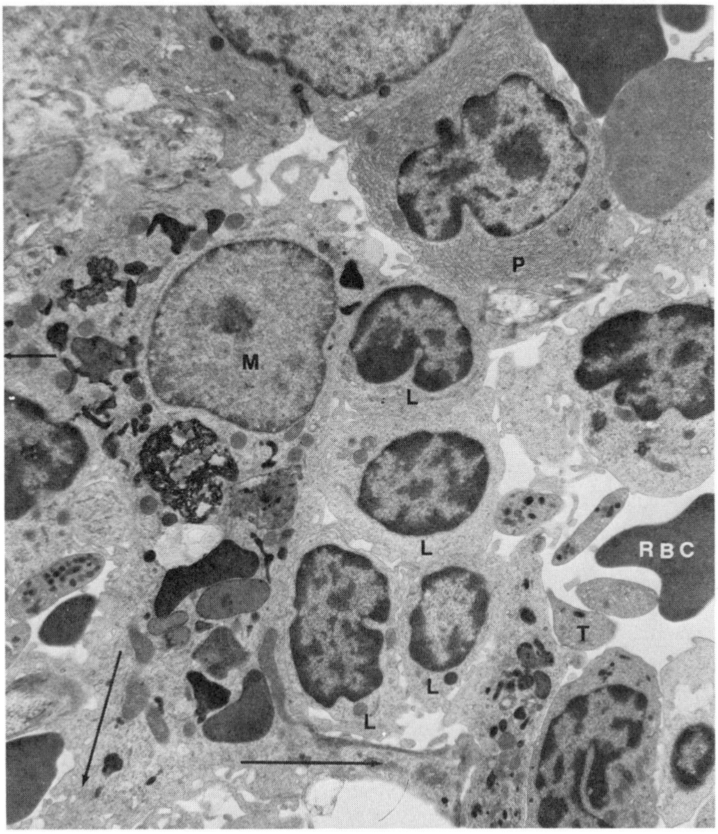

Figure 2-1 Transmission electron micrograph of a rat spleen, showing some of the cells responsible for immune responses; P = plasma cell, M = macrophage (arrows show its cytoplasmic extensions), L = lymphocyte, T = thrombocyte, RBC = red blood cell. Magnification × 5600; taken by the author.

not phagocytic cells. They are motile and are capable of passage through endothelium and its basement membrane. Studies of surface structure by scanning electron microscopy have shown T cells with a fairly smooth surface but B cells studded with numerous villous projections. Surface structure in scanning electron microscopy may be influenced by the method of preparation of the specimen. Lymphocytes vary in size and are often referred to as small, medium, and large lymphocytes. Lymphocytes of peripheral blood are mainly T lymphocytes and are small (about 10 μm). Lymphocytes are not end cells but are capable of multiplication. Before division they become enlarged. Lymphocytes may be stimulated to multiply on exposure to antigens or to mitogens. Stimulation by mitogens such as phytohemagglutinin (PHA), concanavalin A (ConA), and pokeweed mitogen (PWM) is nonspecific but is used in diagnostic tests as an indication of the ability of lymphocytes to be activated. A lymphocyte which can be activated by mitogens is considered immunocompetent. Lymphocytes which have been stimulated to divide are known as *blast cells*.

2-11 Both B and T cells contain histocompatibility antigens on their surface. Much research on histocompatibility antigens in mice has been done; they are designated H-2 antigens and are the counterpart of HLA antigens in human beings. T cells of mice possess a theta (θ), or T, antigen which has not been identified on human lymphocytes; however, a brain-specific antigen on T lymphocytes has been identified. Both B and T cells have surface receptors for antigen. The exact nature of antigen receptors on T cells is not known. The fact that antigen receptors on B cells are immunoglobulins which can be easily detected is used for recognition of B cells by immunoflourescent techniques (Secs. 2-16 and 2-23). Immunoglobulin receptors have been designated as membrane-bound (M-Ig) or as surface immunoglobulins (S-Ig). Most but not all B cells have Fc receptors. Fc receptors react with the Fc portion of IgG immunoglobulins (see Sec. 3-15 on the structure of immunoglobulins). IgG appears to react more firmly with Fc receptors if IgG is aggregated or in combination with antigen. Some B cells also have receptors for the C3 complement component. Both Fc and C3 receptors have been found on non-B cells. Human T cells have receptors for sheep red blood cells (rbc), and this fact is frequently used for the recognition and separation of T cells. Sheep red blood cells stick to the surface of T cells to form what has been described as E-rosette formation, where the E stands for erythrocyte (see Fig. 2-2). B cells which have Fc receptors for immunoglobulins will form rosettes with erythrocytes coated with antibody (called EA rosettes or Fc rosettes, but not with untreated sheep erythrocytes as T cells do. Some lymphocytes are called *null cells* because they cannot be distinguished as B or T cells on the basis of surface markers. It has been shown that the number of T, B, and null cells in a preparation accounts for 100 percent of the lymphocytes.

Maturation and Commitment of B and T Cells

2-12 Maturation of B cells takes place in the bursa of Fabricius of chickens and the equivalent bursa structure of human beings, while maturation of T cells occurs in the thymus. The bursa and thymus are termed *primary* or *central lymphoid organs*. B and T stem cells or precursor cells are derived from

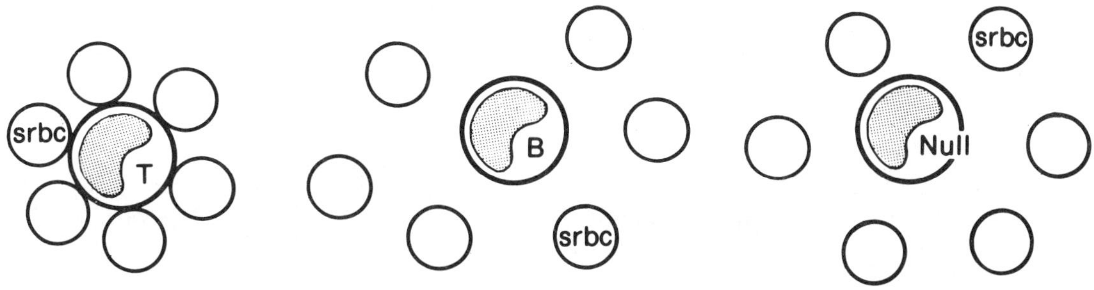

Figure 2-2 Separation of human T lymphocytes from B lymphocytes and null cells by E-rosette formation of T cells with untreated sheep red blood cells (srbc).

yolk sac or fetal liver depending upon the stage of development of the fetus; in the latter stages of development, B and T cells come from bone marrow. Precursor cells, or stem cells, are known as uncommitted cells or antigen-insensitive cells because they are not committed to perform any special function or to respond to any particular antigen. In the bursa, B cells become committed to produce antibody; in addition there is evidence that each B cell is committed or programmed to respond only to a certain antigen. Likewise in the thymus, T cells are committed to cell-mediated or delayed-type hypersensitivity functions with commitment to specificity determined at this time.

2-13 After commitment, B and T lymphocytes proliferate in the bursa and thymus, respectively. After proliferation, committed cells leave the bursa and thymus to seed secondary or peripheral lymphoid structures such as spleen and lymph nodes. When B and T cells seed peripheral lymphoid tissue, they localize in different areas of the lymphoid structure. In the spleen, which is made up of red and white pulp, the T cells are found mainly around central arteries of the white pulp in an area designated the *periarterial lymphatic sheath*. B cells are found mainly in the mantle area surrounding germinal centers of nodules in the white pulp. In lymph nodes, B cells are found in germinal centers, or follicles, while T cells are found in the deeper paracortical areas, which are called *thymus-dependent areas*. Figure 2-3 shows a diagram of a lymph node. Antigens enter lymph nodes by way of the afferent lymphatic vessels; in different parts of the nodes, B and T cells are activated by antigens to form blast cells and to proliferate. Proliferation results in clonal expansion. In immunodeficiency diseases in which antibody production is decreased or lacking, examination of stained sections of lymph nodes shows poorly developed germinal centers or an absence of germinal centers; when cell-mediated immunity is affected, the sections show a marked depletion of lymphocytes in the thymus-dependent paracortical areas.

Distribution of Lymphoid Tissue and Recirculation of B and T Lymphocytes

2-14 Lymphoid tissue is distributed throughout the body so that it is exposed to foreign substances which gain entrance to the body. Probably the main peripheral lymphoid organ is the spleen, which, along with the liver, is responsible for removal of foreign substances from the blood. Lymph nodes are found along the main blood vessels and are widely distributed through the body in the neck, axilla, thorax, abdomen, and groin. Lymphoid nodules are round but nonencapsulated; they are found in loose connective tissue lying beneath and supporting the wet epithelial membranes lining areas like the respiratory, digestive, and genitourinary tracts, where foreign substances may enter.

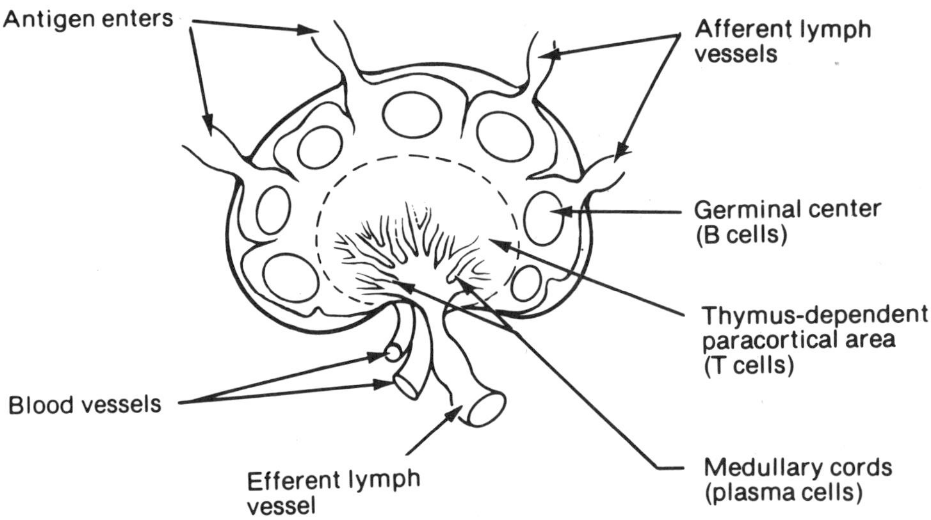

Figure 2-3 Diagram of a lymph node, showing different areas seeded by B and T lymphocytes. Antibody secreting plasma cells are found in medullary cords.

Contact with foreign substances is assured not only by the wide distribution of lymphoid tissue in nodes and nodules but also by the continual recirculation of B and T cells through lymph, peripheral lymphoid tissue, and blood. Lymphocytes do not recirculate through the thymus. When recirculating B or T cells come in contact with antigen, they undergo proliferation on return to lymphoid tissue and there produce plasma cells or sensitized lymphocytes, respectively. Plasma cells are much larger than B cells before activation by antigen and are rarely found in peripheral blood. Large lymphocytes are found in lymphoid tissue but do not recirculate. Large lymphocytes are usually thought of as being B cells, but both B and T cells become enlarged (blast cells) before proliferation. Recirculating lymphocytes are small. Both B and T cells are found in peripheral blood, but the majority (about 75 percent) are T cells. Recently it has been shown that B and T cells of the mother are present in human colostrum in addition to antibodies. The B and T cells in colostrum are immunocompetent cells and may serve to protect the newborn infant against infection.

2-15 Studies with germ-free animals, i.e., those taken by caesarean section, maintained in an environment free of living microorganisms, and fed sterilized food, show that proliferation of lymphoid cells after birth depends largely on exposure to antigens (or immunogens). The amount of peripheral lymphoid tissue present in a germ-free guinea pig is much less than that in a guinea pig of the same age maintained outside, where exposure to living microorganisms occurs. Also the amount of gamma globulin in the serum of a germ-free animal is much less. Immune responses may take place to a very limited extent in germ-free animals because even sterilized material contains some antigens. However, when an animal is taken out of his germ-free environment, within several days there is a rise in serum gamma globulin (antibodies) and a marked increase in peripheral lymphoid tissue.

Antibody Production

Antigen Recognition and Activation of B Lymphocytes by Combination of Surface Receptors with Antigen

2-16 B lymphocytes react specifically with antigens because these lymphocytes have preexisting specific receptors on their surfaces. The receptors are immunoglobulins and after activation by antigen are believed to produce the type of antibodies which served as surface receptors. This is true not only with regard to specificity but also the class of immunoglobulin produced, for example IgM and IgG. In Fig. 2-4 antibody molecules which serve as surface receptors have been drawn with a wish-

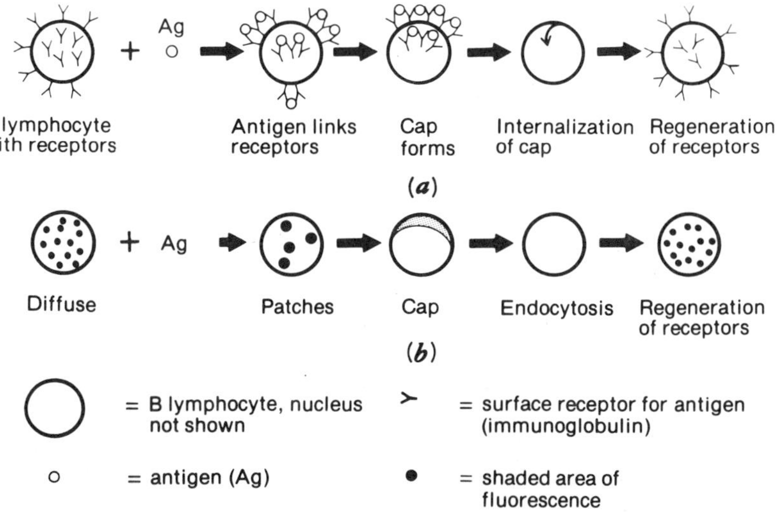

Figure 2-4 Antibody production: antigen recognition and activation of B lymphocyte by combination of surface receptors with antigen. (*a*) diagrammatic representation; (*b*) reactions of cells in (*a*) as they appear in immunofluorescence.

bone, or Y, structure with two combining sites for antigens, one located at the end of each arm of the Y structure. The detailed structure of immunoglobulins is taken up in Chap. 3. It has been estimated that B lymphocytes have about 10^5 surface receptors distributed over their surface. Since the membrane of lymphocytes is in a fluid state, the surface receptors are not fixed but can change position. When receptors on B lymphocytes combine with antigen, cross linkage occurs, so that clusters or patches of receptors can be observed. Cross linkage occurs because antigens are multivalent and receptor immunoglobulins are divalent. The mobility of a lymphocyte and the movement of its membrane mean that patches or groups of immunoglobulin receptors in combination with antigen move to one pole of the cell and coalesce to form a *cap* or *polar cap*, so named because of its appearance on lymphocytes studied by immunofluorescent techniques (Chap. 4). The cap is internalized by the B cell by endocytosis and degraded into fragments. Since the cap was made up of surface receptors, the cell loses its receptors when capping and endocytosis occur. It has been shown experimentally by immunofluorescent studies that surface receptors may be regenerated.

Proliferation (Clonal Expansion) of Antigen-activated B Cells with Differentiation to Form Antibody-producing Plasma Cells and Memory Cells

2-17 Combination of antigen with surface receptors of B cells, just described (Sec. 2-16), triggers blast formation; however, the exact mechanisms by which B cells are activated have not been clarified. There is evidence that mechanisms in addition to capping and internalization of the cap are required for activation of B lymphocytes. Therefore, the number of signals required for activation is not known. It has been established that exposure of B lymphocytes to certain antigens known as *T-cell-dependent antigens* does not result in antibody production unless T cells enter into the reaction. In this situation, T cells are known as *helper T cells*, and their function is discussed next with the interaction of macrophages. Before blast transformation, B lymphocytes appear small, but after transformation they enlarge. Those which are to become plasma cells develop internal structures characteristic of secretory cells. As shown in Fig. 2-5, after blast transformation, B cells go through several divisions and finally differentiate into plasma cells and memory cells. Plasma cells have a very characteristic cytoplasm and secrete antibodies (see the plasma cell in Fig. 2-1). During secretion of antibodies, the cisternae (saclike structures) become enlarged. Plasma cells are end cells and survive for only about 2 weeks. Memory cells have the same appearance as small lymphocytes. Exactly how they arise is not known. After stimulation by antigen large lymphocytes may revert back to small lymphocytes or memory cells. They are responsible for the anamnestic response or more rapid production of antibody on reexposure to antigen. Some investigators believe that proliferation and differentiation of B cells to form plasma cells and memory cells take place in a stepwise manner and that each step is antigen-driven.

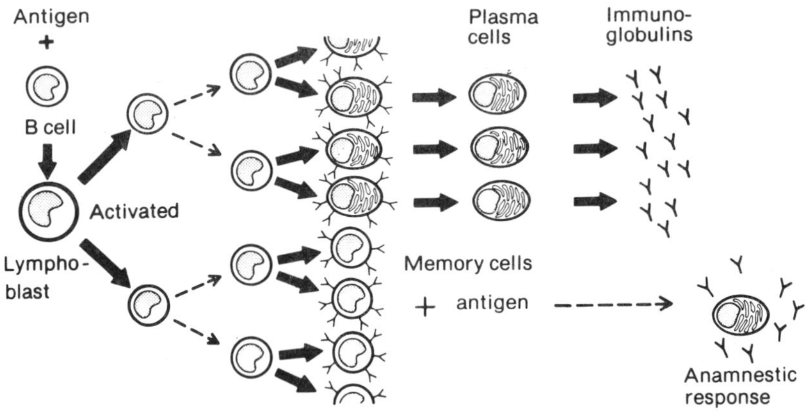

Figure 2-5 Antibody production: proliferation (clonal expansion) of an antigen-activated B cell and differentiation to form antibody-producing plasma cells and memory cells.

Interaction of B Cells with Macrophages and T Cells

2-18 Macrophages may play a number of different roles in antibody formation. It is a well-known fact that macrophages take up antigens. Macrophages may process antigens and pass them on to B lymphocytes in a form which can react with surface receptors for antigen to bring about activation of B lymphocytes; or macrophages may concentrate antigens at their surface and present them to B lymphocytes in sufficient quantity to react with surface receptors for antigen and cause activation of B lymphocytes. Several different types of in vitro reactions between antigens, macrophages, and B cells have been described but will not be presented here. Some antigens may require interaction between macrophages, B cells, and also T cells; several mechanisms postulated for their interaction will be described later. In contrast to the above interactions, which bring about antibody formation, macrophages may inhibit antibody formation by quickly ingesting antigen, degrading it, and causing it to be eliminated from the body, so that the period of antigenic stimulation is shortened.

2-19 In Sec. 2-17 it was pointed out that T cells are necessary in addition to B cells for the production of antibody to certain antigens. The T cells are designated helper cells and the antigens are known as T-cell-dependent antigens or immunogens. Assistance from T cells is not required by immunogens which are large polymers with many copies of the same determinant group per molecule, e.g., pneumococcal polysaccharide. T-cell-independent antigens appear to induce only IgM antibodies. T-cell-dependent immunogens such as some serum proteins are not large polymers although they have a fairly large molecular weight and do have determinant groups of more than one specificity per molecule. T-cell-dependent immunogens induce both IgM antibody formation and IgG, which appears after IgM. Haptens coupled to carrier particles have been used experimentally in an attempt to elucidate the mechanism of action of helper T cells. A hapten is an incomplete antigen or chemical grouping which directs the specificity of the antibody molecules; haptens do not stimulate antibody production unless they are coupled to a protein carrier. T-cell receptors combine specifically with the protein carrier; B-cell receptors combine specifically with the hapten. This interaction between T and B cells brings about activation of the B cells, with the end result that antibodies are formed. One mechanism whereby T cells are proposed to serve as helper cells to B lymphocytes is diagrammed in Fig. 2-6. Antibody production does not take place unless cross linking of receptors on B cells occurs; cross linking occurs when the hapten is bound to a carrier which reacts with T cells; T cells help by presenting the hapten to B cells. For example, sensitization of an individual to penicillin, a hapten, is believed to be caused by the binding of penicillin (or a derivative) to tissue components of the body which serve as carriers. Adherence to the surface of macrophages facilitates the specific interaction between B and helper T cells. In this case the action of macrophages would be nonspecific. Note the close association of the macrophage with the cluster of lymphocytes in Fig. 2-1.

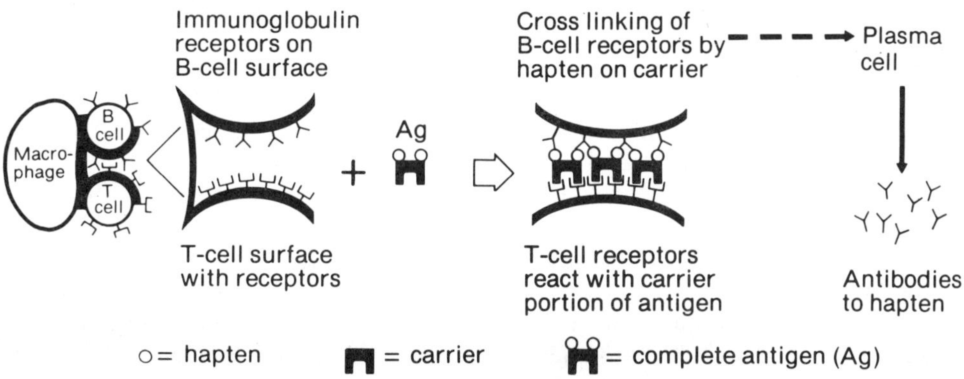

Figure 2-6 Antibody production with helper T-lymphocyte contact. Presentation of antigen to B lymphocytes by helper T cell attached to carrier for hapten. Note the cross linkage of B-cell receptors by hapten held by carrier. The reaction is facilitated by nonspecific adherence of B and T cells to the macrophage surface.

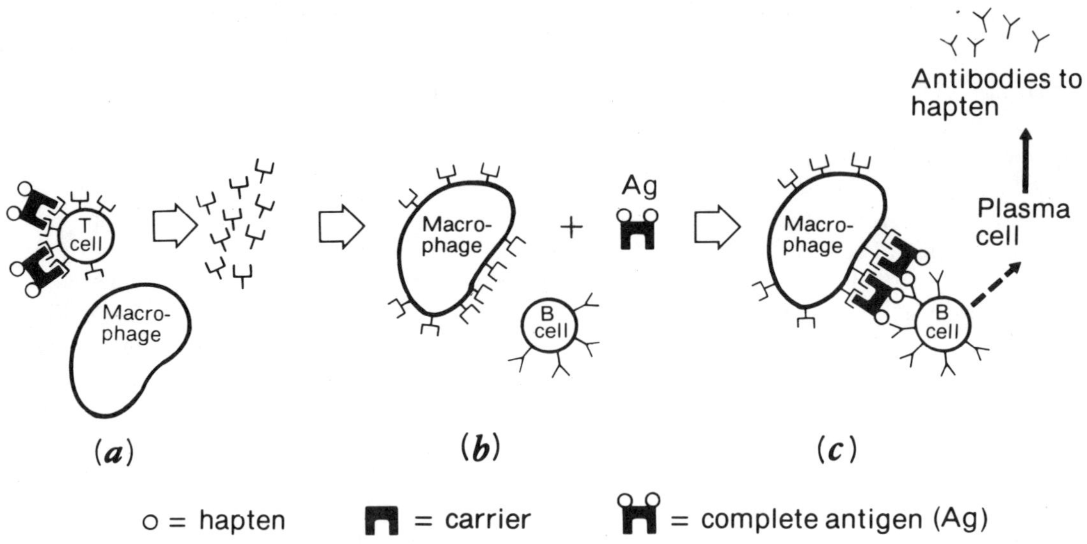

Figure 2-7 Antibody production with helper T lymphocyte diffusible factor. Release of a diffusible immunoglobulinlike factor from antigen-stimulated helper T cells and subsequent interaction with macrophages and B cells. (*a*) Reaction of antigen with T-cell receptors followed by release of soluble receptorlike protein; (*b*) soluble receptorlike protein from T cell adheres to adjacent macrophage; (*c*) cross linking of B-cell receptors by hapten on carrier held by macrophage.

2-20 Another mechanism proposed for helper-T-cell function for which there is some evidence is that helper T cells exert their effect through the release of diffusible factors which act on surrounding B cells. Two diffusible factors have been reported to be released by T cells after reaction with immunogen. One factor is a low-molecular-weight dialyzable substance which is nonspecific. It enhances the activity of B lymphocytes. The other factor, a high-molecular-weight nondialyzable substance, is specific in that it can react only with the immunogen which stimulated its release from T cells. This substance is bound by macrophages and then serves to bind antigen specifically to the macrophage surface in sufficient quantities to react with B-cell receptors. Figure 2-7 shows a diagram of this mechanism; helper T cells react with antigen and produce a soluble substance with immunoglobulinlike properties which sticks to the surface of macrophages and binds antigen to react with B cells to stimulate antibody production.

2-21 T lymphocytes participate in many immunologic functions. Some of the mechanisms whereby T cells exert a helper effect in antibody production have just been discussed. It is important for the proper functioning of the body to be able not only to turn a reaction on but also to turn it off. It has been established experimentally that the injection of specific antibody by passive immunization temporarily inhibits active immunization with antigen of the corresponding specificity. This type of homeostatic control is known as *feedback inhibition*. T cells appear to assume a regulatory role and to function not only as helper cells in antibody formation but also as suppressor cells. The suppressor role of T cells is now under intensive investigation. The mechansim of action may be by cell contact or by elaboration of a soluble factor. Recently it has been reported that a factor which acts as a suppressor was extracted from mouse thymocytes or spleen cells. This factor did not resemble an immunoglobulin; its molecular weight was no higher than 55,000 daltons; it suppressed the helper T cell with the same carrier specificity for antigen but did not act on the hapten-specific B cell.

2-22 In order to observe the normal in vivo interaction of macrophages, B cells, and helper T cells and the suppressor effect of T cells experimentally it is necessary to work with syngeneic cells and not allogeneic cells. *Syngeneic cells* are cells which have the same histocompatibility antigens. Syngrafts contain syngeneic cells and are not rejected. *Allogeneic cells* are cells with histocompatibility antigens different from those of the host. Allografts (*allo-* means "other") contain allogeneic cells and are rejected. On the other hand, injection of allogeneic cells may cause a graft-versus-host reaction (Chap. 1). In this case, the graft acts against the host. Syngeneic cells must be used in leukocyte transfusion of human beings, not just to prevent rejection or destruction of cells but to obtain the interaction of white blood cells which approximates that of the normal host, just described. In human beings, leukocyte transfusions are currently given (1) for restoration of normal immune responses, (2) for granulocytopenia when there is a neutrophil deficiency, and (3) for experimental immunotherapy of tumors. Often no attempt is made to transfuse granulocytes of the same HLA type because allogeneic granulocytes appear to be effective and because they do not cause a graft-versus-host reaction. However, for lymphocyte transfusion, HLA antigens must be matched. (HL stands for human leukocyte.) To date the results observed after transfusion of lymphocytes of a healthy noncancerous person into a patient with cancer have been disappointing (Chap. 10).

B-Lymphocyte Membrane-surface Receptors for Antigen

2-23 The antigen receptors on B lymphocytes are immunoglobulins and can be recognized by immunofluorescent tests. It was pointed out earlier that plasma cells which develop from B lymphocytes are believed to produce the kind of immunoglobulin which served as antigen receptors at the time of activation of B lymphocytes, and this appears to be true not only with regard to specificity but also the class of immunoglobulin produced, for example IgM or IgG. At any one time, an individual cell makes only one kind of antibody with regard to specificity and immunoglobulin class. After primary immunization in the whole animal, IgM antibodies appear first in the serum and then IgG antibodies. There is some evidence that the class of immunoglobulin being made by a single cell may shift, so that later this cell makes antibody of the same specificity for antigen but of a different immunoglobulin class. Several studies indicate that immunoglobulin of the IgM class is the earliest kind found on fetal cells. IgM receptors are monomeric. Studies on a number of animals, including human beings, revealed that other classes of immunoglobulin receptors are found on B lymphocytes before birth; this is interpreted by some investigators to mean that the appearance of different immunoglobulin class receptors does not depend on exposure to antigen. This may not necessarily be true in view of the fact that such animals as mice and human beings have "leaky" placentas, at least during certain stages of gestation. Germ-free colostrum-deprived piglets have been obtained by aseptic hysterectomy 3 to 5 days before term from the Minnesota miniature sow and have been found to be immunologically virgin. These piglets seem to provide an excellent opportunity for tracing the development of the immune system. In contrast to other germ-free animals, the piglets have a nonleaky six-layered epithelial and mesenchymal placenta that provides a barrier between sow and piglet and also provides freedom from antigen exposure during fetal development. It has been reported that their serum does not contain any gamma globulin and that their lymphocytes do not have immunoglobulin receptors. In these piglets, immunoglobulin receptors were reported to develop only after exposure to antigen. This is in contrast to reports on other animals that fetal cells contain IgM membrane receptors before known exposure to antigen. The latter finding would support the idea that these receptors are genetically determined.

2-24 Recently it has been reported that IgD is on 14.5 percent of lymphocytes of newborn babies as determined by examination of cord-blood lymphocytes. Other values reported for receptors in the newborn were IgM, 8.5 percent; IgG, 2.9 percent, and IgA, 0.8 percent. The finding that IgD receptors are prevalent on blood lymphocytes in the newborn is not understood. The function of IgD immunoglobulin in serum has not been elucidated although the presence of this immunoglobulin in small quantities in human serum was recognized many years ago. Although newborn infants have IgD as lymphocyte receptors, IgD is not usually detectable in their serum. There is no quantitative correlation at birth or in adult life between the immunoglobulin class found as receptors for antigen on B lymphocytes and the immunoglobulin class present in serum. IgG is present in the greatest concentration (about 75 percent) in the serum of normal individuals. The amount of IgD in adult serum is about 0.2 percent. The percentage of lymphocytes in adult peripheral blood showing IgD receptors is about 3 percent, in contrast to 14.5 percent of cord blood. It has been reported that only about 15 percent of lymphocytes of cord blood contain immunoglobulin receptors. Since 15 percent was about the same percentage of lymphocytes in cord blood reported to have IgD receptors, it was concluded that some lymphocytes of the newborn have IgD receptors in addition to receptors of another immunoglobulin class. Patients with chronic lymphatic leukemia have some B lymphocytes with both IgM and IgD antigen receptors on the same cell; it has been shown that both receptors have the same specificity. In immunofluorescent studies on Ig antigen receptors, it is important to be sure that immunoglobulins (Ig) in labeled antiserum do not react with Fc receptors on B lymphocytes and lead to erroneous results.

Clonal-Selection Theory of Antibody Formation

2-25 The clonal-selection theory of antibody formation proposed in 1959 by Burnet and modified somewhat since then seems to fit our present knowledge of induction and secretion of antibodies best. The theory assumes that the mutation rate of genes involved in immunoglobulin synthesis is very high in fetal life, so that mutation causes many clones of lymphoid cells to arise which are capable of producing different kinds of antibodies. It is estimated that about 100,000 or more clones arise during prenatal life. Burnet's theory proposes that clones of lymphoid cells which come in contact with antigen during fetal life are destroyed or suppressed; after birth, lymphoid cells which encounter antigen are stimulated to proliferate and differentiate into antibody-secreting cells. According to this theory, the antigens encountered during fetal life would be self antigens and would cause destruction or inhibition of clones of cells which could cause autoimmunization. Burnet's theory has some similarities to Ehrlich's side-chain theory, proposed around 1900. Ehrlich hypothesized that cells of the body possess side chains or surface receptors to capture nutrients from the blood and tissue fluid, that combination of antigen with these receptors would cause later shedding of the receptors and budding of new ones, and that any excess would be secreted into the circulation as free antibody. The side chains, or receptors, were assumed to be chemical groups which combined with antigens depending on their structure. Both Burnet's and Ehlrich's theories are based on selection of antibody by antigen. Before the general acceptance of Burnet's theory, another, the template theory, was popular around 1940 to 1960. It was based on instruction or direction of antibody synthesis by antigen. The template theory proposed that antibody specificity with two specific reactive sites was due to the tertiary structure acquired by folding of the antibody molecule around antigen, which served as a template. This theory is no longer tenable. It has been established that antibody specificity for antigen is determined by the composition and sequence of amino acids in the variable region of the immunoglobulin molecule (see Chap. 3). The general hypothesis of direction or instruction of antibody synthesis by antigen has not been completely excluded by all investigators.

Questions for Secs. 2-10 to 2-25

19. (*a*) Name two substances which activate lymphocytes or stimulate them to divide. (*b*) Why do lymphocytes vary in size (small, medium, and large)? (*c*) What are blast cells? (*d*) Where are B and T lymphocytes mainly found in the body?

20. (*a*) Give one method for separation of human T cells from B cells and null cells. (*b*) Do B cells form rosettes with sheep erythrocytes? (*c*) What known surface receptor allows differentiation of B cells from T cells?

21. (*a*) Where do the maturation and commitment of B and T cells take place? (*b*) What is meant by a committed B cell? (*c*) If a child has a B-cell deficiency, what area of the lymph node would you expect to be affected if stained tissue sections of a node are examined? (*d*) What would be observed in stained tissue sections of a node taken from a child with a T-cell deficiency? (*e*) Are lymph nodes and spleen considered primary (central) or secondary (peripheral) lymphoid structures? (*f*) By what route do antigens in lymph enter lymph nodes?

22. (*a*) Are both B and T cells found in the peripheral blood, and if so, is one kind found in greater numbers than the other? (*b*) Are large lymphocytes and plasma cells found in peripheral blood? (*c*) Name one important function performed by recirculation of lymphocytes. (*d*) Where do proliferation and differentiation of activated B lymphocytes into plasma cells take place?

23. (*a*) What are germ-free animals? (*b*) How does the amount of gamma globulin in the blood and the amount of peripheral lymphoid tissue of germ-free animals compare with that of animals rasied under the usual laboratory conditions? (*c*) When animals are removed from their germ-free environment, what is the effect on serum gamma globulin and peripheral lymphoid tissue? (*d*) Why might the piglets of the Minnesota miniature sow be considered better than the usual laboratory animals for the study of the immune status of germ-free animals before exposure to immunogen?

24. (*a*) What are the composition and specificity of the surface receptors for antigen on B cells? (*b*) How can antigen receptors on B cells be detected? (*c*) Briefly describe what happens on the surface of B lymphocytes during capping. (*d*) What happens to the polar cap? (*e*) What happens to the receptors for antigen? (*f*) Can B cells regenerate their surface receptors for antigen?

25. (*a*) Does reaction of antigen with surface receptors of B cells followed by capping and endocytosis bring about activation of B cells? (*b*) How many signals are necessary for the induction of antibody? (*c*) After activation of B cells, what events take place before antibody is produced? (*d*) Are plasma cells capable of multiplication? (*e*) Approximately how long do plasma cells survive?

26. (*a*) What is the function of macrophages in antibody formation? (*b*) Do T cells produce antibody? (*c*) What role(s) do T cells have in antibody formation?

27. (*a*) What is the difference between T-cell-independent immunogens and T-cell-dependent immunogens? (*b*) What class or classes of immunoglobulins are induced by each kind of immunogen? (*c*) Through what mechanisms might T cells act as helpers in antibody formation? (*d*) Is cross linking of surface receptors for antigen required for activation of B cells?

28. (*a*) When fetal cells are examined for Ig receptors for antigen, what Ig class seems to appear first during ontogeny? (*b*) Does a single cell at any given time produce more than one kind of antibody? (*c*) Can a single cell produce another kind of antibody at a later date? (*d*) Is there any correlation quantitatively between the class of Ig receptors on peripheral blood lymphocytes and the class of immunoglobulins present in serum?

29. (*a*) In general, what is known about IgD in serum? (*b*) Is IgD found as a surface receptor on the cells of normal individuals? If your answer is yes, give an example. (*c*) Name one disease in which IgD has been observed as an Ig receptor on B cells. (*d*) Does more than one class of Ig receptor ever occur on the same cell? If your answer is yes, give an example.

30. (*a*) From what is known about antibody formation, do antigens appear to play a role of instruction or selection? (*b*) Of all the theories proposed for antibody formation, which one appears best supported by present knowledge of antibody formation? (*c*) Who proposed the clonal-selection theory? (*d*) What early theory of antibody formation is similar to the clonal-selection theory? (*e*) Why is the template theory considered untenable?

Answers

19. (*a*) Antigens (immunogens) and mitogens can cause activation of lymphocytes. (*b*) Resting lymphocytes are small, but when they become activated they enlarge before they begin to divide; some lymphocytes, e.g., B cells, differentiate into large forms with secretory function, e.g., plasma cells. (*c*) Blast cells are activated lymphocytes or lymphocytes which have been stimulated to divide; they become enlarged before division. (*d*) B and T lymphocytes are mainly found in blood, lymph, lymphoid tissue, and connective tissue (Sec. 2-10.)

20. (*a*) Human T lymphocytes can be separated from B lymphocytes and null cells because the T lymphocytes form rosettes with untreated sheep red blood cells (srbc). These rosettes are called E (erythrocyte) rosettes to distinguish them from other kinds of rosettes which may be formed under different conditions. Other steps in the procedure for separation of T cells which form E rosettes were not described but can be found in the references. (*b*) B cells do not form rosettes with untreated srbc as human T cells do; however, B cells do form rosettes with srbc which have reacted with antibodies. These rosettes are called EA rosettes or Fc rosettes. (*c*) B cells of human beings and experimental animals tested have surface receptors which are immunoglobulins; these surface immunoglobulin (Ig) receptors are present in sufficient quantities to be easily detected by immunofluorescent tests. Whether or not T cells have Ig receptors has not been definitely determined. If T cells have Ig receptors, they are not present in quantities or in a form which can be readily detected, as Ig on the surface of B cells can. (Sec. 2-11.)

21. (*a*) The maturation and commitment of B cells take place in the bursa of Fabricius for chickens and for other animals in a structure equivalent to the bursa; for human beings, the equivalent structure was once thought to be gut-associated lymphoid tissue (GALT), but now bone marrow is believed to be the site. Maturation and commitment of T cells takes place in the thymus. (*b*) B-cell commitment means that the function of a precursor bone-marrow stem cell has been determined to be antibody formation of a certain specificity. (*c*) If a child has a B-cell deficiency, stained sections of the child's lymph nodes would be expected to show a lack of germinal centers. (*d*) Stained sections of lymph nodes from a child with a T-cell deficiency would be expected to show a lack of lymphocytes in the paracortical area. (*e*) Lymph nodes and spleen are secondary (peripheral) lymphoid structures. (*f*) Antigens in lymph enter lymph nodes by way of afferent lymphatic vessels. (Secs. 2-12 and 2-13.)

22. (*a*) Both B and T cells are found in peripheral blood, but about 75 percent of the lymphocytes in peripheral blood are T cells. (*b*) The lymphocytes in peripheral blood are small lymphocytes; large lymphocytes and plasma cells are not found in peripheral blood but in lymphoid tissue such as lymph nodes. Of course, antibodies secreted by plasma cells are in peripheral blood. (*c*) Recirculating lymphocytes reach all areas of the body and react with foreign substances (antigens or immunogens) to activate immune systems. (*d*) Proliferation (clonal expansion) and differentiation of activated B lymphocytes into plasma cells usually takes place in lymph nodes or other lymphoid tissue. (Sec. 2-14.)

23. (*a*) Germ-free animals are animals taken at time of birth by caesarean section and raised in an environment free from living microorganisms. (*b*) The amount of peripheral lymphoid tissue and gamma globulin in the blood of germ-free animals is very much smaller than that of an animal raised under ordinary laboratory conditions. (*c*) When germ-free animals are removed from their germ-free environment, the amount of peripheral lymphoid tissue and serum gamma globulin increases markedly. (*d*) The Minnesota miniature sow has a six-layered placenta, which is considered much more impervious to transplacental passage of immunogens than the placenta of animals like mice and guinea pigs. (Secs. 2-15 and 2-23.)

24. (*a*) The receptors for antigens on B cells are immunoglobulins (Ig), and their specificity corresponds to that of the antigen which reacts with them and that of the antibody subsequently produced. (*b*) Ig receptors for antigen can be detected by immunofluorescent tests. (*c*) Before capping, membrane Ig receptors combine with antigen; at first, reaction of antigen takes place with receptors in different areas of the membrane to form clumps or patches; the fluid state of the membrane means that the receptors are not stationary, so that the patches coalesce into one compact area known as a polar cap. (*d*) The polar cap is taken inside the cell (internalized or interiorized) by endocytosis. (*e*) Since the receptors along with antigen formed the polar cap, the receptors are removed by capping, (*f*) Yes, B cells can regenerate surface receptors for antigen. (Sec. 2-16.)

25. (*a*) Reaction of antigen with surface receptors of B cells is believed to trigger activation of B cells, but other signals may be required for activation. (*b*) The exact number of signals required for induction of antibody is not known. It is believed that induction requires at least two signals. A second signal may occur when helper T cells enter the system. (*c*) After activation of B cells, they proliferate and differentiate into plasma cells, which secrete antibodies. Memory cells are also formed at this time. (*d*) Plasma cells do not multiply. (*e*) Plasma cells survive for about 2 weeks. (Sec. 2-17.)

26. (*a*) Macrophages may function in different ways. They may process antigen and pass it on to B lymphocytes. They may concentrate antigen on their surface and present it to B lymphocytes in such a way as to bring about cross linkage of antigen receptors to trigger activation. Macrophages may interact with B cells and T cells nonspecifically or specifically to bring about induction of antibody. These are only some of the ways in which macrophages may act during antibody formation. (*b*) T cells do not produce antibody. (*c*) T cells may act either as helpers or suppressors of antibody formation, depending on the situation and signals received. It is important to be able to turn a reaction both on and off. (Secs. 2-18, 2-19, 2-21.)

27. (*a*) T-cell-independent antigens do not require help from T cells for antibody production. T-cell-independent antigens are large polymers such as polysaccharide which have many copies of the same determinant group per molecule. T-cell-dependent antigens require helper T cells for antibody production. These antigens are not large polymers. They have at least two different specificities per molecule. When haptens are combined with carrier particles and used for immunogens, the hapten determines antibody specificity and reacts with the B cell. The carrier particle has the same specificity as the helper T cell and reacts with T cells. (*b*) T-cell-independent antigens appear to induce only IgM antibodies. T-cell-dependent antigens induce both IgM and IgG and other classes of immunoglobulins. (*c*) Two mechanisms proposed to explain how T cells help in antibody formation are based on (1) contact by T cells and on (2) elaboration of a diffusible substance produced by T cells. Review Fig. 2-6 and 2-7. With regard to the mechanism based on contact, T-cell receptors react with carrier joined to hapten and in this way present a number of hapten particles to the B cell so that cross linking of B-cell receptors can occur. The reaction is facilitated by nonspecific adherence of B and T cells on the surface of macrophages. The diffusible factor is released by T cells after reaction of T cells with antigen. The diffusible factor adheres to the surface of macrophages and subsequently combines with the carrier portion of antigen, so that the hapten portion can be presented to B cells. (*d*) Yes, it is believed that cross linking of Ig receptors on the surface of B lymphocytes is required for activation. This process leads to capping. (Secs. 2-19 and 2-20.)

28. (*a*) Fetal cells appear to form IgM receptors before those of any other class. (*b*) Most evidence indicates that at a given time a single cell produces only one kind of antibody with regard to Ig class and specificity for antigen. (*c*) It may be possible for a single cell at a different time to produce antibody of another Ig class but specificity for antigen does not change. (*d*) There is no correlation quantitatively between Ig class of lymphocyte receptors and Ig class in serum. (Secs. 2-23 and 2-24.)

29. (*a*) Very little is known about serum IgD. Although some investigators have reported that it has antibody activity, this has not been established unequivocally. (*b*) Yes, IgD is prevalent as an Ig receptor on cord-blood lymphocytes. (*c*) IgD has been observed as an Ig receptor on lymphocytes of patients with chronic lymphatic leukemia. (*d*) Yes, IgM and IgD have been found on the same lymphocytes in patients with chronic lymphatic leukemia. Some B lymphocytes from cord blood of normal infants have IgD receptors and receptors of another Ig class. (Sec. 2-24.)

30. (*a*) According to our present understanding of antibody formation, antigens appear to play a role of selection. (*b*) The clonal-selection theory seems to fit best. (*c*) Burnet proposed the clonal-selection theory. (*d*) Ehrlich's side-chain theory is similar to the clonal-selection theory. (*e*) The template theory is based on instruction or direction by antigen. This theory is untenable because it proposes that antibody specificity is determined by folding of the antibody molecule in the presence of antigen. It has been established that antibody specificity is determined by the composition and sequence of amino acids in the variable region of the immunoglobulin molecule. (Sec. 2-25.)

Cell-mediated Immunity and Delayed-Type Hypersensitivity

Antigen Recognition by T Cells and Activation of T Lymphocytes Followed by Clonal Expansion

2-26 T lymphocytes are believed to have surface receptors for antigen whereby antigen recognition takes place and activation of T cells is triggered. T-cell receptors, which are discussed in Sec. 2-29, seem to differ somewhat from the receptors on B cells. It is not clear whether T-cell receptors are immunoglobulins or not; specificity of T-cell receptors would be easier to understand at present in terms of immunoglobulinlike receptors. The number of signals required for T-cell activation has not been determined. Certain antigens, e.g., those present in tubercle bacilli, induce specific cell-mediated responses which involve T cells. After reaction of antigen with a certain population of T cells, activation takes place. T lymphocytes become enlarged to form blast cells (lymphoblasts), which undergo proliferation or clonal expansion so that the number of activated or sensitized T lymphocytes is greatly increased (see Fig. 2-8). Activated or sensitized T lymphocytes are also known as effector cells of cell-mediated immunity or delayed-type hypersensitivity. Due to clonal expansion, when antigen is again encountered, activated T lymphocytes produce lymphokines in amounts large enough to cause amplification of specific cell-mediated reactions. The lymphokines are discussed in Sec. 2-27. Effector cells may also react directly with target cells to bring about destruction of the target cells. Specific surface receptors on the T cells bind antigens on the target cells. Examples of target cells would be tumor cells and cells of an organ transplant (allogeneic cells). Sensitized T cells which destroy target cells, especially tumor cells, are sometimes referred to as *killer cells*. Cells other than T lymphocytes after reaction with specific antibodies are also able to destroy tumor cells and other cells and are frequently referred to as killer or K cells.

Production of Lymphokines (Soluble Mediators) by Activated T Cells

2-27 It was pointed out above that sensitized T lymphocytes may combine directly with target cells to bring about their destruction. Another mechanism in specific cell-mediated reactions is the release of soluble mediators called lymphokines by activated T cells on reencounter with antigen.

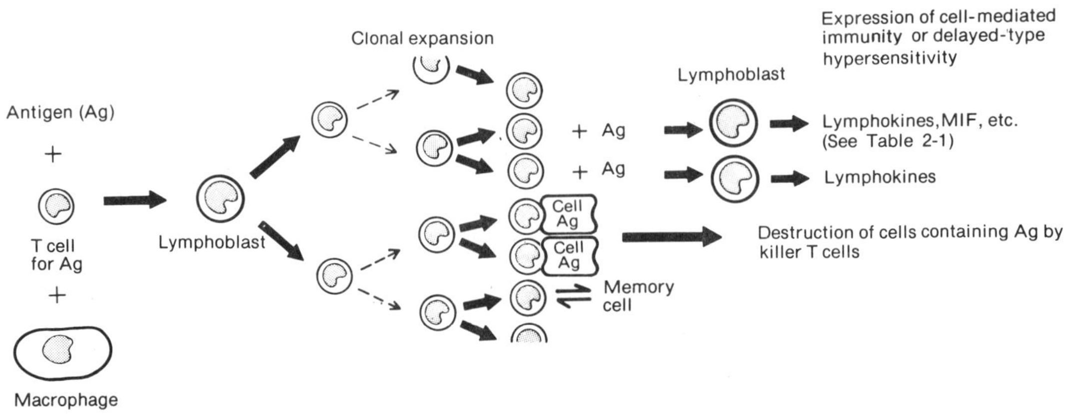

Figure 2-8 Activation of a T lymphocyte by antigen to form an expanded clone of sensitized T cells and production of soluble lymphokines by sensitized T cells on encounter and reaction with antigen.

Table 2-1 Lymphokines: Some of the Soluble Mediators Produced by Activated T Lymphocytes and Demonstrable in vitro or in vivo.

Name	Cells affected
Migration-inhibition factor (MIF)	Macrophages
Macrophage-activating factor	Macrophages
Macrophage-aggregation factor	Macrophages
Macrophage chemotactic factor (MCF)	Macrophages
Macrophage-disappearance factor	Macrophages in vivo
Monocyte chemotactic factor	Monocytes
Blastogenic factor (BF) or mitogenic factor (MF)	Lymphocytes
Potentiating factor (PF)	Lymphocytes
Transfer factor	Lymphocytes in vivo
Neutrophil chemotactic factor	Neutrophils
Eosinophil chemotactic factor	Eosinophils
Eosinophil-stimulation promoter (ESP)	Eosinophils
Interferon	Tissue cells
Lymphotoxin (LT) (cytotoxic factor)	Tissue cells
Proliferation-inhibition factor (PIF)	Tissue cells
Lymph-node-permeability factor (LNPF)	Tissue cells in vivo
Skin reactive factor	Tissue cells in vivo

The lymphokines have different kinds of biological activity and act on different types of cells. The names of some of the lymphokines are self-descriptive. Table 2-1 includes a list of lymphokines and the cells on which they act. Table 2-2 summarizes the events which lead to the release of lymphokines. Recently it has been reported that some lymphokines, e.g., migration-inhibition factor (MIF), may be produced not only by activated T cells but also by activated B cells. Other lymphokines such as lymphocyte mitogenic factor (LMF) are produced only by activated T cells.

Lymphokines and Macrophages

2-28 In histological sections of delayed-type hypersensitivity reactions, mononuclear cells (macrophages and lymphocytes) are characteristically observed at the height of the reaction. This is in contrast to immediate-type hypersensitivity reactions, in which polymorphonuclear leukocytes (granulocytes) are the most characteristic cells present. Since macrophages seem to play a dominant role in the production of cell-mediated immunity and delayed-type hypersensitivity, the lymphokines

Table 2-2 Specific Cell-mediated Reactions: Summary of Events Leading to Release of Lymphokines by T Lymphocytes

T cell specific for antigen (Ag) enters circulation
↓
T cell encounters and combines with Ag
↓
T cell becomes activated by Ag
↓
Activated T cell returns to lymphoid tissue
↓
Proliferation (clonal expansion) of T cells for Ag occurs
↓
T cells for Ag enter circulation in relatively large numbers
↓
Some T cells from expanding clone contact Ag and react with it
↓
Lymphokines (soluble mediators) are released
↓
Lymphokines contribute to production of cell-mediated immunity or delayed-type hypersensitivity

which act on macrophages will be discussed. The macrophage chemotactic factor (MCF) attracts macrophages to the area. Macrophage-activating factor leads to the *activation* of macrophages. Activated macrophages are larger and more phagocytic than nonactivated macrophages and have an increased ability to destroy phagocytized material. These macrophages are sometimes called "angry" macrophages. Tubercle bacilli usually are not destroyed within phagocytes, but they are phagocytized and destroyed by angry macrophages. The migration-inhibition factor (MIF) keeps macrophages from leaving the area after they have been attracted to it. The interaction of MCF, MIF, and activating factor with macrophages helps clear up infections which are not affected by opsonins and neutrophils (discussed in Chap. 1). The release of MIF is currently used in an in vitro test for specific cell-mediated reactions (see Fig. 2-9). The release of MIF has been shown to be both carrier- and hapten-specific. Although the release of lymphokines is specific, once released, their action is nonspecific. For example, macrophages activated by lymphokine released by reaction of sensitized T cells with tubercle bacilli would more actively phagocytize not only tubercle bacilli but also other microorganisms. The release of lymphokines may cause beneficial effects, like those just described for tuberculosis, or they may cause harmful effects, e.g., the destruction of tissue. Lymphotoxin has been shown to be cytotoxic for various tissue-cultured cells. Lymph-node permeability factor can be extracted from lymph-node cells and is capable of increasing vascular permeability. This factor can be detected in skin sites undergoing delayed-type hypersensitivity reactions. When skin reactive factor is injected intradermally, it causes an inflammatory reaction.

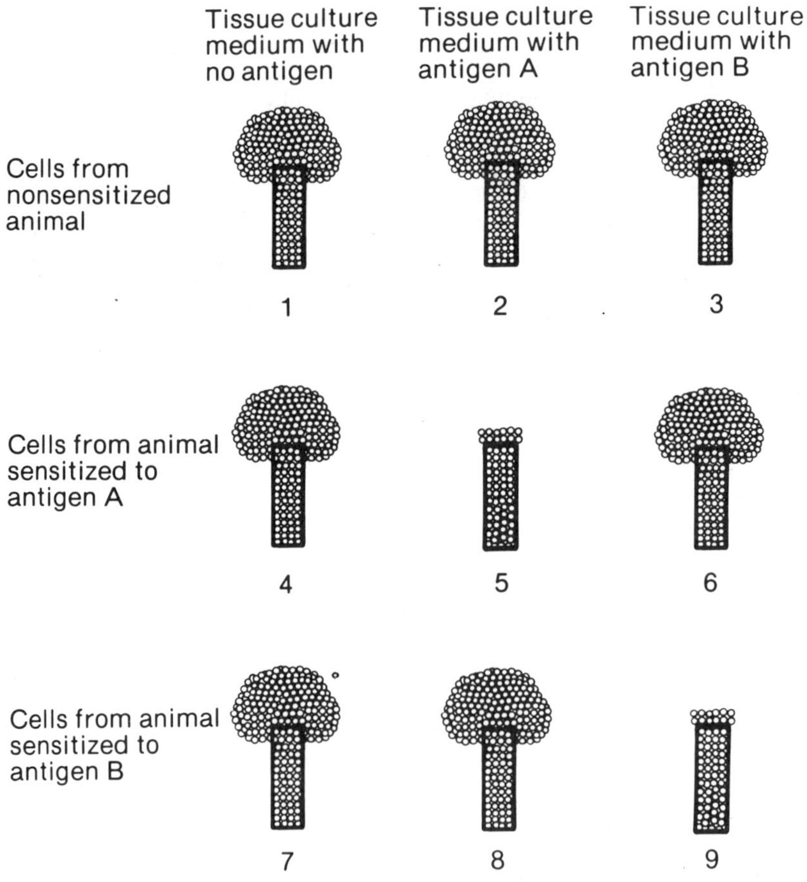

Figure 2-9 Test for migration-inhibition factor (MIF). Cells, predominately macrophages and lymphocytes, in capillary tubes are placed in tissue-culture containers with tissue-culture medium in a CO_2 atmosphere. Sensitized lymphocytes react with antigen and produce migration-inhibition factor (MIF), which inhibits spread of macrophages from mouth of capillary tube. MIF was produced in tubes 5 and 9.

T-Cell Surface Receptors for Antigen

2-29 The specific reaction of T lymphocytes with antigen described in Sec. 2-26 indicates that T cells have surface receptors for antigen recognition; however, the nature or composition of these receptors has not been resolved. T-cell receptors appear different from B-cell receptors. That B cells have immunoglobulin receptors was discussed in Sec. 2-23. By employing anti-immunoglobulin antibodies which cross-link the immunoglobulin receptors on B cells the existence of these receptors can easily be demonstrated by immunofluorescence. Activation of B cells is also triggered by serum containing anti-immunoglobulin antibodies which cross-link receptors as antigens do. It has been reported that immunoglobulin receptors can be demonstrated on T cells if extremely sensitive methods are employed. Ig receptors for antigen should not be confused with Fc receptors reacting with Ig. The number of immunoglobulin receptors on T cells appears to be very small. Some investigators have postulated that immunoglobulin receptors may be present on the surface of T cells but are partially buried in the membrane and therefore difficult to demonstrate. Recent experiments support a T-cell receptor consisting of a single antigen-binding site, which appears to be a site of relatively large extent involving multiple subsites. The antigen-binding receptor on T cells seems to differ in some fundamental way from that on B cells. It was proposed that antigen recognition by T cells is mediated by an immunoglobulin heavy-chain variable region that is not paired with an immunoglobulin light-chain variable region, as in the pairing of heavy and light chains for B-cell receptors. See Chap. 3.

2-30 Since T cells play an important role in specific cell-mediated reactions like graft rejection, some investigators believe that T-cell receptors must be related in some way to antigens responsible for graft rejection, e.g., the human histocompatibility antigens (HLA). Several groups of researchers have recently reported that a microglobulin called *β_2-microglobulin* and the structure carrying HLA antigenic activity are closely associated in their native form in the lymphocyte membrane, so that the β_2-microglobulin–HLA complex might serve as T-cell receptors for cell-mediated immunity. β_2-microglobulin had formerly been demonstrated in such human biological fluids as urine, serum, spinal fluid, and colostrum. β_2-microglobulin, which has a molecular weight of about 11,800 daltons and is a subunit of HLA antigens, may exist free or bound to HLA. It is reported to be present on both B and T cells and on cultured cells. There is similarity in amino acid sequence between β_2-microglobulin and a domain of the constant part of an immunoglobulin heavy chain. T cells are optimally activated by intact cell antigens and are dependent on surface presentation. The gene products of immune-response (Ir) genes appear to function primarily in T cells, so that there may be a relationship between Ir genes and T-cell receptors. It has been determined that Ir genes are closely linked to genes controlling histocompatibility antigens. The real nature of receptors for antigen on T lymphocytes remains to be elucidated.

Activation of B and T Lymphocytes by Mitogens

2-31 Mitogens, in contrast to antigens, are nonspecific substances which bring about the activation of lymphocytes. The plant mitogens phytohemagglutinin (PHA), concanavalin A (ConA), and pokeweed mitogen (PWM) were cited in Sec. 2-10, where it was pointed out that mitogens are capable of nonspecifically activating lymphocytes. This capability is used for in vitro diagnostic tests for immunocompetent lymphocytes. Mitogens have also been used extensively in the investigation of basic underlying mechanisms of lymphocyte activation. Plant mitogens are often referred to as *lectins*. Besides plant mitogens, other mitogens are antisera, which have antibodies to combine with surface receptors; chemical substances, e.g., sodium periodate and dextran sulfate; enzymes, e.g., trypsin; and substances extracted from bacteria, e.g., lipopolysaccharide or endotoxin of gram-negative bacilli. Antisera are considered nonspecific mitogens because the antibodies recognize only the chemical composition of the receptors and not the specificity of the antigen with which the receptors are capable of combining to trigger specific activation of the lymphocytes.

2-32 Lymphocytes were considered end-stage cells until Nowell (1960) described the transformation of a resting lymphocyte into a blast cell with subsequent proliferation after culture in the

Table 2-3 Mitogens for Activation of Lymphocytes

For T cells	For B cells	For B and T cells
Phytohemagglutinin* (PHA)	Lipopolysaccharide† (LPS)	Pokeweed mitogen (PWM)
Concanavalin A (ConA)	Dextran sulfate	Anti-lymphocyte serum (mitogen in vitro)
Sodium periodate	Trypsin	
	Anti-immunoglobulin	

*Soluble PHA and ConA activate T lymphocytes; PHA and ConA insolubilized by adsorption on the surface of Sephadex beads will activate B lymphocytes.

†Lipopolysaccharide is endotoxin from gram-negative bacilli.

presence of an extract of red kidney beans. The extract is now known as phytohemagglutinin (PHA). PHA, ConA, and sodium periodate are T-cell mitogens. These plant mitogens bind to cell receptors; however, binding of the mitogens to cells does not ensure activation. Activation of T lymphocytes occurs when PHA combines with a receptor containing *N*-acetylgalactosamine. Receptors for ConA contain methyl-α-D-mannoside or methyl-α-D-pyranoside. These chemicals compete with the binding of PHA or ConA to lymphocytes and inhibit their proliferation. Although PHA and ConA bind avidly to other cells, e.g., red blood cells and even B lymphocytes, PHA and ConA appear to exhibit exquisite specificity in the type of lymphocyte they activate. PHA and ConA in their soluble form will activate only T lymphocytes and not B lymphocytes, despite the fact that these lectins clearly bind to both types of cells. Recently it has been shown that if PHA and ConA are adsorbed onto insoluble particles such as Sephadex beads, activation of B lymphocytes occurs. The adsorption of mitogens onto a solid surface probably allows a mechanism of presentation of the mitogens to B lymphocytes which does not occur with these mitogens in solution. Table 2-3 summarizes some of the commonly used mitogens and the type of lymphocyte(s) they activate.

2-33 The DiGeorge syndrome and Bruton's type of agammaglobulinemia, both of which are congenital immunologic deficiency disorders, were described in Sec. 2-9. By using lymphocytes from these patients and B and T cell mitogens, it has been shown that lymphocytes from children with DiGeorge syndrome (thymic agenesis) have defective in vitro lymphoproliferative reactions to T-cell mitogens such as PHA and ConA. Patients with Bruton's type of agammaglobulinemia have defective in vitro lymphoproliferative reactions to B-cell mitogens such as LPS. Many patients with acquired (and some with congenital) hypogammaglobulinemia also have impaired in vitro lymphoproliferative reactions to T-cell mitogens. With regard to reactivity to mitogens in acquired diseases associated with immunodeficiency, it could be shown that patients with advanced Hodgkin's disease have relatively greater defective in vitro lymphoproliferative reactions to T-cell mitogens than to B-cell mitogens. The lymphocyte reactivity of animals and patients bearing sizable nonlymphoid neoplasms is often partially defective. Tumor removal frequently corrects the altered reactivity of lymphocytes. Other acquired conditions besides cancer which have been reported to affect the ability of T cells to react with mitogens are malnutrition, aging, and infectious and autoimmune diseases. Recent studies with human lymphocytes have shown that the maximal response of normal controls to PHA is at ages 11 to 15. This response decreases progressively to the age of 45. From 45 until 70, the reaction to PHA remains at a plateau at about one-half the maximal response.

Subpopulations of B and T Cells

2-34 In the foregoing description of how lymphocytes function they have been divided into B and T lymphocytes. For the most part, B and T resting lymphocytes are indistinguishable on the basis of structure, as observed by light microscopy and transmission electron microscopy. When they are activated, they both become enlarged to form blast cells, which metabolically show an increase in DNA synthesis and an increase in protein synthesis. Metabolically active lymphocytes incorporate tritiated thymidine, which is an isotope; the extent of its uptake can be measured. B and T cells cannot be differentiated on the basis of size before the differentiation of B cells to form plasma cells. After activation and blast formation T cells return to their former small size. B and T cells cannot be separated on the basis of life-span or their ability to recirculate, although, as stated previously, the majority of recirculating lymphocytes are long-lived T lymphocytes. B cells may also be long-lived memory cells. T and B cells can be differentiated on the basis of surface receptors discussed in Secs. 2-11, 2-23, 2-24, 2-29, and 2-30. Null lymphocytes are lymphocytes which cannot be separated into B or T lymphocytes on the basis of surface markers.

2-35 It is becoming increasingly apparent that subpopulations of both T and B cells exist. For example, virgin B cells which have not previously encountered antigen are renewed continually about every 48 h. Virgin B cells appear to be associated with solid lymphoid tissue and not to recirculate from blood to lymph. In constrast, memory B cells, which are formed after interaction with antigen, have a much longer life-span and recirculate. It has been reported that their surface appears changed with an increase in the quantity of surface immunoglobulins. Subpopulations of B cells appear to exist with regard to their capacity to be activated by such mitogens as dextran sulfate, lipopolysaccharide, and purified protein derivative of tubercle bacilli (PPD). To emphasize the existence of subpopulations of B cells, designations B_1 to B_5 have been used. B_1 is a *postbursal* immature committed cell incapable of producing antibody; it has not yet reacted with antigen. B_2 is the immunoblast formed after reaction with antigen. The immunoblast undergoes clonal expansion to form lymphocytes, some of which become memory cells, designated B_3 cells, and lymphocytes, designated B_4, which have surface Ig and differentiate into plasma cells, B_5 cells. Plasma cells secrete immunoglobulins (antibodies) of the same kind as the surface Ig on B_4 cells. Plasma cells lack surface Ig. Review Fig. 2-5.

2-36 T cells participate in many immunologic functions. They act as both helper and suppressor cells for antibody formation; they act directly on target cells and are cytotoxic; they release lymphokines in delayed-type hypersensitivity reactions; and they act as memory cells. Whether these are functions of the same or different T-cell populations is now being studied. It is fairly clear, however, that certain subpopulations or subsets of T cells do exist. It was early shown with mice that subpopulations or subsets of T cells and T-cell precursors can be recognized by their surface antigens. Immature thymus cells (thymocytes) of mice and T_1 and T_2 cells can be distinguished on the basis of their surface antigens, as shown in Table 2-4. T_1 cells are reported to be found mainly in the spleen. It has been postulated that after leaving the thymus, T_1 cells may undergo further maturation in the spleen to become T_2 cells, which are immunologically competent and recirculating cells. T_2 cells are found mainly in blood, thoracic duct, and lymph nodes. On encountering antigen, T_2 cells become memory cells or effector (or amplifier) cells of cell-mediated immunity. Review Fig. 2-8. A thymic hormone appears to influence differentiation of T_1 cells to T_2 cells.

Questions for Secs. 2-26 to 2-36

31. (*a*) Are B or T lymphocytes considered the lymphocytes responsible for cell-mediated immunity? (*b*) Do macrophages play an important role in cell-mediated immunity? (*c*) What triggers activation of lymphocytes responsible for cell-mediated immunity? (*d*) What reactions and signals are responsible for activation? (*e*) List the events which follow activation.

Table 2-4 Change in Surface Antigens on Mouse Thymocytes and T Lymphocytes

Surface antigen*	Thymocytes →	T_1 lymphocyte →	T_2 lymphocyte
TL	+	—	—
(θ)	++++	++	+
MPLA	—	+	+
H-2	+	++	++++

*TL = thymus leukemia antigen; MPLA = mouse-specific peripheral lymphocyte antigen; H-2 = major histocompatibility antigen in mice.

32. (*a*) What are T cells called when they have reacted with antigen and undergone clonal expansion? (*b*) What are T killer cells? (*c*) Do any other cells besides T cells act as killer cells? (*d*) After reaction with specific antigen how do sensitized T lymphocytes cause amplification of cell-mediated responses?

33. (*a*) What are lymphokines? (*b*) What type of cells are affected by lymphokines? (*c*) Are lymphokines produced by both B and T cells? If your answer is yes, explain.

34. (*a*) What is the main cellular response observed in specimens from patients with delayed-type hypersensitivity or cell-mediated immunity? (*b*) Is the release and action of lymphokines specific? (*c*) Are lymphokines beneficial or harmful to the host? (*d*) Name two lymphokines which probably contribute to the skin reaction seen in a positive delayed-type hypersensitivity skin test.

35. (*a*) Describe how the lymphokines, macrophage chemotactic factor (MCF), macrophage-activating factor, and migration-inhibition factor (MIF), may act to clear up an infection like that caused by tubercle bacilli. (*b*) Would the lymphokines released by tuberculin-sensitive T cells act on macrophages so that they would destroy *Listeria monocytogenes* if these organisms were present? (*c*) For tubes 1 to 6 in the table for an in vitro test for cell-mediated immunity based on release of MIF, state whether the macrophages in the capillary tubes would fan out from the mouth of the capillary tubes or have their migration inhibited.

Peritoneal exudate cells* in capillary tubes	Tube number of tissue-culture medium containing		
	Hapten A with		Hapten B with
	Carrier Z	Carrier Y	carrier Z
Nonsensitized animal control	1	2	3
Animal sensitized to hapten A with carrier Z	4	5	6

*Peritoneal exudate cells contain macrophages and lymphocytes.

36. (*a*) Do T cells have receptors for antigen? (*b*) Are T-cell receptors immunoglobulins like those of B cells? Explain your answer. (*c*) What is β_2-microglobulin, and how is it related to HLA antigens? (*d*) What is the Ir gene, and what important antigens are controlled by it? (*e*) What is thought to be the nature of T-cell receptors?

37. (*a*) What are mitogens? (*b*) Name two mitogens which activate T lymphocytes. (*c*) Name two mitogens which activate B lymphocytes. (*d*) Name two mitogens which activate both B and T cells. (*e*) Do all mitogens which bind to the surface of lymphocytes cause their activation? Explain. (*f*) Why are anti-immunoglobulin antibodies considered nonspecific mitogens with regard to activation of B cells?

38. (*a*) If lymphocytes are immunocompetent, are more lymphocytes involved in the in vitro response to a mitogen or to an antigen? Explain your answer. (*b*) What is the in vitro response of lymphocytes of children with the DiGeorge syndrome to PHA and LPS? (*c*) What is the in vitro response of lymphocytes from patients with acquired hypogammaglobulinemia to LPS and ConA? (*d*) What types of acquired diseases have been shown to cause defective in vitro lymphoproliferative reactions to PHA and ConA?

Answers

31. (*a*) T lymphocytes are the lymphocytes responsible for cell-mediated immunity. (*b*) Macrophages play a necessary part in cell-mediated immunity; T lymphocytes appear to be activated only when macrophages are present. (*c*) Reaction of antigen with specific

T-cell receptors is believed to trigger activation. (*d*) It appears that a number of reactions and signals are responsible for activation. Several theories based on experimental evidence are now under investigation. (*e*) Following activation, T cells may become sensitized lymphocytes or memory cells. Sensitized lymphocytes may react directly with cells containing antigen and destroy them, or they may release lymphokines, which have many different biological activities associated with cell-mediated reactions. (Sec. 2-26.)

32. (*a*) T cells which have reacted with antigen and undergone clonal expansion are known as activated or sensitized cells or effector cells of cell-mediated immunity or delayed-type hypersensitivity. (*b*) T killer cells are sensitized T lymphocytes which are capable of reacting with and destroying target cells, especially tumor cells. (*c*) Yes, other cells after reaction with specific antibodies (antibody-dependent) may act as killer cells. (*d*) Sensitized T lymphocytes may react with antigen to cause the release of substances with many different kinds of biological activities associated with cell-mediated reactions. These substances are known as lymphokines. (Sec. 2-26.)

33. (*a*) Lymphokines are substances with different kinds of biological activities which are released by reaction of sensitized T lymphocytes with antigen. (*b*) Lymphokines act on lymphocytes, macrophages, and other cells of myeloid origin such as neutrophils and eosinophils. They also act on tissue cells in culture and in vivo. (*c*) Some lymphokines such as MIF are released by both B and T cells. Other lymphokines such as LMF are produced only by T cells. (Sec. 2-27.)

34. (*a*) The main cellular response observed in histological specimens from patients with cell-mediated immunity or delayed-type hypersensitivity is a response involving mainly mononuclear cells such as macrophages, monocytes, and lymphocytes. (*b*) The reaction of antigen with T-cell receptors to trigger activation and release of lymphokines is specific; the action of lymphokines is not specific for the antigen which brought about their release. (*c*) Lymphokines may be beneficial or harmful, depending on the circumstances and the target cells involved. (*d*) LNPF increases permeability of tissue in vivo; skin reactive factor causes an inflammatory skin reaction in vivo. (Sec. 2-28.)

35. (*a*) MCF attracts macrophages into an area, e.g., where there is an infection with microorganisms such as tubercle bacilli; MIF keeps the macrophages from leaving the area; macrophage-activating factor causes macrophages to take on the properties of angry killer cells, which phagocytize and destroy the tubercle bacilli. Tubercle bacilli are not destroyed by other types of cells after phagocytosis. (*b*) Other microorganisms such as *Listeria monocytogenes, Brucella abortus*, etc., would be destroyed if they happened to be present. (*c*) The reaction expected in the in vitro test described would be as follows: macrophages fan out from all tubes except 4, where migration is inhibited. The reaction is both carrier- and hapten-specific. (Sec. 2-28.)

36. (*a*) Yes, T cells have receptors for antigen. (*b*) The answer to the question has not been resolved. T cells may have immunoglobulin receptors, but if they are immunoglobulins, something about them is different from B-cell immunoglobulin receptors because the latter are easily demonstrated. (*c*) β_2-microglobulin has a molecular weight of about 11,800 daltons and a structure similar to that of the constant region of the heavy chain of immunoglobulins. It appears to be a subunit of HLA antigens. (*d*) Ir stands for immune response; Ir genes control certain immune responses associated with T cells; Ir genes control HLA antigens. (*e*) The nature of T-cell receptors is not clear. Immunoglobulins in very small amounts have been demonstrated on the surface of T cells, but whether or not they act as receptors has not been clarified. A β_2-microglobulin-HLA antigen complex demonstrated on the surface of lymphocytes is under investigation now with respect to its relationship, if any, to T-cell receptors. (Secs. 2-29 and 2-30.)

37. (*a*) Mitogens are substances which can activate lymphocytes to undergo proliferative changes in vitro such as incorporation of tritiated thymidine. (*b*) Phytohemagglutinin (PHA) and concanavalin A (ConA) activate T lymphocytes. (*c*) Lipopolysaccharide (LPS)

and dextran sulfate activate B lymphocytes. (*d*) Pokeweed mitogen (PWM) and antilymphocyte serum activate both B and T cells. (*e*) No, not all mitogens which bind to lymphocytes activate them. PHA and ConA activate T lymphocytes by binding to certain chemical groups on their surface. (*f*) Anti-immunoglobulins activate B lymphocytes by cross-linking their surface immunoglobulin receptors. The antibodies are specific for the immunoglobulin nature of the receptors but not for the antigens with which the receptors are capable of reacting, and therefore they are considered nonspecific mitogens. (Secs. 2-31 and 2-32.)

38. (*a*) The response induced in a lymphocyte by an antigen is stronger than that induced by a mitogen, but the number of lymphocytes involved in response to mitogen is greater because mitogen is not specific. Many T cells with receptors for different antigens would be activated by PHA, but only the T cells specific for a particular antigen would be activated by that antigen. (*b*) Lymphocytes from children with the DiGeorge syndrome show defective in vitro lymphoproliferative responses to PHA but normal responses to LPS. (*c*) Lymphocytes from patients with acquired hypogammaglobulinemia show defective in vitro lymphoproliferative responses to LPS and may also show abnormal responses to ConA. (*d*) Patients with Hodgkin's disease, cancer, or autoimmune disease may show a defective in vitro lymphoproliferative reaction to PHA and ConA. Elderly patients and patients suffering from malnutrition often show defective in vitro lymphoproliferative responses to T-cell mitogens. (Sec. 2-33.)

REFERENCES

Abramoff, P., and M. LaVia (1970): "Biology of the Immune Response," McGraw-Hill, New York.

Amos, B. (ed.) (1971): Progress in Immunology, 1st *Int. Cong. Immunol.*, Academic, New York.

Baker, P. J. (1975): Homeostatic Control of Antibody Responses: A Model Based on the Recognition of Cell-associated Antibody by Regulatory T cells, *Transplant. Rev.*, **26**:3-20.

Bellanti, J. A. (1971): "Immunology," Saunders, Philadelphia.

Bloom, B. R., and P. R. Glade (eds.) (1971): "*In Vitro* Methods in Cell-mediated Immunity," Academic, New York.

Boyse, E. A., and H. Cantor (1977): Surface Characteristics of T-Lymphocyte Subpopulations, *Hosp. Pract.*, **12**(4):81-88.

Brock, T. D. (1961): "Milestones in Microbiology," American Society for Microbiology, Washington, D.C.

Bruton, O. C. (1952): Agammaglobulinemia, *Pediatrics*, **9**:722-728.

Burnet, F. M. (1959): "The Clonal Selection Theory of Acquired Immunity," Cambridge University Press, London.

Campbell, P. A. (1976): Immunocompetent Cells in Resistance to Bacterial Infection, *Bacteriol. Rev.*, **40**:284-313.

Cantor, H., and I. Weissman (1976): Development and Function of Subpopulations of Thymocytes and T Lymphocytes, *Prog. Allergy*, **20**:1-64.

Catalona, W. J., W. F. Sample, and P. B. Chretien (1973): Lymphocyte Reactivity in Cancer Patients: Correlation with Tumor Histology and Clinical Stage, *Cancer*, **31**:65-71.

Chase, M. W. (1945): The Cellular Transfer of Cutaneous Hypersensitivity to Tuberculin, *Proc. Soc. Exp. Biol. Med.*, **59**:134-135.

Chess, L., and S. F. Schlossman, (1976): Methods for the Separation of Unique Human Lymphocyte Subpopulations, pp. 77-80 in N. R. Rose and H. Friedman (eds.), "Manual of Clinical Immunology," American Society for Microbiology, Washington, D.C.

Claman, H. N., and E. A. Chaperon (1969): Immunologic Complementation between Thymus and Marrow Cells: A Model for the Two-Cell Theory of Immunocompetence, *Transplant. Rev.*, **1**:92-113.

Cohen, I. R., and S. Livnat (1976): The Cell-mediated Immune Response: Interactions of Initiator and Recruited T Lymphocytes, *Transplant. Rev.*, **29**:24-58.

Cooper, M. D., D. H. Raymond, M. A. South, and R. A. Good (1966): The Functions of the Thymus System and the Bursa System in Chicken, *J. Exp. Med.*, **123**:75-102.

Coutinko, A., and Goran Moller (1975): Thymus-independent B-Cell Induction and Paralysis, *Adv. Immunol.*, **21**:113-236.

Cunningham, B. A. (1976): Structure and Significance of β_2-Microglobulin, *Fed. Proc.*, **35**:1171-1176.
Davis, B. D., R. Dulbecco, H. N. Eisen, H. S. Ginsberg and W. B. Wood (1973): "Microbiology," 2d ed., Harper & Row, Hagerstown, Md.
Dennert, Gunther (1976): Thymus Derived Killer Cells: Specificity of Function and Antigen Recognition, *Transplant. Rev.*, **29**:59-88.
DiGeorge, A. M. (1965): Discussion, *J. Pediat.*, **67**:907-908.
Dutton, R. W. (1975): Suppressor T Cells, *Transplant. Rev.*, **26**:39-55.
Feldman, M., and G. J. V. Nossal (1972): Cellular Basis of Antibody Production, *Q. Rev. Bio.*, **47**:269-302.
Felsburg, P. J., R. Edelman, and R. H. Gilman (1976): The Active E Rosette Test: Correlation with Delayed Cutaneous Hypersensitivity, *J. Immunol.*, **116**:1110-1114.
Finkelman, F. D., J. A. van Boxel, R. Asofsky, and W. E. Paul (1976): Cell Membrane IgD: Demonstration of IgD on Human Lymphocytes by Enzyme-catalyzed Iodination and Comparison with Cell Surface Ig of Mouse, Guinea Pig, and Rabbit, *J. Immunol.*, **116**:1173-1181.
Fishman, M., and F. L. Adler (1967): The Role of Macrophage RNA in the Immune Response, *Cold Spring Harbor Symp. Quant. Biol.*, **32**:343-347.
Forman, J. (1976): The Specificity of Thymus-derived T-Cells in Cell-mediated Cytotoxic Reactions, *Transplant. Rev.*, **29**:146-163.
Gershon, R. K. (1975): Immunoregulation by T Cells, pp. 267-288 in E. E. Smith and D. W. Ribbons (eds.) Molecular Approaches to Immunology, *Miami Winter Sym.* vol. 9, Academic, New York.
Glick, B., T. S. Chang, and R. G. Jaap (1956): The Bursa of Fabricius and Antibody Production, *Poult. Sci.*, **35**:224-225.
Good, R. A., and D. W. Fisher (eds.) (1971): "Immunobiology," Sinauer, Stamford, Conn.
Greene, B. M., and D. G. Colley (1976): Eosinophils and Immune Mechanisms, III: Production of the Lymphokine Eosinophil Stimulation Promotor by Mouse T Lymphocytes, *J. Immunol.*, **116**:1078-1083.
Gronowicz, E., and A. Coutinko (1975): Functional Analysis of B Cell Heterogencity, *Transplant. Rev.*, **24**:3-40.
Janeway, C. A., Jr. (1976): The Specificity of T Lymphocyte Responses to Chemically Defined Antigens, *Transplant. Rev.*, **29**:164-188.
Janossy, G., and M. Greaves (1975): Functional Analysis of Murine and Human B Lymphocyte Subsets, *Transplant. Rev.*, **24**:177-326.
Katz, D. H. (1977): Genetic Controls and Cellular Interactions in Antibody Formation., *Hosp. Pract.*, **12**(2):85-99.
——and D. Armerding (1976): The Role of Histocompatibility Gene Products in Lymphocyte Triggering and Differentiation, *Fed. Proc.*, **35**:2053-2060.
Kim, Y. B. (1973): Developmental Immunity in the Piglet, pp. 549-557 in D. Bergsma, R. A. Good, J. Finstad, and N. W. Paul (eds.), "Immunodeficiency in Man and Animals," Sinauer, Sunderland, Mass.
Kruyff, R. H., D. G. Gilmour, and G. J. Thorbecke (1975): Migratory Patterns of B Lymphocytes, III: Inhibition of Splenic Follicular Localization of Transferred Chicken Bursa Cells by Preincubation with Anti-Ig, *J. Immunol.*, **114**:1700-1704.
Lachmann, P. J., and H. E. Amos (1971): Soluble Factors in the Mediation of the Cooperative Effect, pp. 65-72 in P. A. Miescher (ed.), Immunopathology, *6th Int. Symp. Grindelwald, Aug. 30-Sept. 5,1970*, Grune and Stratton, New York.
Landsteiner, K., and M. W. Chase (1942): Experiments on Transfer of Cutaneous Sensitivity to Simple Compounds, *Proc. Soc. Exp. Biol. Med.* **49**:688-690.
Lawrence, H. S. (1954): The Transfer of Generalized Cutaneous Hypersensitivity of the Delayed Tuberculin-type in Man by Means of Constituents of Disrupted Leukocytes, *J. Clin. Invest.*, **33**:951-952.
——(1974): Transfer Factor: Initiation and Augmentation of Cell-mediated Immunity, pp. 289-329 in R. T. McCluskey and S. Cohen (eds.), "Mechanisms of Cell-mediated Immunity," Wiley, New York.
Leibowitch, J., and J. R. David (1972): Lymphocyte-Macrophage Interaction in Resistance to *Listeria monocytogenes, Fed. Proc.*, **31**:610.
McCluskey, R. T., and S. Cohen (eds.) (1974): "Mechanisms of Cell-mediated Immunity," Wiley, New York.
Miescher, P. A. (ed.) (1971): Immunopathology, *6th Int. Symp.*, Grune and Stratton, New York.
Miller, J. F. A. P. (1961): Immunological Function of the Thymus, *Lancet*, **2**:748-749.
Mitchison, N. A. (1971): Cell Cooperation in the Immune Response: The Hypothesis of an Antigen

Presentation Mechanism, pp. 52-64 in P. A. Miescher (ed.), Immunopathology, *6th Int. Symp., Grindelwald, Aug. 30–Sept. 5, 1970,* Grune and Stratton, New York.

Nowell, P. C. (1960): Phythohemagglutinin: An Initiator of Mitosis in Culture of Normal Human Leukocytes, *Cancer Res.,* **20**:462–466.

Nussenzweig, V. (1974): Receptors for Immune Complexes on Lymphocytes, *Adv. Immunol.,* **19**:217-258.

Oppenheim, J. T., and D. L. Rosenstreich (1976): Signals Regulating *in vitro* Activation of Lymphocytes, *Prog. Allergy,* **20**:65-194.

Owen, J. J. T. (1972): The Origins and Development of Lymphocyte Populations, pp. 35-64 in Ontogeny of Acquired Immunity, *Ciba Found. Symp.,* Associated Scientific Publishers, Amsterdam.

Park, B. H., and R. A. Good (1974): "Principles of Modern Immunobiology: Basic and Clinical," Lea & Febiger, Philadelphia.

Parmley, M. J., A. E. Beer, and R. E. Billingham (1976): *In Vitro* Studies on the T-Lymphocyte Population of Human Milk, *J. Exp. Med.,* **144**:358-369.

Petranyi, G. G., and G. Janossy (1974): The Cellular Basis of Immunological Processes (Immunocytes and Macrophages), pp. 169-202 in E. Rajka and S. Korossy (eds.), "Basic Concepts in Experimental Immunology," vol. 1, Plenum, London.

Porter, R., and J. Knight (eds.) (1972): Ontogeny of Acquired Immunity, *Ciba Found. Symp.,* Elsevier, Amsterdam.

Raff, M. C. (1973): T and B Lymphocytes and Immune Responses, *Nature,* **242**:19-23.

——and H. Cantor (1971): Subpopulations of Thymus Cells and Thymus-derived Lymphocytes, pp. 81-93 in B. Amos (ed.), Progress in Immunology, *1st Int. Cong. Immunol.,* Academic New York.

Rocklin, R. E., R. P. MacDermott, L. Chess, S. F. Schlossman, and J. R. David (1974): Studies on Mediator Production by Highly Purified Human T and B Lymphocytes., *J. Exp. Med.,* **140**:1303-1316.

Roelants, G. E. (1975): Recognition of Antigen by T Lymphocytes, pp. 55-78 in E. E. Smith and D. W. Ribbons (eds.), Molecular Approaches to Immunology, *Miami Winter Symp.,* Academic, New York.

Rose, N. R., and H. Friedman (eds.), (1976): "Manual of Clinical Immunology," American Society for Microbiology, Washington, D.C.

Rowe, D. S., K. Hug, and W. P. Faulk (1973): IgD on the Surface of Peripheral Blood Lymphocytes of the Human Newborn, *Nature New Biol.,* **242**:155-156.

Scher, I., S. O. Sharrow, R. Wistar, Jr., R. Asofsky, and W. E. Paul (1976): B-Lymphocyte Heterogeneity: Ontogenic Development and Organ Distribution of B-Lymphocyte Populations Defined by Their Density of Surface Immunoglobulin, *J. Exp. Med.,* **144**:494-506.

Sercarz, E. E., A. R. Williamson, and C. F. Fox (eds.) (1974): The Immune System: Genes, Receptors, Signals, *3d ICN-UCLA Symp. Molec. Biol.,* Academic, New York.

Shortman, K., H. von Boehmer, J. Lipp, and K. Hopper (1975): Subpopulations of T-Lymphocytes: Physical Separation, Functional Specialization and Differentiation Pathways of Sub-sets of Thymocytes and Thymus-dependent Peripheral Lymphocytes, *Transplant. Rev.,* **25**:163-210.

Singer, S. J. (1974): Molecular Biology of Cellular Membranes with Applications to Immunology, *Adv. Immunol.,* **19**:1-66.

Smith, E. E., and D. W. Ribbons (eds.) (1975): Molecular Approaches to Immunology, *Miami Winter Symp.,* vol. 9, Academic, New York.

Solkeim, B. G. (1974): Association between the β_2-m/HL-A Molecule and the Membrane Structures Responsible for Lymphocyte Activation, *Transplant. Rev.,* **21**:35-52.

Stout, R. D., S. D. Waksal, and L. Herzenberg (1976): The Fc Receptor on Thymus-derived Lymphocytes, III: Mixed Lympholytic Reactivity of Fc^- and Fc^+ T Lymphocytes, *J.Exp. Med.,* **144**:54-68.

Strober, S. (1975): Immune Function, Cell Surface Characteristics and Maturation of B Cell Subpopulations, *Transplant. Rev.,* **24**:84-112.

Taniguchi, M., T. Tada, and T. Tokuhisa (1976): Properties of the Antigen Specific Suppressive T-Cell Factors in the Regulation of Antibody Response of the Mouse, III: Dual Gene Control of the T-Cell Mediated Suppression of the Antibody Response, *J. Exp. Med.,* **144**:20-31.

Waksman, B. H., and H. Ozer (1976): Specialized Amplification Elements in the Immune System, *Prog. Allergy,* **21**:1-113.

Warner, N. L. (1974): Membrane Immunoglobulins and Antigen Receptors on B and T Lymphocytes, *Adv. Immunol.,* **19**:67-216.

Wedner, H. J., and C. W. Parker (1976): Lymphocyte Activation, *Prog. Allergy,* **20**:195-300.

3
Antigens, Immunoglobulins, and Complement

PROPERTIES OF ANTIGENS AND ANTIBODIES

Definition of Antigen, Immunogen, and Hapten

3-1 The term antigen has been in Chaps. 1 and 2. Antigen was defined as a substance which has the two following outstanding characteristics:

1. An antigen induces antibody formation and/or cell-mediated immune responses (mediated by sensitized T lymphocytes).
2. An antigen reacts very specifically with the antibody or sensitized T lymphocytes formed to it.

The term immunogen was used in Chaps. 1 and 2 when emphasis was on the immunogenicity of the substance, i.e., on the induction of an immune response, either humoral or cell-mediated. Some investigators prefer to use the term immunogen for induction of immune responses, i.e., to emphasize the first function listed above for antigen, and reserve the term antigen for specific reaction with antibody, i.e., the second function listed above. This restriction for the term antigen is not generally accepted. The term antigen was derived from antisomatogen. Although the term immunogen appears to have been introduced more recently than antigen, Deutsch referred to immunogens or antigens in 1899.*

3-2 The specificity of antibody molecules is directed by determinant groups of the antigen. Antigenic determinants are chemical groups on the antigen and in some cases may be of very small molecular size. Haptens, which have been called *partial antigens*, contain the determinant groups, but the hapten is unable to stimulate antibody production unless it is combined with a carrier, e.g., a protein molecule. The hapten is capable of combining very specifically with antibody produced by the complete antigen. Complex haptens give a visible precipitation reaction with antibody. They contain more than one determinant group. Simple haptens do not give a visible reaction with antibody but tie up the antigen binding sites on the antibody molecules. It can be ascertained that a reaction has taken place because after reaction with simple haptens the antibody molecules fail to react with the complete antigen. The term *ligand* is sometimes used to refer to antigens and haptens when it is not important to make a distinction between the two. Recently, the term *epitope* has also been used to refer to the determinant group. Landsteiner contributed greatly to our understanding of specificity by artificially coupling very simple chemical substances (haptens) with serum proteins. For coupling, Landsteiner used a diazo linkage, so that these artificial antigens were called *diazotized* or *conjugated proteins.* There are other methods now for coupling haptens to proteins. After injection of these conjugated proteins into experimental animals, it was shown that the antibody produced was specific for the hapten conjugated to the serum protein. Landsteiner's work helped us understand how simple haptens like aspirin and penicillin cause hypersensitivity. They sensitize the host by combining with proteins of the host to form complete antigens. The term *sensitize* is often used instead of immunize when exposure to the antigen causes an unfavorable reaction in the host. Penicillin sensitivity is discussed in Chap. 5.

Characteristics of Antigens Influencing Antibody Production

3-3 In order to be antigenic, a substance must be recognized by the host as being nonself or foreign. We shall see in Chap. 6 that under certain circumstances the body fails to recognize a substance as self, so that sensitization occurs to one or more components of the host's own tissue and may lead to disease states such as rheumatoid arthritis, lupus erythematosus, etc. Under normal conditions, several kinds of tissue specificity can be detected, e.g., species specificity, specificity within a species related to different blood groups, individual specificity, and organ specificity. With regard to species specificity, the tissue or body fluids from another species such as horse serum is antigenic for people. The dangers of sensitization to horse serum used for passive immunization were discussed in Chap. 1, where it was recommended that, if possible, human gamma globulin should be used for passive immunization. Sometimes a person may become sensitized to human tissue or cells because some antigens are possessed by certain members of the population but not all. These antigens are called *isoantigens* or *alloantigens* (newer term). Examples of alloantigens are blood-group antigens A and B and the Rh factor. Erythroblastosis fetalis results from an incompatibility in Rh factor between the mother and fetus and is discussed in Sec. 3-6. Individual tissue specificity is important in skin grafts and organ transplantation. Individual specific antigens are the HLA antigens of human beings. They are alloantigens but are usually referred to as *transplantation* or *histocompatibility antigens.* Organ-specific antigens exist between the organs even of different species, so that cross reactions between species can be observed. In Chap. 1, encephalitis following immunization with the Pasteur vaccine was cited. One of the theories given to account for this type of reaction was that a cross reaction between human and rabbit brain tissue occurred following sensitization of human beings to rabbit brain in the vaccine. The duck-embryo vaccine for rabies immunization does not contain brain tissue. When the Salk vaccine containing poliomyelitis virus grown in monkey kidney tissue and given by parenteral injection was first tested, it was feared that sensitization to monkey kidney tissue might occur due to organ specificity and possibly lead to nephritis, but fortunately this did not occur.

Ann. Inst. Pasteur*, **13: 689–727 (1899).

A parenteral (*par-* means "beside") injection is an inoculation by routes other than the intestinal tract, e.g., subcutaneous or intramuscular injections.

3-4 Antigens are usually high-molecular-weight proteins; high-molecular-weight polysaccharides are also antigenic for human beings but not all animal species. Lipids are not antigenic unless they are coupled to a protein carrier. Low-molecular-weight proteins such as insulin (MW 5700) and gelatin (MW 10,000) are not antigenic or only weakly antigenic. It appears, however, that the amino acid composition is just as important as the molecular weight. This has been demonstrated by synthesizing antigens known as *synthetic antigens* made up of different combinations of amino acids. One synthetic polypeptide which was antigenic had a molecular weight of 4100 and the following percentage composition of amino acids with the L configuration: alanine 38, glutamic acid 52, and tyrosine 10. Immunochemical studies have shown that polymers composed of only one amino acid are not antigenic regardless of their molecular weight. Polypeptides composed of only two amino acids are usually poor antigens.

Induction of Antibody by Antigens or Immunogens

3-5 Antigens are associated with the afferent limb of the immune response as in antigen recognition and triggering of immune responses by reaction of antigen with B or T lymphocytes. Antibody reactions or specific cell-mediated reactions are associated with the efferent limb of the immune system. Figure 3-1 shows the kind of primary and secondary antibody responses which usually occur following injection of an antigen. Injection of an antigen brings about active immunization, discussed in Chap. 1. After first exposure to the antigen, a week or longer is required to obtain a significant level of antibody. When the antigen is injected again after 30 days, there is a much more rapid rise in antibody titer than after the first exposure. The secondary phase is called the anamnestic or memory response. Antibody titer also persists at a higher level after the secondary response. The anamnestic response is the basis for the booster injection. Figure 3-1 also shows that the first serum antibodies to appear after immunization are IgM. IgG antibodies are formed later during the primary response and continue to increase as the level of IgM antibodies decreases. The main kind of antibody produced during the secondary response is IgG. IgM is believed to be the most primitive kind of antibody. If an infection occurs in utero, IgM is produced first. For example, the presence of IgM antibodies to the spirochete of syphilis in the serum of a newborn child is evidence of infection in utero rather than transplacental passage of a syphilitic mother's antibodies since IgM antibodies do not pass the placenta as IgG do. When antibody production reaches a certain level, homeostatic control mechanisms temporarily shut off further antibody production. That suppressor T cells may have a role in controlling antibody production was discussed in Sec. 2-21. It was also pointed out

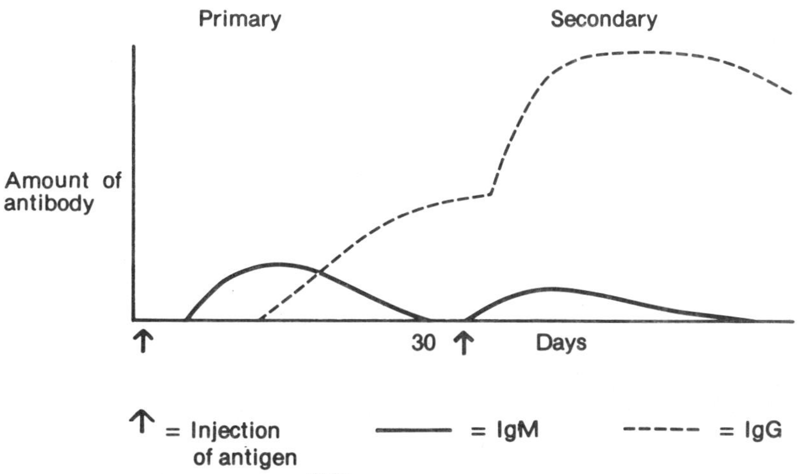

Figure 3-1. Primary and secondary responses with formation of IgM and IgG immunoglobulins (antibodies).

that injection of a fairly large amount of a specific antibody temporarily inhibits active immunization with antigen of the corresponding specificity. This type of suppression of antibody formation is known as feedback inhibition.

Transplacental Passage of IgG Antibody and Erythroblastosis Fetalis due to Rh Incompatibility between Mother and Fetus

3-6 In Sec. 3-3 it was pointed out that alloantigens are antigens possessed by some members of a species but not all. The Rh blood-group antigens are alloantigens (isoantigens) which may cause significant medical problems, related mainly to transfusion reactions and to erythroblastosis fetalis, a hemolytic disease of the newborn. The term Rh is derived from rhesus (monkey). It was reported by Landsteiner and Wiener (1940) that about 85 percent of the population possess an antigen which is also present in the red blood cells of Rhesus monkeys, while about 15 percent do not have this antigen and are called Rh-negative. Erythroblastosis fetalis had been recognized for some time before 1940, but its cause was not known. Levine and coworkers (1941) presented evidence based on previous cases of erythroblastosis fetalis that this condition occurs when the mother is Rh-negative and the child and father are Rh-positive. During pregnancy, Rh-positive cells from the child may enter the mother's circulation and cause the production of antibodies to the Rh antigen; IgM antibodies, which are produced first, do not cross the placenta, but IgG antibodies, which appear later, do. However, the greatest chance of sensitization occurs at parturition, when the placental barrier is more permeable. After sensitization of the mother, antibodies to Rh-positive cells would be transferred across the placenta during subsequent pregnancies and would react with the child's cells, if Rh-positive, and lead to their eventual destruction, e.g., after removal by phagocytosis in the spleen. The term erythroblastosis was given to this condition because as the fetal cells are destroyed, the fetus tries to compensate by pouring out erythroblasts (immature erythrocytes) into the blood. There are at least 27 distinct antigenic determinants which have been described for the Rh blood-group system. Three different types of nomenclature have been proposed. The Rh antigen which causes most medical problems is known as Rh_0 or D (and sometimes RH_1, but at present the RH_1 designation is used infrequently). If an Rh-positive father is heterozygous rather than homozygous for the Rh_0 (D) antigen, the child may not be positive for this antigen, so that erythroblastosis would not occur.

3-7 RhoGAM is the commercial name of human gamma globulin containing antibodies to Rh_0 (D) antigen; it has proved quite effective in the prevention of erythroblastosis fetalis due to Rh_0 incompatibility between mother and fetus. RhoGAM is also used to try to prevent sensitization when an Rh_0-negative patient is wrongly transfused with Rh_0-positive blood. RhoGAM must be given within 72 h after delivery or after a transfusion accident; within this time RhoGAM has been fairly effective in preventing sensitization to the Rh factor. A number of observations led to the development of RhoGAM. It was observed that erythroblastosis fetalis due to Rh incompatibility usually did not occur until the second or third pregnancy. It was determined that sensitization may occur during the last stages of pregnancy and especially at parturition. The observation that Rh sensitization occurs less frequently when there was also ABO blood-group incompatibility between mother and child led investigators to postulate that specific antibodies were combined with the offending Rh-positive erythrocytes, facilitating their rapid removal by phagocytes so that sensitization did not occur. It has been shown experimentally that red blood cells with attached antibodies are rapidly phagocytized by macrophages and degraded. Some endocytosed antigens may escape complete degradation and become accessible for immunological recognition; however, if antibodies are present to react with any antigen released from the macrophages, which happens to be the case here, the released material cannot stimulate antibody production. When RhoGAM is given, the mechanism of feedback inhibition may serve, in addition to the above mechanism, to depress antibody formation to the Rh_0 (D) antigen. Blocking or nonagglutinating antibodies, first recognized in connection with the Rh factor, are detected by special procedures described in Secs. 4-14 and 4-15.

3-8 Erythroblastosis fetalis due to ABO blood-group incompatibility between mother and fetus rarely occurs, but when it does, the mother is usually group O with a high titer of anti-A or anti-B isoantibodies of the IgG class and the fetus has an A or B phenotype inherited from the father. In contrast to Rh, the naturally occurring isoantibodies anti-A and anti-B are found in serum when A or B antigens are absent, as in a group O individual. A and B blood-group antigens are polysaccharides; it was pointed out in Chap. 2 that polysaccharides are T-cell-independent antigens and stimulate mainly IgM antibodies. IgM antibodies usually do not pass the placenta unless it has been damaged. If IgG antibodies to A and B blood-group substances are present and pass the placenta, their effect is usually less damaging to red blood cells than anti-Rh_0 antibodies because A and B blood-group antigens are found not only on red blood cells but also in tissue. Some persons, known as *secretors*, also have A and B antigens in body secretions. A and B antigens in tissue and body secretions react with anti-A or anti-B antibodies if these antibodies pass the placenta and help to protect the red blood cells. Rh antigens are confined to red blood cells, so that erythrocytes receive the full damaging effect of Rh antibodies. Hemolytic disease of the newborn due to ABO blood-group incompatibility between mother and fetus may occur during the first pregnancy. This is in contrast to what is usually observed with Rh incompatibility since antibodies to the Rh factor are present in serum only as a result of sensitization. If an Rh-negative woman had previously been sensitized by transfusion with Rh-positive blood, erythroblastosis fetalis would probably occur during the first pregnancy.

Characteristics of Antibodies

3-9 Antibodies have the structure of immunoglobulins (Ig), described beginning with Sec. 3-11. Antibodies which have been recognized have been designated IgG, IgM, IgA, and IgE. They are mainly gamma (γ) globulins. One of the characteristics of antibodies in general is that they react very specifically with the antigen which stimulated their production. Reaction between antibodies and their antigens can be demonstrated by a number of different kinds of tests, including agglutination, precipitation, complement fixation, immunofluorescence, and other methods described in Chap. 4. Antibodies formed early during the immune response are highly specific. As immunization continues, the antibodies produced appear less specific but form a stronger union with antigen. The firmness of the union reflects the avidity of the antibody.

3-10 Antibody which reacts with soluble antigen to cause precipitation has been termed *precipitin*, while antibody which reacts with particulate antigen to cause agglutination has been called *agglutinin*. Precipitins and agglutinins are not always different kinds of antibodies, in some cases being different manifestations of the same kind of antibody. For example, an antiserum containing antibodies specific for pneumococcal capsular polysaccharide type I will agglutinate virulent type I pneumococci which possess a capsule of type I polysaccharide. If the type I pneumococci are treated so that the capsular material is removed and purified, the polysaccharide will react to cause precipitation with the above antiserum. In this case, the precipitins for polysaccharide are believed to be the same kind of antibodies as the agglutinins causing agglutination when the antiserum is mixed with intact type I encapsulated pneumococci. If the antiserum is mixed with either type I pneumococci or type I pneumococcal polysaccharide, complement, if present, will be fixed in the reaction between specific antibody and antigen. The unitarian hypothesis of antibody formation, proposed many years ago, states that precipitins, agglutinins, complement-fixing antibodies, etc., are different manifestations of the same kind of antibody. With our knowledge of the heterogeneity of antibodies reflected in numerous classes and subclasses, we know that the unitarian hypothesis is not true in many cases.

Questions for Secs. 3-1 to 3-10

1. What is the difference between an antigen and an immunogen?
2. (*a*) What is meant by the determinant group of an antigen? (*b*) What did Landsteiner's experiments with conjugated proteins show about specificity of an antigen?
3. (*a*) Do haptens stimulate antibody production? (*b*) Do haptens react with antibody to give a visible reaction? Explain your answer. (*c*) Do haptens coupled to large protein molecules such as serum albumin stimulate antibody production? (*d*) How does a person

become sensitized to nonantigenic substances such as penicillin and aspirin?

4. What are some of the outstanding characteristics of an antigen?

5. Answer yes or no to the following questions: (*a*) Is goat serum antigenic if it is injected parenterally into human beings? (*b*) Is goat serum usually antigenic when ingested by human beings? (*c*) Do most individuals of the same blood group have identical tissue antigens? (*d*) Would rabbit brain tissue injected into another animal species like the dog be expected to show both species specificity and organ specificity?

6. What are the differences between the afferent and the efferent branches of the immune system?

7. (*a*) What kind of antibody (immunoglobulin) is produced first in response to an infection in utero? (*b*) What kind of antibody is considered the most primitive phylogenetically? (*c*) What antibody is produced first during the primary response of immunization? (*d*) What antibody is produced in the greatest amount during the secondary response? (*e*) On what type of expected response is the booster injection for immunization based?

8. (*a*) What is an alloantigen? (*b*) What is an isoantigen? (*c*) What is erythroblastosis fetalis? (*d*) What has been shown to be the mechanism of erythroblastosis fetalis due to the Rh blood group? (*e*) What Rh antigen is clinically the most important? (*f*) There are three different methods of classification or three different designations for this antigen. What are they? (*g*) With regard to this antigen, about how many people in the general population are Rh-negative? (*h*) Does a father who is positive for Rh_0 (D) antigen always have a Rh_0-positive (D-positive) child? Explain.

9. (*a*) What is used to prevent erythroblastosis fetalis? (*b*) What is the mechanism of prevention? (*c*) When must it be given in order to be effective?

10. (*a*) Why would a group O Rh_0-negative mother who has a group A, Rh_0-positive child be less likely to become sensitized to Rh_0 antigen than a group A Rh_0-negative mother who has a group A Rh_0-positive child? (*b*) Why does erythroblastosis due to ABO blood-group incompatibility between mother and child rarely occur or occur less frequently than that due to Rh?

11. (*a*) What are some of the tests used for demonstration of antibodies? (*b*) What are the antibodies called which react with soluble polysaccharide to give a flocculent material? (*c*) What are the antibodies called which cause clumping of intact pneumococci? (*d*) What is the unitarian hypothesis of antibody formation? (*e*) Is it still valid? (*f*) What is meant by avidity of an antibody molecule?

Answers

1. The terms antigen and immunogen are often used synonymously. Both terms are used to refer to substances which induce immune responses. Antigens are defined as substances which (1) induce antibody production or specific cell-mediated responses and (2) react very specifically with antibody or sensitized lymphocytes induced by the antigen. For immunogen, emphasis is on the first function of antigen stated above. (Sec. 3-1.)

2. (*a*) The determinant group is the chemical group on the antigen which determines the specificity of the antigen or the antibodies formed in response to the antigen. (*b*) Landsteiner's work with conjugated proteins showed that a small chemical group conjugated to a large protein molecule can change the antigenic specificity of the latter. (Sec. 3-2.)

3. (*a*) No. (*b*) Haptens composed of more than one determinant group (of the same specificity) can react with specific antibodies to give a visible precipitation reaction. Haptens containing only a single determinant group per molecule combine with specific antibodies, but precipitation does not occur; however, it can be shown that they did react with antibodies in the serum since when the complete antigen is mixed with the serum, precipitation does not occur as expected because the antibody combining sites have already been saturated by molecules of the hapten. (*c*) Yes. (*d*) By combination of penicillin or aspirin with tissue proteins to form complete antigens. (Sec. 3-2.)

4. Antigens must be recognized as nonself. The host recognizes microorganisms as foreign and also tissue or serum from a different animal species. Antigens are usually proteins of high molecular weight; however, high-molecular-weight polysaccharides may also be antigenic. Large synthetic polymers showing no complexity of structure are not antigenic. (Secs. 3-3 and 3-4.)

5. (*a*) Yes. (*b*) No. (*c*) No. (*d*) Yes. (Sec. 3-3.)

6. The afferent branch of the immune system is concerned with exposure to antigen or antigen recognition. The efferent branch of the immune system is concerned with events which happen after antigen recognition, e.g., reaction of antibodies produced with antigens or the occurrence of specific cell-mediated reactions. (Sec. 3-5.)

7. (*a*) IgM. (*b*) IgM. (*c*) IgM. (*d*) IgG. (*e*) Anamnestic or memory response. (Sec. 3-5.)

8. (*a*) An alloantigen (*allo-* means "other") is an antigen which is present in the tissue or blood of some individuals of a species but not all. (*b*) Isoantigen is an older term formerly used for alloantigen (isoantigen is still frequently used with blood groups). (*c*) Erythroblastosis fetalis is a hemolytic disease of the newborn. Erythroblasts are immature red blood cells present in blood of the infant at birth because of previous destruction of red blood cells. (*d*) Erythroblastosis fetalis due to the Rh blood group usually occurs when the mother is Rh-negative, the father is Rh-positive, and the fetus is Rh-positive. The mother becomes sensitized to Rh-positive cells, usually at the time of delivery, when the placenta is more permeable, and Rh-positive cells gain entrance to the mother's circulation. During the next or subsequent pregnancies the mother's antibodies formed to the Rh-positive cells may cross the placenta and cause destruction of the child's red blood cells if the child is Rh-positive. (*e*) Rh_0 (D). (*f*) Rh_0, D, Rh_1. (*g*) 15 percent. (*h*) No, if the father is heterozygous, i.e., has one chromosome with the gene for Rh_0 (D) and one without, the child may receive the chromosome without the gene for Rh_0 (D) antigen. (Secs. 3-3 and 3-6.)

9. (*a*) Antibodies to the Rh_0 (D) antigen. Serum containing these antibodies is fractionated so that only gamma globulin is injected. The commercial name for this preparation is RhoGAM. (*b*) Antibodies to Rh_0 (D) react with red blood cells containing these antigens which may gain entrance to the mother's circulation. This causes these red blood cells to be phagocytized and degraded so that sensitization of the mother does not occur. (*c*) RhoGAM must be given within 72 h after delivery or a transfusion accident. (Sec. 3-7.)

10. (*a*) Because this group O mother has naturally occurring antibodies to group A antigens, so that these antibodies react with any of the child's red blood cells which gain entrance into her circulation and cause them to be destroyed before they can cause sensitization to Rh. (*b*) Group A and B antigens are polysaccharides and T-cell-independent antigens and mainly induce only IgM antibodies, which do not pass the placenta. In some cases, the mother has a high titer of anti-A or anti-B antibodies of the IgG class, which may cross the placenta. The child has A or B antigens, depending on the blood group, not only on the red blood cells but also in tissue, and these tissue antigens react with antibodies which cross the placenta and help to protect the red blood cells. In contrast, the Rh antigen is found only on the red blood cells; therefore, these cells show the full effect of anti-Rh antibodies which cross the placenta. (Sec. 3-8.)

11. (*a*) Precipitation, agglutination, and complement-fixation tests. (*b*) Precipitins. (*c*) Agglutinins. (*d*) The unitarian hypothesis states that precipitins, agglutinins, complement-fixing antibodies, etc., are not different antibodies but the same antibodies demonstrated by different types of tests. (*e*) The unitarian hypothesis of antibody formation does not hold for all antibodies. In some cases it appears to be true. (*f*) Capacity to bind firmly with antigen. (Secs. 3-9 and 3-10.)

Immunoglobulins with and without Apparent Antibody Activity

3-11 There is evidence that all immunoglobulins may have antibody activity. This has been more apparent with some immunoglobulins than with others. For human beings, five classes of immunoglobulins have been recognized, namely, IgG, IgM, IgA, IgE, and IgD. All except IgD definitely have been shown to act as antibodies. There are claims that IgD also has antibody activity, but this matter is still not clear. It was pointed out in Chap. 2 that B lymphocytes may have immunoglobulin receptors of the IgD class in addition to others; the significance of this finding remains to be elucidated. Compared with what all is known about the four other immunoglobulin classes, very little is known about the biological function of IgD. *Pathological immunoglobulins* or *paraproteins* are immunoglobulins which are produced as a result of a plasma-cell tumor. The tumor usually affects a single clone, so that these immunoglobulins are also called *monoclonal* or *M proteins.* The plasma-cell tumor eventually results in the secretion of immunoglobulins in uncontrollable quantities. Because a single clone is affected, these immunoglobulin molecules are very homogeneous. It is not easy to pinpoint the antigen for which these pathological immunoglobulins are specific; however, recent evidence indicates that they generally possess antibody specificity. It was pointed out in Chap. 2 that a single clone makes only one kind of antibody with regard to specificity although there may be a switch in immunoglobulin class, e.g., from IgM to IgG. Pathological immunoglobulins are associated with such diseases as multiple myeloma and Waldenström's macroglobulinemia. Pathological immunoglobulins belonging to all of the five classes have been recognized. Because these pathological immunoglobulins are produced in large amounts, and because they are homogeneous, they have been used for study of the structure of immunoglobulins. It is difficult to study the structure of immunoglobulins with serum containing antibodies of many different specificities and therefore constituting a very heterogeneous group. If antibodies in serum could be separated according to specificity, they would appear fairly homogeneous. It is important to understand at this point that microorganisms, red blood cells, tissue cells, etc., may contain many different antigens which bring about the formation of antibodies with many different specificities.

Physical Properties of Immunoglobulins

3-12 All proteins contain radicals which dissociate to give positive and negative ions like $-NH_3^+$ and $-COO^-$. The particle charge is affected by pH and electrolyte in the suspending medium. When proteins like serum-containing antibodies are placed in an electric field at a given pH, the components of serum move in a distinctive path according to their electric charges. On the alkaline side of the

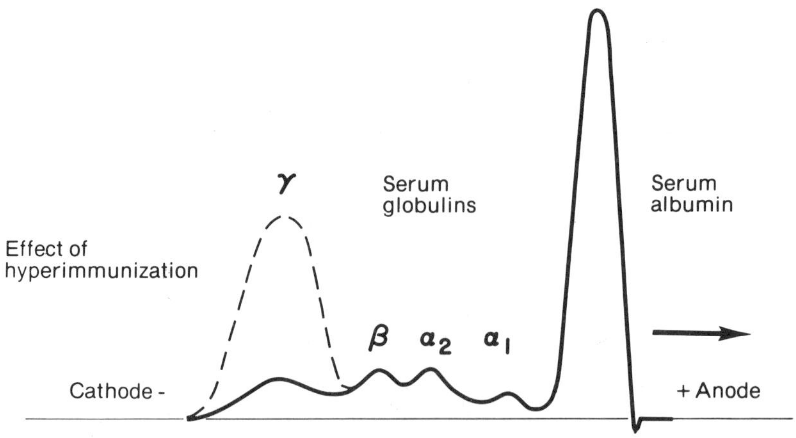

Figure 3-2 Electrophoresis of normal serum, showing a moving boundary in pH 8.5 buffer. Broken lines show increase in gamma globulin occurring in the serum of a hyperimmunized animal.

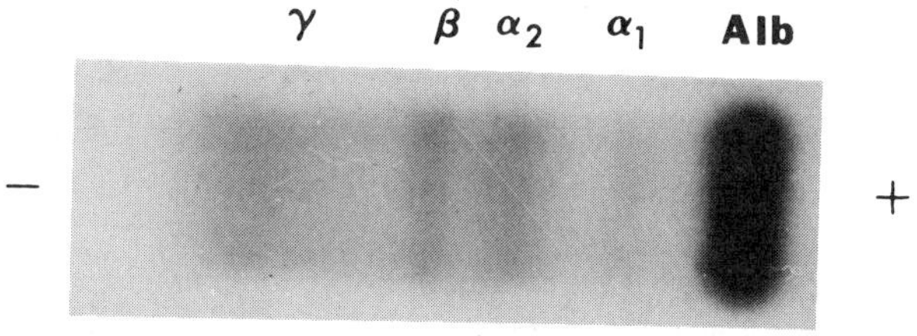

Figure 3-3 Electrophoresis of normal serum on a cellulose acetate filmstrip. After electrophoresis, the strip was stained; Alb = albumin. (*Courtesy of B. P. Barton, Department of Pathology, Medical College of Georgia.*)

isoelectric point at a buffered pH of 8.5, all serum components are negatively charged and move to the anode, as shown in Fig. 3-2. Albumin has the greatest charge and is the fastest-moving component; gamma globulin is the slowest. The rate of migration is also affected by the molecular weight. Albumin has a molecular weight of 69,000, while globulin consisting of a family of globulins has a molecular weight of 150,000 daltons or greater. Also the height of the peaks shows that albumin is present in normal serum in the greatest concentration. The approximate normal values for human serum are albumin, 55 percent; alpha 1 (α_1) globulin, 4 percent; alpha 2 (α_2) globulin, 9 percent; beta (β) globulin, 17 percent; and gamma (γ) globulin, 15 percent. Tiselius and Kabat (1939) demonstrated by electrophoresis that antibody activity is associated with the gamma-globulin fraction of serum. When an animal is hyperimmunized, the amount of gamma globulin may be greatly increased, as shown by the broken lines in Fig. 3-2. Zone electrophoresis is the migration of one or more substances in an electric field through a supporting medium such as paper, cellulose acetate, agar, or starch gel. Figure 3-3 shows zonal electrophoresis of normal serum on a stained cellulose acetate filmstrip. The strip also shows that albumin is the fastest-moving component and is present in the largest amount, as reflected by its position in the strip and its intensity of staining in comparison with other separated components. Analysis of all the electrophoretic components for antibody activity shows that IgG activity is mainly in the gamma-globulin fraction but that the other immunoglobulins overlap into the beta and alpha 2 fractions. Except for electrophoretic methods such as disc electrophoresis employing polyacrylamide gel, which acts as a molecular sieve, electrophoresis allows only a crude separation of serum fractions.

3-13 Studies with the serum of germ-free animals, e.g., guinea pigs, show that these animals have a very low level of gamma globulin, which could be antibodies formed to antigens present in their sterile environment such as those in food. When these animals are removed from a sterile environment, there is a marked increase in serum gamma globulin (Sec. 2-15). It has been reported that germ-free piglets from the Minnesota miniature sow, which has a six-layered, almost impervious placenta, do not have any serum gamma globulin (Sec. 2-23). The gamma-globulin fraction can be separated out of serum by nonspecific precipitation with chemicals like ammonium sulfate or ethanol. Serum fractions containing antibodies are used for passive immunization, as discussed in Chap, 1, and also for diagnostic tests, discussed in Chap. 4. For experimental purposes specific antibodies to an antigen can be obtained by specific precipitation or agglutination. Since antigen and antibody reactions are reversible under certain conditions, the specific aggregate can be separated and washed and specific antibodies obtained by dissociation from antigen after increasing the salt concentration, raising the temperature, or changing the pH. Depending on the nature of the antigen, antibodies dissociated from antigen and antibody complexes can be further separated by gradient centrifugation, electrophoresis, gel filtration, or ion-exchange chromatography. Only antibodies belonging to classes IgG, IgA, and IgM can be separated by specific precipitation or agglutination since the other immunoglobulins are not known to cause these reactions.

Structure of IgG and Basic Structural Unit of Other Immunoglobulins

3-14 Different classes of immunoglobulins have somewhat different structures, as is evident from their molecular weights and sedimentation coefficients. For example, IgG has a molecular weight of about 150,000 daltons, while IgM has a molecular weight of about 900,000 daltons. By ultracentrifugation and measurement in Svedberg (S) units, IgG has a sedimentation coefficient of 7S and IgM a sedimentation coefficient of 18 to 19S. Although antibodies have been described above as being heterogeneous, all antibodies share certain similar structural features. All consist of one or more basic units composed of four polypeptide chains held together by disulfide bonds. Two of the chains are called *heavy chains* because of their greater molecular weight; the other two chains are termed *light chains* (see Figure 3-4*a*). The heavy (H) chains possess antigens which allow human immunoglobulins to be differentiated into classes, IgG, IgM, IgA, IgE, and IgD; the heavy chains of these immunoglobulins are designated by the Greek letters gamma (γ), mu (μ), alpha (α), epsilon (ϵ), and delta (δ) respectively. On the basis of minor structural differences in the heavy chains, IgG is divided into four subclasses; IgA has two subclasses. Light chains do not contain the antigens which allow differentiation of classes, but they do contain antigens for two distinct antigenic types, kappa (κ) and lambda (λ). Kappa and lambda light chains are found in all five immunoglobulin classes; however, any given immunoglobulin molecule has either kappa or lambda light chains but never both, i.e., never one of each type. Therefore, a molecule of IgG would have a formula for its four chains of either $\gamma_2\kappa_2$ or $\gamma_2\lambda_2$. Both heavy and light polypeptide chains have constant (C) and variable (V) regions with regard to amino acid composition and sequence. The variable region is responsible for antibody specificity.

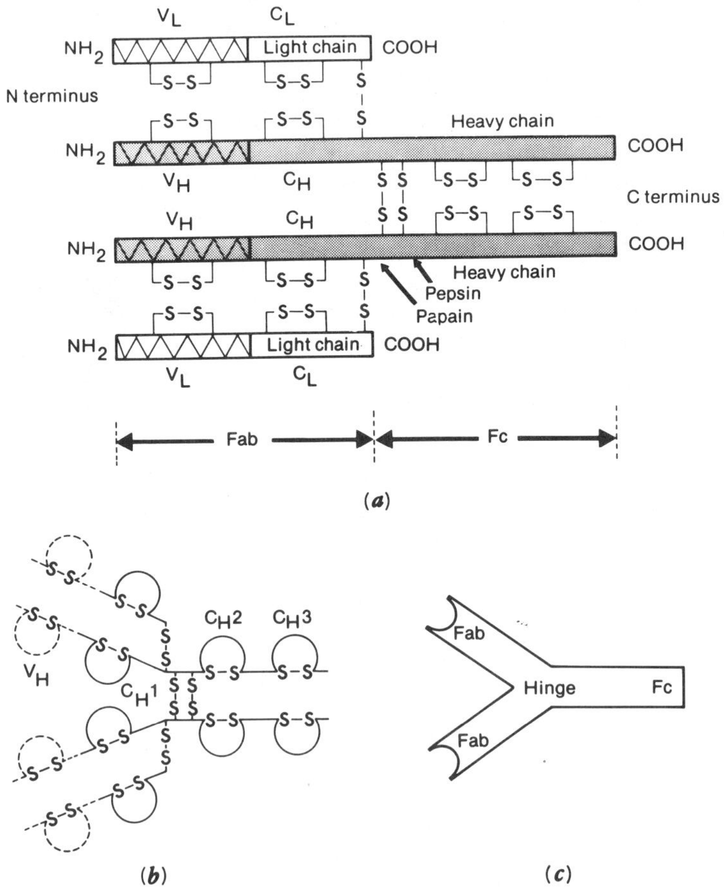

Figure 3-4 (*a*) Diagrammatic representation of the composition of immunoglobulin IgG. Arrows show where papain and pepsin split the chain; Fc does not remain intact with pepsin but is digested into smaller fragments not represented here. Fab = fragment antigen-binding; Fc = fragment crystallizable; C = constant; V = variable; H = heavy; L = light. (*b*) Diagrammatic representation of structure of IgG showing domains of heavy chains. (*c*) Wishbone, or Y, representation of IgG showing hinge region.

3-15 Pioneers in immunoglobulin structure have been Porter and Edelman in England and the United States, respectively. Antibody molecules have been studied (dissected) by treatment with proteolytic enzymes like pepsin and papain. Arrows in Fig. 3-4*a* show where papain and pepsin split the molecule. The IgG molecule split by papain can be shown to have two antigen-binding sites designated Fab (fragment antigen-binding). Fab is composed of one light chain and part of a heavy chain and also of both variable and constant regions, V_H, V_L, C_H, and C_L. The variable region is the terminal half of Fab. The Fc component of IgG split off by papain stands for fragment crystallizable and consists only of part of the constant region of the heavy chains. Since the amino (NH_2), or N terminus, of both the heavy and light chains is at the variable end of the Fab component, the carboxyl (COOH), or C terminus, of the heavy chain is at the end of the Fc region. Several biological functions are associated with the Fc region, including transplacental passage of IgG, attachment of IgG to phagocytes (macrophages and neutrophils), fixation of complement by IgG and IgM, and attachment of IgE to tissue mast cells and blood basophils. In addition to the interchain disulfide bonds, which hold light and heavy chains together, there are also intrachain disulfide bonds for both light and heavy chains, as shown in Fig. 3-4*a*. Figure 3-4*b* shows the heavy and light chains of IgG not as straight chains, as they were represented in Fig. 3-4*a*, but with the chains looped and held by disulfide bonds. The heavy chains are divided into different domains designated C_H1, C_H2, and C_H3, where C stands for constant region and H for heavy chain. In order to diagram antigen and antibody reactions, IgG is sometimes described as having a wishbone, or Y, structure, represented in Fig. 3-4*c*. When antibody combines with antigen, it appears that the arms of the wishbone or Y may open out at a region designated the *hinge region.*

3-16 If an animal is simultaneously immunized with more than one antigen, e.g., antigens A and B, it will form antibodies specific for antigen A and antibodies specific for antigen B. Under natural conditions of antibody formation, a single antibody molecule apparently cannot have combining sites specific for more than one antigen. However, it has been shown that bispecific antibodies, called *hybrid antibodies,* can be formed artificially using two different antisera. After treatment with papain, Fab fragments from each are reassembled artificially in vitro to form single antibody molecules with two different specificites. Hybrid antibodies are used in research to link two unrelated antigens together.

Structure of IgM and IgA

3-17 The basic structural units of IgM and IgA are very similar but not identical to IgG. For example, IgM heavy chains are longer and have more oligosaccharide branches and a higher carbohydrate content. IgM immunoglobulins have a molecular weight of approximately 900,000 daltons and a sedimentation constant of 18 to 19S. They are pentamers (*penta-* means "five") and are composed of five identical subunits or IgM monomers. The monomers are assembled in the star-shaped configuration shown in Fig. 3-5. This star- or spider-shaped molecule can be observed by electron microscopy if the resolving power of the microscope is sufficiently large. The IgM monomers are held together in the Fc region by disulfide bonds. A single J chain (J for "joining") has been shown to be attached to the pentamer by disulfide bridges. Although IgM antibodies occur only as pentamers, the monomeric form of IgM is found as immunoglobulin receptors on B lymphocytes, as described in Chap. 2. IgM monomers do not have J chains. The IgM pentamer has ten combining sites (two for each subunit), but usually only five sites are demonstrable, probably because half the combining sites are blocked from combining with antigen as a result of steric hindrance. IgM is very efficient in bringing about agglutination and precipitation since a single molecule has several combining sites.

3-18 IgA was recognized as a separate immunoglobulin class of human serum using immunoelectrophoresis techniques, described in Chap. 4. Immunoelectrophoresis combines the techniques of electrophoresis and precipitation. Separation of serum components in agarose gel is accomplished by electrophoresis; the separated components are recognized and identified by specific precipitation in agarose gel. The importance of IgA in secretions and in local immunity has already been pointed out (Chap. 1). IgA may exist in several forms, i.e., as a monomer, dimer, trimer, and sometimes even tetramer. Human IgA in the blood is usually in the form of a monomer, while IgA in secretions from

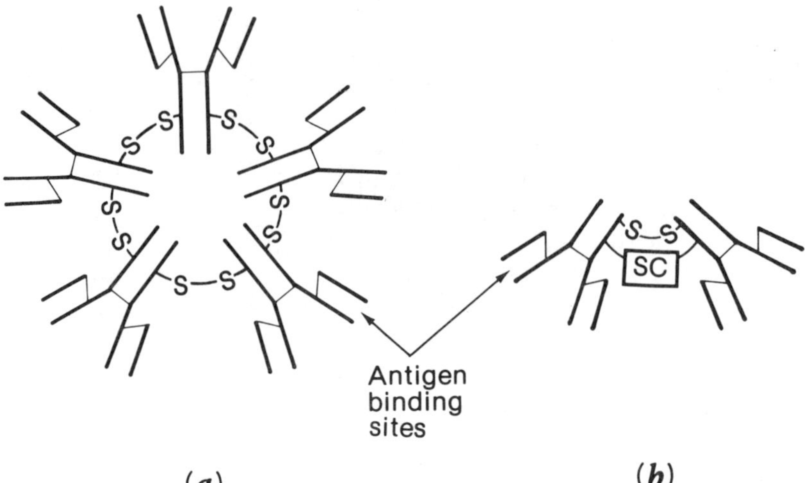

Figure 3-5 Structure of (*a*) IgM pentamer and (*b*) secretory IgA dimer.

exocrine glands occurs mostly as a dimer. The dimer form of IgA is shown in Fig. 3-5. Like IgM, it contains a J, or joining, chain. In addition, it contains a secretory piece or secretory component (SC), once known also as a transport (T) piece. IgA with J chain is formed by plasma cells, but the secretory component is produced in epithelial cells of the exocrine glands before secretion of IgA. The function of the secretory component is not clear; it appears to be responsible for resistance of secretory IgA to proteolysis and presistence in tissue. Production of IgA in the intestinal tract was discussed in connection with the Sabin vaccine in Chap. 1.

Questions for Secs. 3-11 to 3-18

12. (*a*) Name five classes of immunoglobulins which have been demonstrated in human serum. (*b*) Which class has not been well characterized with regard to biological function? (*c*) What is the origin of pathological immunoglobulins? (*d*) What are two other names by which these pathological immunoglobulins are known? (*e*) What two characteristics of pathological immunoglobulins produced by a single clone make them suitable for the study of the structure of immunoglobulins?

13. (*a*) What five components of serum can be recognized by electrophoresis? (*b*) What charge do proteins have in a buffer with a pH above their isoelectric point? (*c*) In an electric field, do negatively charged proteins move to the anode or cathode? (*d*) What is the fastest-moving component of serum? Why? (*e*) In what fraction(s) of serum are immunoglobulins found? (*f*) What fraction is greatly increased when animals are hyperimmunized?

14. (*a*) How is gamma globulin separated from other serum fractions? (*b*) Does this gamma-globulin fraction contain a mixture of antibodies with regard to class and specificity? (*c*) How can a fairly pure preparation of antibodies specific for a certain antigen be prepared? (*d*) What three immunoglobulins are mainly separated by the method described in part (*c*)?

15. (*a*) What are the approximate molecular weights of IgG and IgM? (*b*) What are the approximate sedimentation coefficients of IgG and IgM? (*c*) With regard to sedimentation coefficients, what does the letter S represent? (*d*) Why does IgM have a much larger molecular weight and greater sedimentation coefficient than IgG?

16. (*a*) Does IgG exist only as a monomer? (*b*) How many polypeptide chains make up IgG? (*c*) How are these chains held together? (*d*) How many heavy chains are in an IgG molecule? (*e*) What are the heavy chains of IgG called? (*f*) What is the approximate molec-

ular weight of the heavy chains? (*g*) How many light chains are in an IgG molecule? (*h*) What two different kinds of light chains may IgG and other immunoglobulins have? (*i*) Does IgG or any other single immunoglobulin molecule ever have more than one kind of light chain? (*j*) Can an individual have some immunoglobulins with kappa light chains and other immunoglobulins with lambda light chains? (*k*) What is the approximate molecular weight of the light chains of IgG? (*l*) Does the total molecular weight of the four chains add up to about 150,000, which is the approximate molecular weight of an IgG molecule? (*m*) Does the structure of the heavy chains or the light chains determine the immunoglobulin class? (*n*) Does the structure of the heavy chains or light chains divide IgG into four subclasses? (*o*) What part of the heavy and light chains is responsible for antibody specificity?

17. Immunoglobulins are protein molecules and can be "dissected" by digestion with proteolytic enzymes such as papain. Papain splits IgG into two Fab fragments and one Fc fragment. Answer the following questions about the structural components of IgG: (*a*) Which part of IgG is responsible for transplacental passage of the mother's antibodies? (*b*) Which part of IgG binds complement? (*c*) Which part of IgG contains specific sites for reaction with antigen? (*d*) What is variable about the variable region? (*e*) Where is the variable region found, and what function does it serve? (*f*) Are the combining sites for antigen found at the carboxyl (C) or amino (N) terminus of the polypeptide chains of immunoglobulins? (*g*) Does the Fab portions of IgG contain both light and heavy chains, and if so, how much of each chain? (*h*) What is the composition of the Fc fragment? (*i*) Does the Fc fragment contain the carboxyl (C) or amino (N) terminal region of the intact heavy chains? (*j*) Is the Fc fragment composed of only the constant regions of the immunoglobulin molecule? (*k*) Where is the hinge region of IgG? (*l*) What is the function of the hinge region?

18. (*a*) What immunoglobulin, according to its structure, has 10 combining sites for antigen? (*b*) Are all of these sites functional? Explain your answer. (*c*) What immunoglobulin(s) contain a J chain? (*d*) Are J chains produced by plasma cells when the immunoglobulin molecules are formed? (*e*) What immunoglobulin(s) contain a secretory component (SC)? (*f*) Is the secretory component produced by plasma cells? (*g*) What is the function of the secretory component? (*h*) What form of IgA is usually found in the blood? (*i*) What form of IgA is usually found in secretions?

Answers

12. (*a*) IgG, IgM, IgA, IgE, and IgD. (*b*) IgD. (*c*) A tumor of a clone of plasma cells. (*d*) Paraproteins and monoclonal, or M, proteins. (*e*) Homogeneous structure and production in large amounts. (Sec. 3-11.)

13. (*a*) Albumin and four globulin fractions, alpha 1, alpha 2, beta, and gamma. (*b*) Negative. (*c*) Anode. (*d*) Albumin, because it carries the greatest negative charge and has a smaller molecular weight. (*e*) IgG is found mainly in the gamma-globulin fraction, but the other immunoglobulins are found in the gamma-, beta-, or alpha 2-globulin fractions. (*f*) Usually gamma globulin. (Sec. 3-12.)

14. (*a*) By nonspecific precipitation with chemicals such as ammonium sulfate or ethanol. (*b*) Yes. (*c*) By specific precipitation or specific agglutination followed by dissociation of antibodies from antigen molecules under appropriate conditions. (*d*) IgG, IgM, IgA. (Sec. 3-13.)

15. (*a*) MW 150,000 for IgG; 900,000 for IgM. (*b*) 7S for IgG; 18 to 19S for IgM. (*c*) Svedberg units. (*d*) IgM is a pentamer; i.e., it is composed of five basic structural units consisting of four polypeptide chains each, while IgG is composed of only one unit. An IgM monomer has longer heavy chains and a slightly larger molecular weight than IgG. (Secs. 3-14 and 3-17.)

16. (*a*) Yes. (*b*) Four. (*c*) By disulfide bonds. (*d*) Two heavy chains. (*e*) Gamma

(γ) chains. (*f*) 50,000 daltons each. (*g*) Two light chains. (*h*) Kappa (κ) and lambda (λ). (*i*) No. (*j*) Yes. (*k*) 25,000 daltons each. (*l*) Yes. (*m*) Heavy chains. (*n*) Heavy chains. (*o*) Variable (V) region. (Sec. 3-14.)

17. (*a*) Fc. (*b*) Fc. (*c*) Fab. (*d*) Amino acid composition and sequence. (*e*) Terminal half of Fab. The variable region is responsible for antibody specificity. (*f*) Amino (N) terminus. (*g*) Yes; Fab is composed of an entire light chain and approximately half of the heavy chain. (*h*) The Fc fragment contains approximately half of the two heavy chains. (*i*) Carboxyl (C) terminus. (*j*) Yes. (*k*) The hinge region is located approximately where papain splits the molecule. (*l*) One of the functions of the hinge region appears to be to allow flexibility of the immunoglobulin molecule for reaction with antigen. (Sec. 3-15.)

18. (*a*) IgM. (*b*) It appears that all ten sites are functional but that only about five are able to enter into a reaction with antigen at any one time probably because of steric hindrance. (*c*) IgM and IgA. (*d*) Yes. (*e*) IgA. (*f*) No, it is produced by epithelial cells of exocrine glands and added on when IgA is secreted. (*g*) At first it was thought that the secretory component was important for transport, but now it appears that the secretory component is concerned with resistance to degradation by enzymes, e.g., by proteolytic enzymes in the intestinal tract. (*h*) IgA monomer. (*i*) IgA dimer with secretory component. (Secs. 3-17 and 3-18.)

Immunoglobulins as Antigen Receptors on B Lymphocytes

3-19 In Chap. 2 it was pointed out that B lymphocytes, which are precursor cells for plasma cells and therefore for antibody production, have immunoglobulins IgG, IgM, IgA, IgE, and even IgD as receptors for antigen. The immunoglobulin receptors are monomers. Antigen recognition triggers the events which lead to antibody production. The specificity of the immunoglobulin receptors in recognizing antigen appears to be the same as antibody specificity discussed in this chapter. The significance of IgD on a large percentage of B cells at birth remains to be clarified. It appears that, in at least some cases, B cells have IgD and another immunoglobulin class as receptors. For a discussion of this subject, refer back to Sec. 2-24. It is believed that plasma cells produce the same class of immunoglobulin as those which served as B-lymphocyte receptors. It was also pointed out in Chap. 2 that the exact nature of T-cell receptors is not known but that a β_2-microglobulin-HLA complex on the surface of lymphocytes might serve as antigen receptors to trigger specific cell-mediated responses (Sec. 2-30). Also there is evidence that T cells, like B cells, have immunoglobulins on their surface but in smaller amounts. Some investigators have speculated that the T-cell receptors may be an unrecognized class of immunoglobulins, referred to as IgX, but so far as is known at present, there are only five classes of immunoglobulins.

Serum Concentration and Metabolism of Immunoglobulins and Their Relationship to Passive Immunization

3-20 The serum concentration and metabolic characteristics of human immunoglobulins are summarized for comparison in Table 3-1. Each class of immunoglobulin differs in the amount synthesized and the amount catabolized per day and consequently is present in serum in different amounts. IgG is present in serum in the largest amount and is catabolized the slowest. However, the rate at which IgG is catabolized rises at high serum levels and falls at low serum levels. Under normal conditions IgG has a half-life of 23 days. When serum is used for passive immunization, it is IgG which contributes the most for protection. The other immunoglobulins are either present in very small amounts or are catabolized too rapidly to be effective for passive immunization except for a short time. The amount of IgA synthesized approaches the amount of IgG synthesized, but apparently a large amount of IgA is lost through secretions. More than half the total body IgG and IgA is found extravascularly in tissues; IgM and IgD are predominantly intravascular. Since IgD is of similar size to IgG and IgA, the fact that 80 percent of IgM is intravascular cannot be attributed entirely to its large molecular size. IgE is about evenly distributed intravascularly and extravascularly.

Table 3-1 Comparison of Serum Concentrations and Metabolism of Human Immunoglobulins

Immunoglobulin	Average serum concentration, mg/ml	Intravascular distribution, %	Synthesis mg/ (kg) (day)	Survival (half-life), days	Fractional catabolic rate, %/day	MW (000)
IgG	12	45	33	23	6.7	150
IgM	1.2	80	6.7	5	18	900
IgA	2.5	42	24	6	25	160*
IgE	0.0003	51	0.02	2.5	89	190
IgD	0.03	75	0.4	3.0	37	180

*Dimer and other polymers have higher molecular weight.

Outstanding Properties of IgG, IgM, IgA, and IgE

3-21 Except for IgE, immunoglobulins are fairly heat-stable in that they are not inactivated by heating serum in a water bath at 56°C for 30 min. Complement, a normal component of the serum of warm-blooded animals, is inactivated by this procedure. IgA and IgE have been reported to lack complement-fixing capacity. Summaries of important characteristics of IgG, IgM, IgA and IgE are given in Table 3-2.

Specificity of Immunoglobulins, Including Isotypes, Allotypes, and Idiotypes

3-22 Immunoglobulin isotypes are antigenic types of immunoglobulins which exist in all members of a species. For example, IgG, IgM, IgA, IgE, and IgD classes are human immunoglobulin isotypes. The four subclasses of IgG, known as IgG_1, IgG_2, IgG_3, and IgG_4, are also isotypes. Different biological functions are associated with these four subclasses. The two subclasses of IgA designated IgA_1 and IgA_2 are isotypes. Kappa and lambda light chains would also be classified as isotypes. It has been reported that of all the immunoglobulin molecules with all classes considered, 60 percent contain kappa light chains and 40 percent contain lambda light chains. Isotypic variants or subtypes of lambda light chains due to variation in the "constant" region have been recognized. Two of these variants are Oz and Kern. An individual may have lambda light chains which are Oz^+, Oz^-, $Kern^+$,

Table 3-2 Properties of IgG, IgM, IgA, and IgE

IgG	IgM	IgA	IgE
Sedimentation coefficient = 7S; MW ≈ 150,000 daltons (IgG has less carbohydrate content than the other immunoglobulins) Constitutes about 75% of total amount of all immunoglobulins in body High concentration in blood (intravascular) and in tissues (extravascular) Catabolism slowest of all immunoglobulins; half-life 23 days; therefore, IgG is immunoglobulin most responsible for protection following passive immunization Passes placenta, responsible for passive immunity of newborn Cytophilic for phagocytes (macrophages and neutrophils) thus aiding in opsonization (Fig. 2-1) Effective against many microorganisms through mechanisms of bacteriolysis, opsonization, virus neutralization, etc.	Sedimentation coefficient = 18 to 19S; MW ≈ about 900,000 daltons Largest of immunoglobulins; pentamer consisting of five subunits First antibody formed after immunization; level of IgM usually falls rapidly after onset of IgG synthesis Carbohydrate or polysaccharide T-cell-independent antigens elicit prolonged production of IgM antibodies rather than usual switchover to IgG Fixes complement and is very efficient in agglutinating bacteria and red blood cells, probably because of many combining sites present on one molecule Mainly found intravascularly	Sedimentation coefficient = 7S to 11S; MW 150,000 to 600,000 daltons, depending on whether or not it is a polymer or contains a secretory component (SC) Present predominantly in saliva and secretions of respiratory tract and gastrointestinal tract as dimer; present in blood usually as monomer In secretions contains secretory piece which makes molecules more resistant to digestion by proteolytic enzymes Important in local tissue immunity, especially to viruses	Sedimentation coefficient = 8S; MW 190,000 daltons Fc portion of the IgE molecule has affinity for surface receptors on tissue mast cells and blood basophils Responsible for certain immediate-type hypersensitivity reactions, e.g., anaphylaxis and atopy Called *reagin* in allergy literature but entirely different from syphilis reagin Heat-labile, unlike other antibodies Must be demonstrated by special techniques since it does not cause precipitation, agglutination, or complement fixation

and Kern$^-$. For example, an Oz^+ chain has lysine at position 193; an Oz^- chain has arginine at position 193. Other lambda-light-chain variants have been reported. The presence of the isotypes cited above with the exception of IgA (especially in IgA-immunodeficient individuals) does not cause sensitization because they are all common to a single individual; therefore, the body does not recognize them as foreign or react to them in any adverse way as long as they are present in normal amounts. Care should be taken not to confuse immunoglobulin isotypes with the term isoantigen applied to blood groups. With blood groups, the term isoantigen or alloantigen is used to refer to antigens present in some members of a species but not all.

3-23 Immunoglobulin allotypes are immunoglobulins with structural differences common to some members of a species but not all. Structural differences in immunoglobulins can be determined by serologic tests or by amino acid sequencing. Allotypes due to structural differences in the constant region of heavy chains of IgG are known as Gm markers (IgG markers). There are 25 Gm allotypes. A Gm allotype is determined by the inheritance of linked genetic units (gene complexes) called *haplotypes.* One haplotype comes from the mother and one from the father. Allotypes due to structural differences in the constant region of heavy chains of IgA_2 are known as Am markers, of which there are two. No allotypes have been observed with IgA_1. Patients with IgA immunoglobulin deficiencies have been reported to develop transfusion reactions due to the presence of antibodies to IgA. These antibodies may have specificities related to the IgA class, to IgA isotypes, or to IgA allotypes. Allotypes due to structural differences in the constant region of kappa light chains have recently been designated Km markers (K for kappa), although they were known for many years as InV markers. There are three recognized Km allotypes. Km is the only system of allelic markers recognized for light chains. Km allotypes are caused by substitution of amino acids at positions 153 and 191 on the kappa light chains. These positions are located on adjacent polypeptide loops of the kappa light chain within 10 angstroms of each other ($1 Å = 10^{-10}$m). In Km(1), (2), and (3) allotypes, the substitutions are

Km(1): 153, valine; 191, leucine

Km(2): 153, alanine; 191, leucine

Km(3): 153, alanine; 191, valine

Antisera for distinguishing these Km markers recognize leucine at position 191 for Km(1), both alanine at 153 and leucine at 191 for Km(2), and alanine at 153 for Km(3).

3-24 If human globulin is injected into rabbits, antibodies are produced which will react with human immunoglobulins and not with antibodies of other animal species. Antibodies to immunoglobulins have been called *anti-antibodies* or preferably *antiglobulin antibodies* and are used in the Coombs test, in immunofluorescent-antibody techniques, etc., described in Chap. 4. For these diagnostic tests, anti-human globulin antibodies are used to determine whether or not antibodies (human) have taken part in the reaction. A true anti-antibody would be one directed to the combining site of the antibody molecule and must be sufficiently sensitive to detect changes in the combining site responsible for antibody specificity or the ability of the antibody to combine with only one certain antigen. Immunoglobulin structure responsible for this type of specificity is called the *idiotype.*

3-25 It is fairly clear now that specificity of antibody molecules for a particular antigen is determined by the variable region of the immunoglobulin molecule (review Fig. 3-4). The polypeptide chains are made up of amino acid residues. Figure 3-6 shows a kappa light chain of IgG_1, which is composed of 214 amino acid residues. For antibodies of different specificities, there is considerable variation in the region of amino acids from 1 to 107, and this variability, along with that in the variable region of the heavy chain, is responsible for the specificity of the antibody combining site. The amino acid residues from position 108 to 214 are almost constant. Substitutions at position 153 and 191 are responsible for Km allotypes formerly known as InV. The Km genetic markers are found on kappa but not on lambda light chains. The heavy chain of IgG is composed of 446 amino acid residues. Beginning with the amino terminal, the first 121 amino acid residues make up the variable

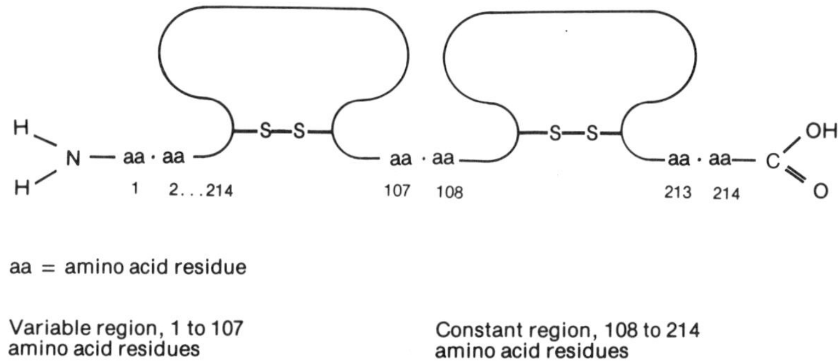

Figure 3-6 Kappa light chain of IgG, showing the number of amino acid residues in the variable and constant regions.

region, which, like the light-chain variable region, determines specificity. The remainder of the chain is homogeneous except for a few substitutions concerned with alloantigens such as Gm. Both light- and heavy-chain variable regions have *hypervariable sites,* or *hot spots,* which make up the antigen-binding site.

Age at Which Human Immunoglobulins Develop and Reach Normal Adult Levels

3-26 When transplacental infection occurs, e.g., with syphilis, the human fetus synthesizes IgM antibodies in utero. The presence of IgM antibodies to *Treponema pallidum* at birth is taken as an indication that the child is infected. If only IgG antibodies to *T. pallidum* are present, they are considered to be the mother's antibodies acquired by transplacental passage. If the mother is adequately treated during the early stages of pregnancy, the child does not become infected but still receives the mother's antibodies to *T. pallidum* as well as to many other organisms. Although the child is able to produce IgM antibodies by about the twentieth week of gestation, the amount of IgM antibodies present at birth is extremely small in the absence of any kind of infection. At birth, however, the child has the normal level of adult serum IgG acquired from the mother. Since the half-life of IgG is about 23 days, the maternal IgG antibodies are dissipated during the first few months. At about 2 months of age the lowest level of immunoglobulins is observed; but at this time the child begins to produce its own antibodies through exposure to various microorganisms or antigenic stimuli in the environment. Since IgM is the earliest kind of antibody produced, the level of IgM at 4 months of age is as great or greater than adult levels. At this time the IgG level is about one-third the normal adult level. The normal adult level of IgG is attained at about 2 to 5 years of age. IgA antibodies are produced at an early age but in small amounts. IgA levels continue to increase at a slow rate until about 8 to 12 years of age.

Disorders of Immunoglobulin Production

3-27 In Chap. 2 the failure of the body to produce antibodies was discussed. Now we shall look at disorders concerned with overproduction of immunoglobulins or pieces of immunoglobulins; for additional information see Chap. 7. When abnormally large amounts of pathological immunoglobulins are produced, the normal production of antibodies is depressed.

Monoclonal proteins Monoclonal proteins are structurally normal immunoglobulins which are produced in excessive amounts by a malignant colony or clone of plasma cells. Monoclonal proteins are very homogeneous with regard to class, subclass, type of light chains, allotype, and idiotype. For a while it was thought that monoclonal proteins lacked antibody specificity. This appears not to be the case, but immunoglobulins from any one clone all have the same specificity. It is very difficult to determine the specificity of pathological immunoglobulins because through natural exposure people come in contact with many different antigenic substances. In order to determine specificity, it might be necessary to test monoclonal proteins against many different antigens.

Multiple myeloma Monoclonal proteins of IgG, IgA, IgD, and IgE classes are associated with multiple myeloma. Bence Jones proteins, which consist only of light chains, are also found in multiple myeloma. As far back as 1846, Bence Jones proteins were recognized in the urine as proteins with unusual thermosolubility properties. They precipitate out when urine is heated at 45 to 60°C, but the precipitate dissolves on further heating to boiling. Bence Jones proteins precipitate again on cooling. Bence Jones proteins were not recognized as light chains of immunoglobulins until 1962. In contrast to the unusual thermosolubility properties of Bence Jones proteins, serum immunoglobulins are coagulated irreversibly by boiling.

Waldenström's macroglobulinemia Monoclonal proteins of the IgM class are responsible for Waldenström's macroglobulinemia. IgM is a large (macro) globulin. It has the structure of a pentamer and a molecular weight of about 900,000. Bence Jones proteins (or light chains) may also be present in this disease.

Heavy-chain disease Heavy-chain disease is caused by lymphoid-cell neoplasia and is characterized by the production of a large amount of immunoglobulin heavy-chain fragments. It was pointed out previously (Sec. 3-14) that there are five classes of heavy chain (gamma, mu, alpha, epsilon, and delta). Heavy-chain diseases with production of gamma, mu, or alpha heavy chains have been recognized. It is presumed that delta and epsilon heavy-chain diseases also occur. The heavy chains have an incomplete structure and are found in serum and/or urine.

Questions for Secs. 3-19 to 3-27

19. (*a*) Are the receptors for antigen recognition on B lymphocytes similar in structure to that of antibodies? (*b*) Have all classes of immunoglobulins been observed as receptors on B cells? (*c*) How do the receptors recognize antigen? (*d*) Are immunoglobulin receptors monomers, or are some polymers? (*e*) Do T lymphocytes have immunoglobulin receptors for antigen recognition?

20. (*a*) What immunoglobulin class is present in serum in the greatest amount? (*b*) What immunoglobulin class is synthesized to the greatest extent? (*c*) What immunoglobulin class is broken down or catabolized the slowest? (*d*) What is the approximate half life of IgG? (*e*) What immunoglobulin of known significance is found mainly intravascularly? Why?

21. (*a*) Name the immunoglobulin class (or classes) transferred across the placenta. (*b*) Name the immunoglobulin class (or classes) which is cytophilic for macrophages and neutrophils and aids in phagocytosis? (*c*) Are all five immunoglobulin classes present in the serum? (*d*) Which one(s) confers the most protection against infection when serum is used for passive immunization? Why?

22. Fill in the blanks with the appropriate immunoglobulin class(es).

______ (*a*) Sedimentation coefficient = 19S
______ (*b*) Is a pentamer with MW 900,000
______ (*c*) In secretions is usually a dimer with a secretory component
______ (*d*) Main response to T-cell-independent antigens such as polysaccharides
______ (*e*) Attaches to tissue mast cells and blood basophils
______ (*f*) Most important in local tissue immunity, especially to viruses
______ (*g*) Fixes complement and is very efficient in agglutination because it has many (more than two) combining sites
______ (*h*) Heat-labile and nonprecipitating
______ (*i*) Called reagin in allergy literature
______ (*j*) Has component which makes it resistant to digestion by proteolytic enzymes

23. (*a*) Check the appropriate answer in the table or fill in the blanks as indicated. (*b*) About how many Gm allotypes have been demonstrated? (*c*) In what type of light chain is the Km marker found? (*d*) Do any of the immunoglobulins in the table cause transfusion reactions? If your answer is yes, state which. (*e*) Are any of the allotypes listed in the table known to cause transfusion reactions? If your answer is yes, state which.

Structural differences in immunoglobulins	Example of		Chain involved		Class of Ig affected
	Isotype	Allotype	Heavy	Light	
IgG, IgM, IgA, IgE					
Kappa					
Lambda					
IgG_1, IgG_2, IgG_3, IgG_4					
IgA_1, IgA_2					
Gm					
Km (formerly InV)					
Am					

24. (*a*) With what kind of immunoglobulins do anti-human globulin antibodies react? (*b*) Assume that you have antibody molecules to antigens A, B, and C produced in rabbits and that they all belong to the same class, subclass, and allotype; would you expect differences between these antibodies in both the variable and constant regions? (*c*) What is the idiotype of an immunoglobulin molecule? (*d*) Can antibodies be produced which are sufficiently sensitive to detect the idiotype of an immunoglobulin?

25. (*a*) What immunoglobulin is usually present at birth in the largest amount? Explain why. (*b*) Why is there a low level of IgG antibodies at about 2 months of age? (*c*) What immunoglobulin is elevated at birth if infection occurred in utero such as syphilitic infections? Explain why. (*d*) IgG, IgM, IgA are important for protection. At what ages do these immunoglobulins reach concentrations usually present in adult serum and then level off?

26. (*a*) What causes immunoglobulins to be produced in abnormally large amounts? (*b*) If at least some of these immunoglobulins are structurally normal, why are they called pathological immunoglobulins? (*c*) Have pathological immunoglobulins been found for all five classes?

27. (*a*) What is multiple myeloma? (*b*) What is Waldenström's macroglobulinemia? (*c*) In what diseases are light chains of immunoglobulins found in the urine? What were they originally called, and how were they detected? (*d*) What is heavy-chain disease?

Answers

19. (*a*) Yes. (*b*) Yes. (*c*) By variable regions or antigen binding sites. (*d*) Monomers, even classes such as IgM. (*e*) The answer to this question is not yet clear. (Sec. 3-9.)

20. (*a*) IgG. (*b*) IgG. (*c*) IgG. (*d*) 23 days. (*e*) IgM. Its large molecular weight of 900,000 daltons may partially account for most of IgM in the body being intravascular; however, since IgD with MW 190,000 (close to the size of IgA) is mainly intravascular, other factors in addition to size must also be responsible for intravascular location. (Sec. 3-20.)

21. (*a*) IgG. (*b*) IgG. (*c*) Yes. (*d*) IgG, because it is present in the largest amount; it has the longest half-life; it is known to act against microorganisms in such mechanisms as bacteriolysis, opsonization, neutralization of viruses, etc. (Sec. 3-21.)

22. (*a*) IgM (*b*) IgM (*c*) IgA (*d*) IgM (*e*) IgE
(*f*) IgA (*g*) IgM (*h*) IgE (*i*) IgE (*j*) IgA

Structural differences in immunoglobulins	Example of Isotype	Example of Allotype	Chain involved Heavy	Chain involved Light	Class of Ig affected
IgG, IgM, IgA, IgE	√		√		IgG, IgM, IgA, IgE
Kappa	√			√	All classes
Lambda	√			√	All classes
IgG_1, IgG_2, IgG_3, IgG_4	√		√		IgG
IgA_1, IgA_2	√		√		IgA
Gm		√	√		IgG
Km (formerly InV)		√		Kappa	All classes
Am		√	√		IgA (IgA_2)

Table 3-3 Summary of Isotypes and Allotypes of Human Immunoglobulins

(Sec. 3-21.)

23. (*a*) See Table 3-3. (*b*) About 25. (*c*) Kappa. (*d*) Yes, IgA (especially in IgA immunodeficient patients). (*e*) Yes, Am (IgA_2). (Secs. 3-21 and 3-22.)

24. (*a*) Human immunoglobulin of all classes. (*b*) No, only in the variable region. (*c*) The idiotype of an immunoglobulin is determined by the difference in sequence of amino acid residues responsible for the specificity of the combining site for antigen. (*d*) Yes, in at least some cases. (Secs. 3-24 and 3-25.)

25. (*a*) IgG. The mother's IgG immunoglobulins pass the placenta and protect the newborn child temporarily. (*b*) At around 2 months of age, the mother's antibodies have begun to disappear, and the baby has just started forming his own. (*c*) IgM; IgM is the first class of immunoglobulins formed in response to infection. (*d*) Serum IgM of a child reaches concentrations as great as that of an adult within a few months; the concentration of IgG reaches that of an adult by 2 to 5 years of age and levels off; IgA continues to slowly increase until 8 to 12 years of age. (Sec. 3-26.)

26. (*a*) The development of a malignant plasma-cell clone. (*b*) Because they are associated with a disease condition. They all have the same specificity and therefore confer very little protection, if any; the elevated level of serum protein causes a depression of the normal antibody response needed for protection. (*c*) Yes. (Sec. 3-27.)

27. (*a*) Disease in which a monoclonal protein is produced in abnormal amounts due to a malignant plasma-cell clone. (*b*) Disease state caused by a tumor of a plasma-cell clone which is producing pathological immunoglobulins of the IgM class. (*c*) Multiple myeloma and Waldenström's macroglobulinemia. Bence Jones proteins (light chains) can be detected by heating urine and observing their unusual thermosolubility properties. (*d*) Disease in which incomplete or abnormal heavy chains are produced in large amounts and are found in serum and/or urine. (Sec. 3-27.)

THE COMPLEMENT SYSTEM

Elucidation of the Nature of Complement

3-28 In 1894 Pfeiffer reported that intraperitoneal injection of cholera vibrios into guinea pigs previously immunized against cholera caused lysis (bacteriolysis) of the vibrios. In 1898 Bordet reported that this type of result is due to two distinct substances, one specific for the bacteria against which the animal was immunized and the other, a nonspecific substance, found in the fresh serum of many animals. The latter was called *alexin* until Ehrlich renamed it *complement*. It was shown by Bordet that red blood cells lyse when serum containing specific antibodies to red blood cells and fresh normal serum containing complement are added to a suspension of red blood cells. In 1901 Bordet and Gengou developed the complement-fixation test, based on the idea that complement which reacts with bacteria and their specific antibodies is the same as complement which reacts with sensitized red blood cells. In 1906 Wassermann used the complement-fixation test for the first serologic test for syphilis (see Chap. 11). Although the Wassermann test is seldom used now, the complement-fixation test has found many other applications (see Chap. 4). The principle of the test is that when complement is present during reaction of certain antibodies with antigen, complement is fixed in the reaction. In order to show whether or not complement has been fixed, red blood cells (usually sheep) and specific antibodies to the red blood cells are added. If a standardized amount of complement is fixed in the first reaction between antigen and antibodies, complement is not available to react with red blood cells and their specific antibodies to cause lysis. Lysis of red blood cells is the indicator system.

3-29 Only in the presence of complement do specific antibodies cause bacteriolysis of many gram-negative bacilli such as the enteric bacilli. Only in the presence of complement are specific antibodies bactericidal for gram-negative diplococci such as meningococci. Specific bacteriolysis of gram-positive bacteria such as pneumococci does not occur, but complement enhances phagocytosis of pneumococci (see Chap. 1). Through the study of *immune adherence* it has been shown that a number of microorganisms in combination with specific antibodies and complement adhere to the surface of macrophages, neutrophils, platelets, red blood cells, and cells with complement receptors. Adherence to the surface of phagocytes probably leads to immediate phagocytosis. Platelets or red blood cells with attached microorganisms appear foreign to the host and are taken up by macrophages. This mechanism is considered to help defend the host and is beneficial provided the destruction of platelets, red blood cells, and other cellular elements is not too great. Another way in which complement aids in phagocytosis is through its chemotactic properties of attracting phagocytes, as discussed in Chap. 1. Complement takes part in many reactions in the body. Some of the reactions in which complement is involved may turn out to be harmful to the host rather than helpful. This often depends on the extent of the reaction. It was recognized quite early that complement is bound by antigen and antibody complexes only when antigen, antibodies, and complement are present in certain proportions. Complement is not fixed when the antibody titer is extremely low in relation to antigen, nor is it fixed when there is an extreme excess of antibodies in relation to antigen. The latter situation, described in 1901 with the serum of hyperimmunized animals, is known as the *Neisser-Wechsberg phenomenon*.

Nature of Complement and Complement Components

3-30 Complement is present in the serum of all warm-blooded animals, and the content of complement in the serum is not increased by immunization. Guinea pig serum is usually employed as a source of complement for complement-fixation tests carried out in the laboratory because of the relatively high amount of complement in serum of this species. Complement is present in serum separated from freshly drawn blood; it is unstable in the refrigerator at 5 to 10°C but is preserved by freezing or by lyophilization. Complement (C′) is composed of nine separate components designated C1, C2, . . . C9. C1 consists of three subcomponents, bringing the total number of complement proteins to 11. The complement components are proteins and move in electrophoresis mainly with the beta globulins except for a few components in the alpha- or gamma-globulin fractions. The subcomponents of C1, termed C1q, C1r, and C1s, are held together in serum by calcium ions, but they can be separated by chromatography and gel-filtration methods. Complement can be inactivated by heating at 56°C for 30 min since certain components of complement (C1, C2, C6, and C8) are heat-labile at this temperature. Complement is important in many immune reactions in vivo. The complement system appears to exist in the body essentially for protective functions, but it is also known to take part in certain pathological conditions, e.g., those associated with immune complex disease and many autoimmune diseases.

Stepwise Activation of Complement

Classical Pathway for Activation of Complement (Complement Cascade)

3-31 Certain immunological reactions require the interaction of all nine components of complement. These include specific bacteriolysis, specific cytolysis or specific hemolysis (red blood cells), and specific cytotoxic destruction of tissue cells. The reaction of the nine components of complement in sequence until lysis occurs is sometimes called the *complement cascade*. Since the first four complement components were described and numbered before the sequence of activation was worked out, activation of these components does not take place in order. After activation by reaction of antibody (IgG or IgM) with antigen, the first component acquires the ability to activate several molecules of the next component, so that at each step in the sequence the reactivity of complement is amplified. A bar across the complement component, as in $C\bar{1}$, denotes that the component(s) has been activated and has acquired enzymic or other biological activity. IgG and IgM are the only immunoglobulins known to bind complement by the classical pathway. It appears that after IgG and IgM react with antigen, conformational changes take place at the C_H2 domain of the Fc region (see Fig. 3-4*b*) so that C1q can be bound at this region. At least two IgG molecules have to attach to a single antigen molecule in close proximity to each other in order to activate C1q, which has two or more separate combining sites. A single IgM molecule, which is a pentamer, will activate complement after reaction with antigen.

3-32 A mixture of antigen (Ag) and antibody (Ab) with fresh guinea pig serum which contains all nine components of complement brings on the sequence of reactions shown below. The complement cascade is initiated when C1q binds to IgG or IgM so that it is activated and activates C1r and C1s. These three subcomponents act as a trimolecular complex known collectively as C1. Activation of components C1 to C9 takes place in five main steps:

$$\text{C1 }(\text{C1q}\cdot\text{C1r}\cdot\text{C1s}\cdot\text{Ca}^{2+}) + \text{Ag} + \text{Ab} \rightarrow \text{AgAb}\cdot\text{C}\bar{1}$$

where $C\bar{1}$ is an esterase;

$$\text{C4} + \text{C2} + \text{Mg}^{2+} + \text{AgAb}\cdot\text{C}\bar{1} \rightarrow \text{AgAb}\cdot\text{C}\bar{1}\cdot\text{C}\overline{4,2}$$

where $C\overline{4,2}$ is the enzyme C3 convertase; $C\overline{4,2}$ is formed from C4b and C2b; and C4a and C2b fragments are released but do not take part in the activation sequence;

$$\text{C3} + \text{AgAb}\cdot\text{C}\bar{1}\cdot\text{C}\overline{4,2} \rightarrow \text{AgAb}\cdot\text{C}\overline{1,4,2,3} + \text{C}\overline{3\text{a}}$$

where $C\overline{4,2}$, or C3 convertase, splits C3 into C3a and C3b; C3b is bound to form $C\overline{1,4,2,3}$; and C3a is not necessary for further activation of complement but is important as an anaphylatoxin;

$$\text{C5} + \text{C6} + \text{C7} + \text{AgAb}\cdot\text{C}\overline{1,4,2,3} \rightarrow \text{AgAb}\cdot\text{C}\overline{1,4,2,3,5,6,7} + \text{C}\overline{5\text{a}}$$

where C5 is split into C5a and C5b; C5b is bound and also C6 and C7; and C5a acts as an anaphylatoxin.

$$\text{C8} + \text{C9} + \text{AgAb}\cdot\text{C}\overline{1,4,2,3,5,6,7} \rightarrow \text{AgAb}\cdot\text{C}\overline{1,4,2,3,5,6,7,8,9}$$

where the binding of $C\overline{8,9}$ causes hemolysis of red blood cells, bacterolysis, or cytotoxic destruction of tissue cells depending on the nature of the antigen. By transmission electron microscopy at high magnification, small holes have been observed in red-blood-cell membranes and bacterial membranes. Since most of the studies with complement have been carried out with erythrocytes, the letters E for erythrocyte and A for antibody are frequently used in some texts to describe the antigen-antibody complex, that is, EA, with which complement reacts. AgAb was used above to designate the complex in order to emphasize that complement is bound in many kinds of antigen and antibody reactions provided the antibodies involved are IgM or IgG. Antibodies of IgG_4 subclass in combination with antigen do not activate complement by the classical pathway.

3-33 Anaphylatoxins C3a and C5a were formed by cleavage of C3 and C5 during activation of complement described in Sec. 3-32. C3a and C5a do not take part in the activation sequence of complement but are released as peptide fragments, which act on mast cells and bring about release of histamine. The release of histamine is associated with anaphylaxis; hence the term anaphylotoxins for C3a and C5a. The release of anaphylatoxins and histamine in small amounts can be beneficial, e.g., in the inflammatory response to infection discussed in Chap. 1. Histamine causes an increase in capillary permeability, which allows bactericidal substances from the blood to enter the area of infection. Anaphylatoxins C3a and C5a have also been reported to have chemotactic properties which would attract phagocytes into an area of infection. If anaphylatoxins are produced in large amounts, e.g., during immune-complex disease, the anaphylatoxins cause reactions which are very harmful to the host. Another activation product which has chemotactic properties in addition to C3a and C5a is $C\overline{5,6,7}$. C3b is associated with both increased phagocytosis (opsonization) and immune adherence.

Alternate Pathway for Activation of Complement

3-34 In Sec. 3-32 the activation of complement was described, beginning with the union of C1q with IgG and IgM antibodies after reaction of antibodies with antigen. Other immunoglobulins do not have receptor sites for C1q. It has been found that in some situations this first step may be bypassed so that activation of the complement system takes place by what is known as the *alternate pathway*, beginning with the activation of the C3 component, which is considered one of the main complement components. In the alternate pathway C1 esterase is not formed, nor is $C\overline{4,2}$, which is C3 convertase in the classical pathway and cleaves C3. The alternate pathway is also called the extrinsic pathway or the C3 shunt. Magnesium ions are required for the alternate pathway but not calcium. It is difficult to define the factors needed to bring about the formation of the C3 activator for cleaving C3 in the alternate pathway. The alternate pathway for complement activation can be triggered by a number of substances, including the following:

1. Polysaccharides: inulin from plants, zymosan from yeasts, endotoxin or lipopolysaccharide (LPS) from gram-negative bacteria, agar from algae
2. Aggregated immunoglobulins, especially IgA but also IgG_4, IgE, and $F(ab)_2$ of immunoglobulins
3. Nephritic factor produced in some forms of glomerulonephritis
4. Factor in cobra venom

After C3 is activated by the alternate pathway, the terminal complement components C5 to C9 are activated. The clinical significance of the alternate pathway is not fully understood. This type of complement consumption occurs in human beings, e.g., in gram-negative septicemias. The alternate pathway seems to be beneficial in resistance to infection, but it also appears to be one of the mechanisms responsible for tissue damage in glomerulonephritis and some other diseases. It is responsible for lysis of red blood cells observed in paroxysmal nocturnal hemoglobuinuria. Techniques are available for the assay of all the complement components in serum. If the C3 component is decreased but the level of C1, C2, and C4 is not affected, activation of complement was by the alternate pathway.

3-35 The alternate pathway for activation of complement is believed to be the same as the properdin system, described by Pillemer and coworkers (1954). Properdin was first described in connection with natural resistance as a high-molecular-weight globulin found in normal serum. It was described as bactericidal for gram-negative enteric bacilli. Besides properdin, other factors present in fresh normal serum were required for demonstration of its activity. Magnesium ions were also required. It has been determined that properdin is not an immunoglobulin and is not a component of complement. When serum components necessary for the properdin system were compared with the serum components necessary for activation of complement by the alternate pathway, the components of the two systems appeared to be the same. A great deal of experimental work has been done on the alternate pathway, the properdin system, and the cobra-venom-factor system. It is always confusing when a number of different terms are used to refer to one substance. The following components appear to take part in the activation of complement component C3 by the alternate pathway:

Factor I, or initiating factor (IF)

Properdin

Factor D (also called C3 proactivator convertase or GBGase)

Magnesium ions

Factor B (also called C3 proactivator or GBG, for glycine-rich β-glycoprotein)

It now appears that properdin does not enter into the alternate pathway immediately. When C5 convertase is formed, this enzyme is stabilized by properdin. Factor I (initiating factor) reacts with the surface of certain bacterial cells, etc., containing polysaccharide or some other structure which causes it to become activated. According to Müller-Eberhard (1976), initiation of the alternate pathway can be represented as

$$\mathrm{IF} + \mathrm{B} + \mathrm{C3} \xrightarrow[\mathrm{D}+\mathrm{Mg}]{\mathrm{S_1}} \overline{\mathrm{IF,B,C3}}$$

$$\mathrm{S_2} + \mathrm{C3} \xrightarrow{\overline{\mathrm{IF,B,C3}}} \mathrm{S_2,\ C3b}$$

where S_1 denotes the site of initiation and S_2 the cite of C3b attachment. Also according to Müller-Eberhard, the processes of formation of the labile C5 convertase C36,B its modulation by properdin, and the function of the stabilized enzyme can be represented as

$$\mathrm{S_2,C3b} + \mathrm{B} \xrightarrow[\mathrm{Mg}]{\mathrm{D}} \mathrm{S_2,C3b,B}$$

$$\mathrm{S_2,\ C3b,\ B} + \underline{\mathrm{P}} \rightarrow \mathrm{S_2,C3b,P,B}$$

$$\mathrm{S_3} + \mathrm{C5} + \mathrm{C6} + \mathrm{C7} + \mathrm{C8} + \mathrm{C9} \xrightarrow{\overline{\mathrm{S_2C3b,P,B}}} \mathrm{S_3,C5b\text{-}9}$$

where S_2 refers to the site of binding of C3b and S_3 to the site of attachment of the C5b-9 membrane attack complex.

3-36 The entire system of C3 cleavage is affected by a positive feedback through C3b. A protein called KAF can inhibit the C3b feedback pathway by degradation of C3b into its inert form, C3bi. In addition to activation of complement by the alternate pathway described above, certain proteases, e.g., those released from lysosomes or those like plasmin involved in blood clotting, may also bring about cleavage of C3 to form C3b and C3a.

Biosynthesis of Complement Components; Regulation of the Complement System

3-37 Very little is known about biosynthesis of the complement components. It has been reported that C1 is synthesized by the intestinal epithelium; C2 and C4 by macrophages; C3, C6, and C9 by the liver; and C5 and C8 by cells of the spleen. How components of the complement system are activated is discussed above. Because of the potent effect of some of these activated components, regulatory mechanisms must exist, including the rapid decay of certain activated components, the loss of binding capacity, the dissociation of components leading to the loss of enzyme activity, and the production of inhibitors or inactivators of certain complement components. A rare disease known as *hereditary angioedema* is caused by the lack of a serum inhibitor for C1 esterase (activated C1). In acute attacks of this disease there are increased levels of C1 esterase in the blood and markedly decreased levels of C2 and C4, the complement components on which C1 esterase acts. The disease is characterized by recurrent episodes of acute edema of the skin, upper respiratory tract, and gastrointestinal tract.

Complement Deficiencies

3-38 The importance of complement to the general defense mechanisms of the host can be appreciated by examining the results of deficiences of one or more complement components. Complement deficiences are either not common in human beings or they have not been detected and reported. Of the complement deficiencies reported, a C3 deficiency seems to have the most adverse effect, causing increased susceptibility to infection. A patient lacking KAF, inactivator for C3b, showed repeated infections because of a low level of C3 brought on by the continual activation of the alternate pathway through the C3b feedback mechanism. One family with a C1r deficiency showed serious infection al-

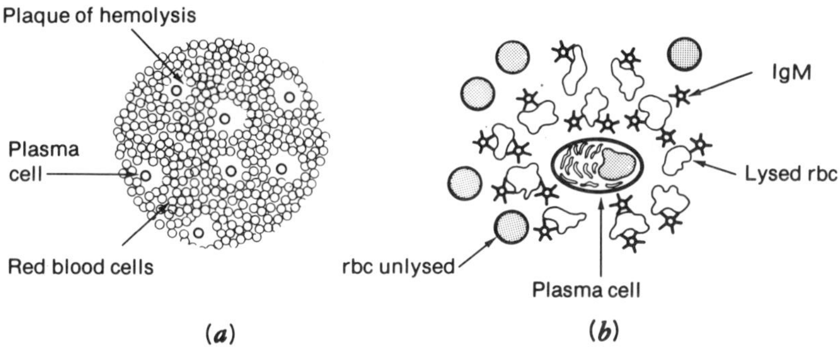

Figure 3-7 (*a*) Jerne technique, showing clear plaques caused by specific hemolysis. Note antibody-synthezing cell in the center of each plaque. (*b*) A single plaque, showing a plasma cell which has excreted IgM antibodies. The IgM antibodies which are specific for sheep rbc have reacted with sheep rbc in the presence of complement so that complement has been fixed and lysis has occurred.

though the alternate pathway for complement activation was intact. It appears that one mechanism for complement activation cannot entirely take the place of the other. Some cases of complement deficiency are caused by hereditary conditions, like those just discussed. Others are due to disease, e.g., immune-complex disease. A low level of complement in the blood is referred to as *hypocomplementemia.* Complement component C6 is required for normal clot formation. Blood from rabbits with a genetic deficiency of C6 clots very slowly; the addition of C6 corrects this defect. A hereditary C6 deficiency described in human beings showed no coagulation abnormality.

Jerne Hemolytic-Plaque Technique

3-39 The Jerne technique is described here because it is a research technique employing specific hemolysis and one which has been extensively used, especially for the study of antibody production by single cells. Animals whose cells are to be examined for antibody production are immunized against sheep red blood cells, which also are used in the test. The lymphoid cells to be tested, e.g., spleen cells containing B lymphocytes, are mixed with sheep red blood cells in soft agar. Tissue-culture medium supports the synthesis and excretion of antibody by antibody-synthesizing cells. After a suitable incubation period, complement (fresh guinea pig serum) is layered onto the surface of the agar. The plate is observed for clear areas of hemolysis, which are called *plaques*. A plaque will be formed if a cell produces antibodies to sheep red blood cells. The antibodies diffuse into the surrounding medium and attach to red blood cells. Lysis occurs because complement is present and is activated by the antigen-antibody reaction. The release of IgM antibodies readily causes lysis because each IgM molecule has several combining sites and readily fixes complement after reaction with antigen (rbc); see Fig. 3-7. If IgG antibodies are produced in the Jerne technique, complement is not fixed because with the small amount of antibodies produced by a single cell, it is unlikely that at least two molecules of IgG will attach to the surface of a red blood cell close enough to each other to fix complement. This obstacle is overcome by adding antibodies to IgG in such a concentration that at least two anti-IgG antibodies will react with an IgG antibody attached to a red blood cell. Complement will be fixed and lysis will occur, indicating that initially IgG antibodies were released from the antibody-forming cell. Each area of lysis represents antibodies produced by a single cell. Production of other classes of immunoglobulins by single cells can be detected by using antisera to the different classes of immunoglobulin.

Questions for Secs. 3-28 to 3-39

28. In each of the following cases state whether or not lysis would occur: (*a*) *Salmonella typhi** + specific antibodies, (*b*) *S. typhi* + specific antibodies + complement, (*c*)

**S. typhi* is a gram-negative bacillus;

sheep rbc + antiserum to sheep rbc, (*d*) sheep rbc + complement, (*e*) sheep rbc + antiserum to sheep rbc + fresh guinea pig serum, (*f*) sheep rbc + antiserum to rabbit rbc + complement, (*g*) *Diplococcus pneumoniae* + specific antibodies + complement, (*h*) *Bacillus anthracis* + specific antibodies + complement, (*i*) tissue cells + complement.

29. (*a*) Does complement have any effect on gram-positive microorganism? Explain. (*b*) Does the amount of antibody in relation to antigen have any effect on whether or not complement will be fixed? Explain.

30. (*a*) What is complement? (*b*) What is a common source of complement? (*c*) How many components of complement are there? (*d*) What is the chemical nature of the components of complement? (*e*) Is complement in serum increased during immunization? (*f*) How is complement usually inactivated?

31. (*a*) Is the activation of complement by the classical pathway initiated only by an immune reaction? (*b*) What immunoglobulins bind complement after reaction with antigen? (*c*) What component of complement is bound first? (*d*) To what area of the immunoglobulin molecule is complement fixed? (*e*) What components of complement form C3 convertase when they are activated? (*f*) What is the action of C3 convertase? (*g*) What activation products of complement are known as anaphylatoxins? (*h*) What biological activities are associated with anaphylatoxins? (*i*) What activation product of complement is associated with immune adherence and enhancement of phagocytosis?

32. (*a*) What complement components are bypassed in the alternate pathway for activation of complement? (*b*) Is the alternate pathway triggered by an immune response? (*c*) Name three substances which might cause activation of the alternate pathway in vivo. (*d*) Experimentally, can aggregates of IgA formed without reaction with antigen cause activation of the alternate pathway?

33. (*a*) Is properdin an antibody? (*b*) With what is the properdin system associated? (*c*) What appears to be the role of properdin? (*d*) What other substances are needed for activation of complement in the alternate complement pathway? (*e*) What enzymes are produced which are responsible for further activation of complement?

34. (*a*) Where is complement synthesized? (*b*) How does the body regulate activation of complement? (*c*) What is the name of the disease caused by the lack of an inhibitor for C1 esterase? (*d*) What is hypocomplementemia? (*e*) Name one kind of disease state which could cause hypocomplementemia. Explain why.

35. Total hemolytic complement screening tests were carried out on the serum of two patients, and abnormal values were obtained. Next, tests for quantitation of C3, C4, and C3 activator were carried out. Using the results for patients *a* and *b*, which follow, for each patient state whether activation of complement appears to be by the classical pathway or alternate pathway: (*a*) low C3; normal C4; low C3 activator; (*b*) low C3; low C4; normal C3 activator.

36. (*a*) What is one advantage of the Jerne hemolytic-plaque technique? (*b*) Explain why one molecule of IgM can bind complement and cause lysis when IgM reacts with antigen on the surface of a red blood cell and why at least two molecules of IgG are required for lysis. (*c*) What additional reagent is used in the Jerne technique to detect production of IgG antibodies by single cells? (*d*) For part (*c*) sketch the reaction which will take place if IgG antibodies are excreted.

Answers

28. (*a*) No lysis. (*b*) Lysis. (*c*) No lysis. (*d*) No lysis. (*e*) Lysis. (*f*) No lysis. (*g*) No lysis. (*h*) No lysis. (*i*) No lysis. (Secs. 3-28 to 3-30.)

29. (*a*) When gram-positive microorganisms combine with specific antibodies, phagocytosis is enhanced if complement is present in the reaction., Gram-positive microorganisms are destoryed by phagocytes when they come in contact with lysosomes. (*b*) Complement is not fixed when there is an extreme excess of antigen in relation to specific antibodies or when there is an extreme excess of antibodies in relation to antigen. (Sec. 3-29.)

30. (*a*) Complement is composed of several proteins which are present in the serum of vertebrates; in the body, complement either is required for certain immune reactions or amplifies them. (*b*) Guinea pig serum. (*c*) 9, C1 to C9; C1 has 3 subcomponents, C1q, C1r, and C1s, making a total of 11 complement proteins. (*d*) Globulins which electrophoretically move mainly with the beta fraction, but a few are found in the alpha and gamma fractions. (*e*) No. (*f*) By heating at 56°C for 30 min. (Sec. 3-30.)

31. (*a*) Yes. (*b*) IgM and IgG. (*c*) C1q. (*d*) Fc region. (*e*) C4 and C2. (*f*) It cleaves C3 into C3a and C3b. (*g*) C3a and C5a. (*h*) They act on tissue mast cells to release histamine. (*i*) C3b. (Secs. 3-31 to 3-33.)

32. (*a*) C1 (C1q·C1r·C1s), C4, and C2. (*b*) No. (*c*) Endotoxin (lipopolysaccharide) from gram-negative bacteria; zymosan in yeast cell walls; nephritic factor. (*d*) Yes. (Sec. 3-34.)

33. (*a*) No. (*b*) The alternate pathway for activation of complement. (*c*) It appears to act as a stabilizer. (*d*) Factor I (initiating factor); two serum factors, factor B and factor D; magnesium ions; complement component C3 and the terminal components of complement, C5 to C9. (*e*) C3 activator and C5 convertase. (Secs. 3-35 and 3-36.)

34. (*a*) Very little is known about the synthesis of complement; synthesis of complement components has been reported to take place in a number of different cells, including macrophages and cells of the liver, spleen, and intestinal epithelium. (*b*) Rapid decay of some components; synthesis of inactivators or inhibitors for activated components. (*c*) Hereditary angioedema. (*d*) Decreased amount of complement in blood. (*e*) Immune-complex disease. In some cases, formation of immune complexes is considerable, and they are formed with antibodies which fix complement. (Secs. 3-37 and 3-38.)

35. (*a*) Alternate pathway. (*b*) Classical pathway. (Secs. 3-32, 3-34, and 3-35.)

36. (*a*) Allows study of antibody production by single cells. (*b*) IgM is a pentamer, and a single molecule has more than one binding site for C1q, which requires binding of at least two receptors for activation of complement by the classical pathway. Two molecules of IgG must react with antigen in very close proximity to each other in order to activate a molecule of C1q. This is not likely to happen when there is a relatively small amount of antibody. (*c*) Anti-IgG. (*d*) See sketch. (Sec. 3-39.)

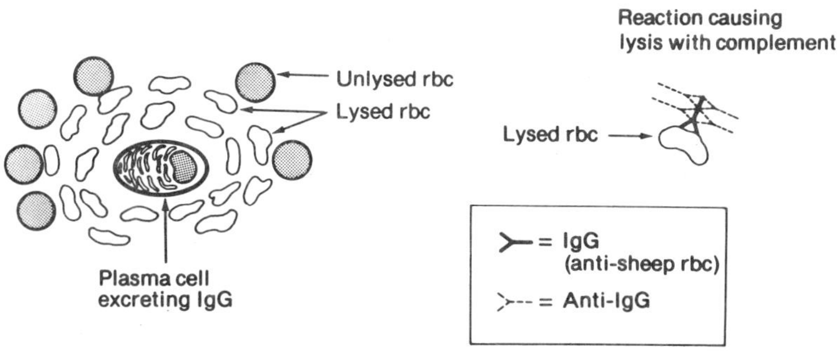

REFERENCES

Amos, B. (ed.) (1971): Progress in Immunology, *1st Int. Congr. Immunol.*, Academic, New York.

Capra, J. D., and J. M. Kehoe (1975): Hypervariable Regions, Idiotypy, and the Antibody-combining Site, *Adv. Immunol.*, **20**:1–40.

Colton, H. R. (1976): Biosynthesis of Complement, *Adv. Immunol.*, **22**:67-118.

——and C. A. Alper (1976): Complement, pp. 387–403, in F. H. Bach and R. A. Good (eds.), "Clinical Immunobiology," vol. 3. Academic, New York.

Fearon, D. T., S. Ruddy, P. H. Schur, and W. R. McCabe (1975): Activation of the Properdin Pathway of Complement in Patients with Gram Negative Bacteremia, *New Eng. J. Med.*, **292**: 937–940.

Freedman, M., R. Merrett, and W. Pruzanski (1976): Human Monoclonal Immunoglobulins with Antibody-like Activity, *Immunochemistry*, **13**:193-202.
Fudenberg, H. H., J. R. L. Pink, D. P. Stites, and A. Wang (1972): "Basic Immunogenetics," Oxford University Press, London.
——E. R. Gold, G. N. Vyas, and M. R. McKenzie (1968): Human Antibodies to Human IgA Globulins, *Immunochemistry*, **5**:203-212.
——D. P. Stites, J. L. Caldwell, and J. V. Wells (1976): "Basic and Clinical Immunology," Lange, Los Altos, Calif.
Joklik, W. K., and H. P. Willett (eds.) (1976): "Zinsser Microbiology," 16th ed., Appleton-Century-Crofts, New York.
Koshland, M. E. (1975): Structure and Function of the J Chain, *Adv. Immunol.*, **20**:41-69.
Lachman, P. J. (1975): Complement, pp. 323-361 in P. H. Gell, R. R. A. Coombs, and P. J. Lachmann (eds.), "Clinical Aspects of Immunology," 3d ed., Blackwell, Oxford.
Landsteiner, K., and A. S. Wiener (1940): An Agglutinable Factor in Human Blood Recognized by Immune Sera for Rhesus Blood, *Proc. Soc. Exp. Biol. Med.*, **43**:223.
Leikola, J., J. Koistinen, M. Lehtinen, and M. Virolainen (1973): IgA-induced Anaphylactic Transfusion Reactions: A Report of Four Cases, *Blood,* **42**:111-119.
Levine, P., E. M. Katzin, and L. Burnham (1941): Immunization in Pregnancy: Its Possible Bearing on the Etiology of Erythroblastosis Fetalis, *JAMA*, **116**: 825-827.
Müller-Eberhard, H. J. (1976): The Serum Complement System, pp. 45-73 in P. A. Miescher and H. J. Müller-Eberhard (eds.), "Textbook of Immunopathology," 2d ed., Grune and Stratton, New York.
——(1977): Chemistry and Function of the Complement System, *Hosp. Pract.*, **120**:33-43.
Naff, G. B. (1975): Role of the Properdin System, pp. 219-222 in D. Schlessinger (ed.), "Microbiology; 1975," American Society for Microbiology, Washington, D.C.
Nisonoff, A., J. E. Hopper, and Susan B. Spring (1975): "The Antibody Molecule," Academic, New York.
Pillemer, L., L. Blum, I. H. Lepow, O. A. Ross, E. W. Todd, and A. C. Wardlaw (1954): The Properdin System and Immunity: Demonstration and Isolation of a New Serum Protein, Properdin, and Its Role in Immune Phenomena, *Science*, **120**:279-285.
Reichlin, M. (1975): Amino Acid Substitution and the Antigenicity of Globular Proteins, *Adv. Immunol.*, **20**:71-123.
Roitt, I. (1977): "Essential Immunology," 3d ed., Blackwell, Oxford.
Rowe, D. S. (1975): Immunoglobulins, pp. 285-307 in P. H. Gell, R. R. A. Coombs, and P. J. Lachman (eds.), "Clinical Aspects of Immunology," 3d ed., Blackwell, Oxford.
Seligmann, M., and J. C. Brouet (1972): Antibody Activity of Human Myeloma Globulins, *Sem. Hematol.*, **10**:163-177.
Solomon, A. (1976): Bence-Jones Proteins and Light Chains of Immunoglobulins, *New Engl. J. Med.*, **294**:17-23, 91-98.
Tiselius, A., and E. A. Kabat (1939): An Electropheretic Study of Immune Sera and Purified Antibody Preparations, *J. Exp. Med.*, **69**:119-131.

4

Antigen-Antibody Reactions and Diagnostic Serologic Tests

ANTIGEN AND ANTIBODY REACTIONS

Serologic Tests

4-1 The many serologic tests used for diagnosis of disease include agglutination, precipitation, complement-fixation, neutralization, and immunomicroscopic tests, e.g., those employing antibody labeled with fluorescent dyes or enzymes. Serologic tests involve a reaction between antigen and antibody. Serum of a patient or a laboratory animal containing antibodies is employed, hence the name serologic. Since serologic tests are highly specific and very sensitive, they are valuable research tools as well as useful diagnostic aids. Emphasis in this section will be on serologic tests commonly used in hospital laboratories for diagnosis of disease. Some methods are more sensitive than others; i.e., they will detect a smaller amount of antibody or antigen in a specimen. Some tests can be carried out more quickly than others and the results reported to the physician sooner. A number of factors such as the physical state of the antigen, the amount of antigen or serum available, the sensitivity of the test, and the time required to perform the tests may determine which test is chosen. The stage of the disease in the patient may also be a determining factor.

Cross Reactions

4-2 Cross reactions occur because of the presence of common or similar antigens in microorganisms, red blood cells, tissue, etc. Cross reactions between closely related species are not surprising; cross reactions between distantly related microorganisms or cells such as pneumococci and sheep red blood cells usually are not expected. Antigens responsible for cross reactions between distantly related species or phylogenetically unrelated substances are called *heterogenetic antigens*, and antibodies to them are called *heterophile antibodies.* One antigen which is responsible for the production of heterophile antibodies, known as the *Forssman antigen*, is widely distributed in nature, being present in some microorganisms, some vegetables, animal tissues, or red blood cells of certain animal species. It is not surprising to find that through natural exposure in their environment people may have antibodies to the Forssman antigen. The Forssman antigen is present in sheep red blood cells, which are used in a number of serologic tests. Usually antibodies to Forssman antigen are not present in large amounts in a patient's serum, but whenever their presence could cause questionable results in a serologic test, these heterophile antibodies must be absorbed or removed before the test is carried out.

Absorption of a Serum to Remove Cross-reacting Antibodies

4-3 A serum can be absorbed with antigen to prevent cross reactions in serologic tests, the antigen employed being the one responsible for the cross reaction. Figure 4-1, which illustrates the principle for absorption of a serum, shows the antigenic composition of a microorganism to which an antiserum has been prepared by injecting a suspension of this organism into rabbits. For illustrative purposes, this microorganism is called bacillus X. The antiserum is found to react not only with bacillus X but also with a closely related species, called bacillus Y, because these two microorganisms have a common antigen D. A suspension of bacillus Y is mixed with antiserum to bacillus X and incubated at 37°C to allow time for antibodies to D antigen to react with this antigen. The tube is centrifuged, and the sediment is discarded. The supernate is the absorbed antiserum and now is specific for bacillus X; it no longer cross reacts with bacillus Y.

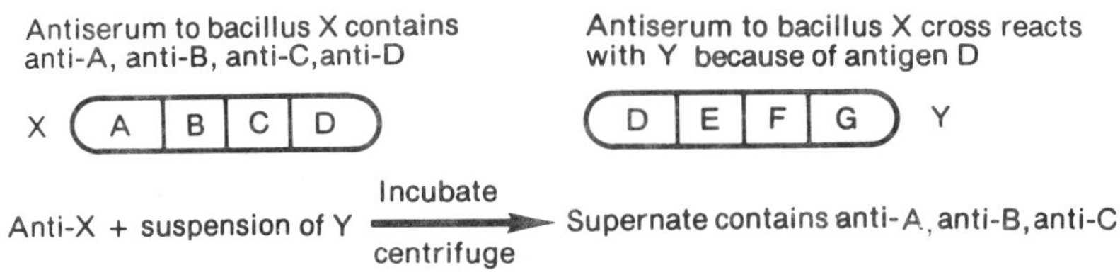

Figure 4-1 Absorption of cross-reacting antibodies.

LABORATORY TESTS USED FOR DIAGNOSIS OF DISEASES

Agglutination

4-4 The agglutination reaction is one of the simplest serologic tests to perform. The antigen is referred to as *particulate* or *cellular*, meaning that it is on a particulate, or cellular, structure. Microorganisms and red blood cells contain many different antigens. The agglutination test is the one most frequently used for the diagnosis of bacterial diseases. It is also used for blood grouping. The agglutination or clumping of the particulate or cellular antigens can be observed macroscopically. The basic agglutination reaction can be modified to include a number of serologic tests, e.g., the antiglobulin test for nonagglutinating antibody and the indirect, or passive, agglutination test. The agglutination reaction takes place in two stages: (1) specific combination occurs between specific groups of the antibody and corresponding groups of the antigen, and (2) the observable reaction of agglutination occurs. Under some conditions, e.g., the absence of salts, the first stage can take place but the second cannot. The first stage usually occurs rapidly and the second sometimes slowly. For all serologic tests, the physical binding of antigen to antibody is called the *primary reaction. Secondary reactions* are antigen-antibody reactions which are observable, e.g., agglutination.

Tube Agglutination Test and Determination of Antibody Titer

4-5 The agglutination test can be performed in a number of ways, depending on the volume and dilution of serum desired. Ten tubes in a rack as shown in Fig. 4-2 are used to determine the antibody titer of a serum. Saline, 0.9 ml, is added to the first tube, and 0.5 ml of saline is added to each of the other nine tubes in the rack. Next 0.1 ml of the serum (antibody) is added to tube 1 to give a total volume of 1.0 ml. The serum (antibody) dilution in tube 1 is 1:10. Serial dilutions of the serum (antibody) are made by pipetting 0.5 ml from tube 1 (1:10) to tube 2, which doubles the dilution of serum in tube 2 to give a dilution of 1:20. The procedure is continued through tube 9, and 0.5 ml of the serum dilution is discarded from this tube. Serum is not added to tube 10 as this tube will be the antigen control and should contain only antigen and saline. The first nine tubes now should contain serial dilutions of serum (antibody) to a final volume of 0.5 ml. Next, 0.5 ml of antigen is added to each tube, including tube 10. For the agglutination reaction, the turbidity of the antigen is standardized. Since an equal volume of antigen was added to each serum dilution, the serum dilution in each tube was doubled. The antibody titer is read after incubation of the rack of tubes in a water bath at 37 to 55°C for 2 to 24 h. The antibody titers is the highest dilution of serum (antibody) giving a visible agglutination reaction. The antibody titer may be read as the original dilution of serum before addition of antigen or as the final dilution after antigen is added. How a particular test is read is standardized for that test.

4-6 The lattice theory of agglutination and precipitation is a simple way of visualizing aggregation of antigen by antibody. This theory assumes that antibodies are at least divalent. IgG is divalent (has two antigen binding sites), and IgM is multivalent in that it has several sites for combination with

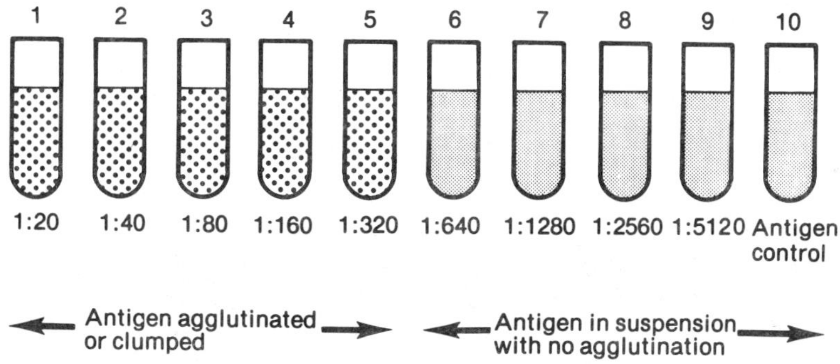

Figure 4-2 Determination of antibody titer by tube agglutination test using serial dilutions of patient's serum. The antibody titer is 1:320.

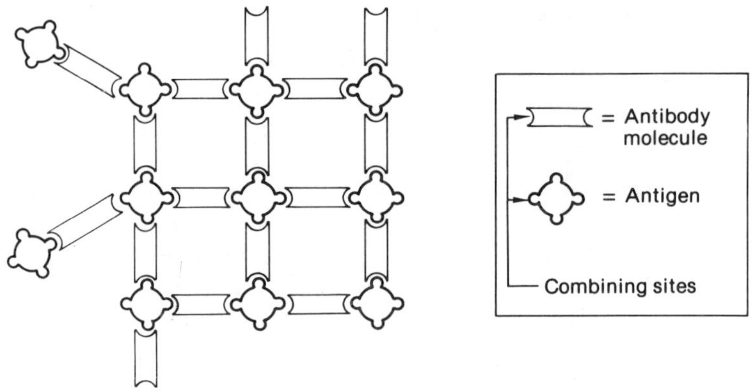

Figure 4-3 Formation of a lattice with agglutination due to reaction between specific antibodies and antigen.

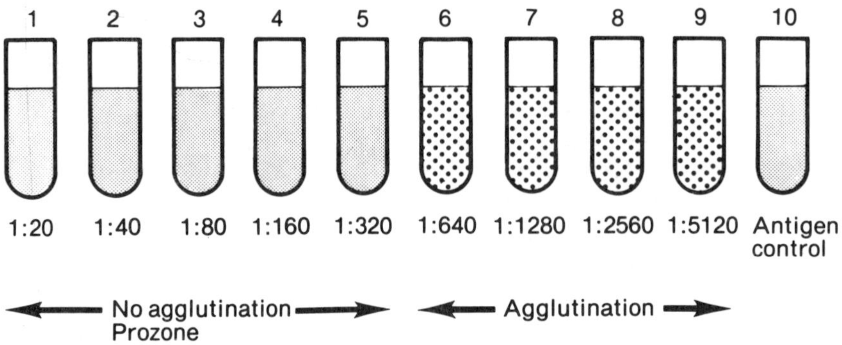

Figure 4-4 Agglutination test on patient's serum showing a prozone reaction.

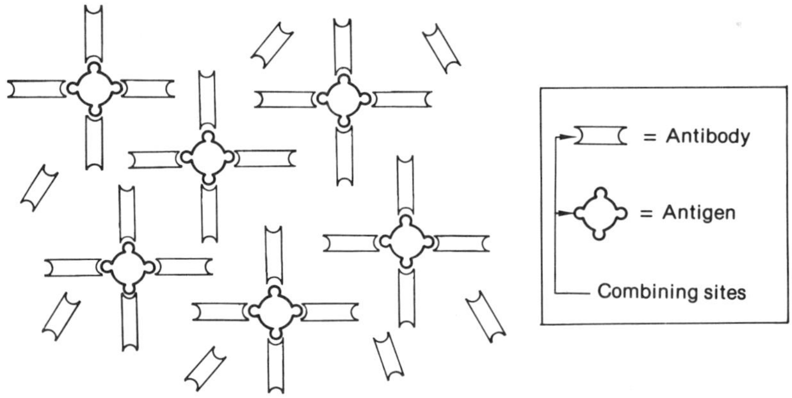

Figure 4-5 Inhibition of agglutination by an excess of antibody in relation to antigen, as in a prozone reaction.

antigen. Figure 4-3 shows the formation of a lattice of the kind formed in agglutination. The antigen molecule, e.g., a bacterial cell, has several combining sites for reaction with antibodies. For convenience instead of the wishbone structure of antibody the simpler symbol shown in Fig. 4-3 was used. Actually, it has been shown that when antibodies combine with antigen, as in the agglutination reaction, the arms of the wishbone may open out very wide at the hinge region.

4-7 A prozone reaction which can sometimes be observed in an agglutination test (Fig. 4-4), occurs when there is an unusually high titer of antibodies in the patient's serum in relation to the amount of antigen. Figure 4-5 diagrams what happens between antigen and antibodies in a prozone reaction.

Even if all the antigen receptors are not completely saturated, steric hindrance prohibits lattice formation. Whenever a prozone reaction occurs, it is necessary to make a greater initial dilution of serum and repeat the test so that an endpoint is obtained.

4-8 It is difficult for a physician to interpret only one antibody titer on the patient unless the titer is extremely high. An agglutination titer on the serum of a patient of 1:40 could be due to an early infection or to a previous subclinical infection or even to exposure to a closely related antigen. To avoid this conflict, physicians should take a specimen of blood as soon as they see the patient and then a week or more later. The paired sera are titrated for antibody, and a rise in titer indicates that the patient has an active infection which is stimulating antibody production. A fourfold rise in antibody titer is considered to be significant, say from 1:40 to 1:160. A twofold rise in titer could be due to technical variation. If the physician does not see the patient soon after onset or fails to collect an early specimen, a high antibody titer (depending on the disease in question) would probably be considered significant. It is better to base a diagnosis on a rise in antibody titer.

The Use of Heterophile Antibodies in Diagnostic Agglutination Tests

4-9 Heterophile antibodies (Sec. 4-2) are cross-reacting antibodies between distantly related or phylogenetically unrelated species or substances. The agglutination test (Sec. 4-4) is one of the simplest of the serologic tests to perform. Use is made of the cross reaction between certain species of *Rickettsia* and strains of *Proteus vulgaris* in a simple agglutination test called the *Weil-Felix test*, a test for rickettsial infections. *P. vulgaris,* a gram-negative bacillus, grows out overnight on simple culture media, whereas *Rickettsia* species require living cells for growth; the method of obtaining the latter is a somewhat tedious technique requiring inoculation of embryonated eggs. Therefore, *P. vulgaris* offers a cheaper source of antigen and an easy method for testing. The Weil-Felix test is a presumptive, not a definitive, test. A definitive test for rickettsial infection is the complement-fixation test employing the specific antigen. Another test based on the presence of heterophile antibodies is the *Paul-Bunnell test* for infectious mononucleosis. Infectious mononucleosis appears to be caused by a virus, probably Epstein-Barr (herpes) virus. Patients with infectious mononucleosis have agglutinins for sheep red blood cells. Antibodies to Forssman antigen also agglutinate sheep red blood cells, but these antibodies are not the same as those found in infectious mononucleosis. To distinguish between the two, a modification of the Paul-Bunnell test by Davidsohn, known as the *Davidsohn differential test*, is used. The serum of the patient suspected of having infectious mononucleosis is absorbed with tissue containing Forssman antigen. Guinea pig kidney is used for this purpose because it absorbs heterophile agglutinins associated with Forssman antigen but not heterophile agglutinins associated with infectious mononucleosis. The later are absorbed by beef or ox cell. A rapid slide test has been developed in which absorption takes place on the slide and centrifugation of absorbed serum is not necessary.

Questions for Secs. 4-1 to 4-9

1. (*a*) What are serologic tests? (*b*) What are heterogenetic antigens? (*c*) What are heterophile antibodies?
2. (*a*) What causes cross reactions in serologic tests? (*b*) How can cross-reacting antibodies be removed from a patient's serum or from an antiserum?
3. (*a*) What kind of antigens are employed in the agglutination reaction? (*b*) Name two main uses for the agglutination test. (*c*) What reagents are necessary for the agglutination test?
4. (*a*) How is the antibody titer determined? (*b*) If agglutination occurs in the antigen control, is the test readable (see Fig. 4-2)? (*c*) If agglutination occurs in the last dilution of serum (tube 9, Fig. 4-2), what is the antibody titer?
5. (*a*) What is a prozone reaction? (*b*) How does the lattice theory of agglutination account for a prozone reaction? (*c*) If no agglutination occurs in a test but from the history of the patient a prozone reaction is suspected, what is done to get rid of the prozone reaction?

6. (*a*) What is meant by paired sera? (*b*) Why does a physician look for at least a fourfold rise in antibody titer?

7. (*a*) What antigen or antigens are used in the Weil-Felix agglutination test? (*b*) What kind of infections are detected by the Weil-Felix test? (*c*) Is the Weil-Felix test a specific serologic test? (*d*) What is used as antigen in the Paul-Bunnell test for infectious mononucleosis? (*e*) How can antibodies to sheep red blood cells associated with infectious mononucleosis be distinguished from sheep red-blood-cell agglutinins associated with the Forssman antigen?

Answers

1. (*a*) Tests based on antigen and antibody reactions; they employ either the patient's serum or a diagnostic antiserum and the appropriate antigen. (*b*) Antigens formed by a variety of phylogenetically unrelated species, e.g., the Forssman antigen. (*c*) Antibodies to heterogenetic antigens. (Secs. 4-1 and 4-2.)

2. (*a*) Antibodies to a common antigen. (*b*) By absorption. (Sec. 4-3.)

3. (*a*) Antigens in a particulate or cellular structure, such as bacteria and red blood cells, which are commonly referred to as particulate antigens. (*b*) Diagnosis of bacterial infections and blood grouping. (*c*) Antiserum, antigen (particulate), and saline. (Sec. 4-4.)

4. (*a*) The antibody titer is determined by making serial dilutions of the serum, allowing each dilution to react with antigen, and then determining the highest dilution of serum which gives a visible reaction, e.g., agglutination. (*b*) No. (*c*) The antibody titer could not be determined by this result. It would be 1:5120 or higher. The serum would have to be diluted further and the test repeated in order to reach an endpoint for the antibody titer. (Sec. 4-5.)

5. (*a*) One in which a visible reaction, e.g., agglutination, does not occur in a serologic test due to an extreme excess of antibody in relation to antigen. (*b*) All combining sites on the antigen molecules are saturated by antibodies so that a lattice does not form, or antibodies react with so many sites on the antigen that steric hindrance occurs and prevents lattice formation; therefore, agglutination does not occur. (*c*) A greater initial dilution of serum antibody is made, and the test is repeated. (Secs. 4-6 and 4-7.)

6. (*a*) Specimens of sera collected on two separate occasions from a patient usually when the doctor first sees the patient and then about a week or more later to allow time for a rise in antibody titer. (*b*) At least a fourfold rise in titer is required for diagnosis because a smaller rise could be due to technical error. (Sec. 4-8.)

7. (*a*) Strains of *Proteus vulgaris*. (*b*) Rickettsial infections. (*c*) No. (*d*) Sheep rbc. (*e*) Sheep rbc agglutinins associated with the Forssman antigen are absorbed by guinea pig kidney, but those associated with infectious mononucleosis are not. (Sec. 4-9.)

Plate or Slide Agglutination Tests

4-10 Antibody titers can be determined not only by tube agglutination tests but also by plate or slide agglutination tests. The latter can be carried out rapidly and are used often in hospital laboratories. A number of bacterial antigens are available commercially for diagnostic purposes, including preparations of *Brucella abortus*, *S. typhi* H and O antigens, and *Proteus* strains OX-19, OX-2, and OX-K for rickettsial infections (review the Weil-Felix test, Sec. 4-9). The H antigen of *S. typhi* is an antigen on flagella, which are responsible for motility. H is derived from the German *Hauch* ("thin layer") associated with the film formed on the surface of agar plates by some motile strains of gram-negative bacilli. Antibody to the H antigen of *S. typhi* is used for diagnosis but is not related to infection. O is for the somatic antigen and is derived from *ohne Hauch* (*ohne* means "without"). Certain strains of *S. typhi* have a polysaccharide envelope called the Vi (for virulence) antigen. The Vi antigen is lost soon after culture. If the Vi antigen completely covers the O antigen, it can interfere with agglutination by anti-O. The O antigen and the Vi antigen are concerned with virulence.

Table 4-1 ABO System

Group	Antigen on red blood cell	Antibody in serum
A	A (A_1 and A_2)	Anti-B
B	B	Anti-A
AB	A and B (A_1B, A_2B)	Neither anti-A nor anti-B
O	Neither A nor B	Anti-A and anti-B

Antibody to the O antigen will cause bacteriolysis in the presence of complement. The agglutination test for typhoid fever employing O and H antigens is known as the *Widal test.* A marked nonspecific increase in O and H agglutinins may sometimes occur as a result of febrile reactions caused by unrelated microorganisms.

Blood Grouping and Cross Matching for Transfusions

4-11 Blood grouping is determined by the agglutination reaction. If anti-Rh_0 serum (antibody to Rh_0 or D antigen) is placed on a slide and a person's red blood cells added, agglutination would show that the person is positive for the Rh_0 or D antigen. This is the Rh antigen, which is responsible for most transfusion reactions due to the Rh factor. Blood grouping for the four main human blood groups, A, B, AB, and O, is similar. Transfusions of blood must use blood of the same group as the recipient's blood. Group O is the most common and group AB the least common. Table 4-1 summarizes the ABO system, showing the antigens on the red blood cells and the antibodies to them in serum. Landsteiner discovered and worked out this human blood-group system. A person's blood group is genetically determined. Genes for A and B antigens are dominant to O. The B phenotype may have genotypes BB or BO. The natural occurrence of antibodies to A and B antigens is not understood but may be caused by natural exposure of those lacking the antigen(s) to A and B antigens in their environment. In contrast, antibodies to the Rh antigens occur only through sensitization, e.g., by blood transfusion of the incorrect Rh type. Figure 4-6 shows results obtained by typing blood of the four groups. Drops of the appropriate typing sera are placed on each side of the slide. A drop of the blood to be typed is added to each, mixed, and observed for agglutination.

4-12 Human red blood cells contain many antigens besides the A, B, or Rh antigens; e.g., Duffy, I, Kell, Kidd, Lewis, Lutheran, M and N, and P. Most of these red-blood-cell antigens do not give rise to as many transfusion reactions as those of the ABO system; however, since these other antigens exist in the red blood cells, a cross match should be carried out after determining the blood type of the patient and obtaining a donor. Minor antigens like Kell and Duffy tend to cause trouble only after repeated transfusions. The patient's serum is incubated with the donor's blood cells in a test tube. After suitable incubation at 37°C, the mixture is observed for agglutination and hemolysis. If there is no agglutination or hemolysis, cells in the test tube are washed 3 times with physiological saline and anti-human globulin serum is added in order to increase the sensitivity of the match. If any antibodies were attached to the donor's cells, they would not have been removed by washing

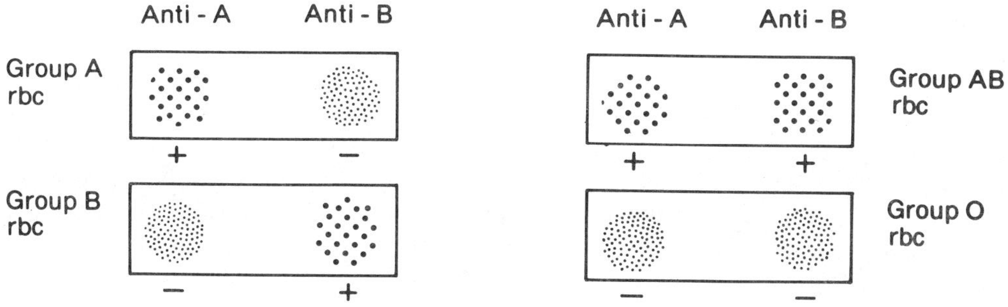

Figure 4-6 Results of blood typing.

but other antibodies and serum components would have been removed. When anti-human globulin antibodies are added, they react with any antibodies attached to the donor's red blood cells and cause agglutination. In cases of extreme emergency, group O blood can be given to anyone since the red blood cells of a group O person contain neither A nor B antigens. For this reason group O individuals were sometimes referred to as universal donors. Anti-A and anti-B antibodies of the group O donor blood (500 ml) are diluted with the patient's blood (about 7 liters) during transfusion to a level where they should not be dangerous. Group O blood with a pretitrated low titer of anti-A and anti-B antibodies should be kept on hand in a blood bank for extreme emergencies. Group O blood with a high titer of anti-A or anti-B antibodies could cause a severe transfusion reaction.

Structural Basis of Blood Groups; H Substance and Blood Group O

4-13 There is considerable evidence that the blood-group molecule of the ABO system is built from a single large glycopeptide onto which various sugars or antigenic determinants are added by enzymes specified by genes corresponding to A, B, and H. The H substance is common to all blood groups A, B, AB, and O. The H gene causes the production of an enzyme which adds L-fucose to the terminal D-galactose of the oligosaccharide chain common to all blood groups. A genes or B genes next produce enzyme transferases which add *N*-acetylgalactosamine (for A gene) or D-galactose (for B gene) to the same terminal D-galactose but at a different point. For AB specificity, both sugars are added. The addition of one or both sugars (or antigenic determinants) causes masking of H specificity. The A_2 gene is less effective in masking H specificity than the A_1 gene. The H substance is not masked in blood-group O cells. The O gene is an *amorph* in that it does not specify an antigenic determinant or particular alloantigen on human red blood cells. The H substance, which is also called O antigen, is present in both human and animal species. H stands for heterogenetic. In some rare-blood-type individuals, first described in Bombay, a defective or absent H gene leads to the absence not only of the H substance but also of A and B antigenic determinants. Bombay-type individuals can form antibodies in high titer to the H antigen of O cells either spontaneously or in response to injection. They also have anti-A and anti-B antibodies in their serum, so that transfusion of a Bombay-type individual would present a great problem.

Antiglobulin Test, a Development Test for Nonagglutinating Antibody

4-14 Soon after recognition of the Rh factor, it was observed that the serum of certain individuals with antibodies to Rh-positive cells fails to cause agglutination. Such nonagglutinating antibodies have been referred to as *blocking, incomplete,* and *functionally univalent antibodies.* The term blocking was originally used with Rh nonagglutinating antibodies, but since then blocking has been used by allergists in connection with a different kind of antibody (see atopy, Sec. 5-22). Antibodies produced during desensitization to allergens in atopy have been called blocking antibodies and should not be confused with blocking nonagglutinating antibodies to the Rh factor. Antibodies to the Rh factor which fail to agglutinate when mixed with Rh-positive red blood cells are of the IgG class. Coombs devised an ingenious method of detecting nonagglutinating antibodies. If an Rh-negative woman becomes sensitized to Rh-positive cells, and if she develops nonagglutinating antibodies to Rh-positive cells, conventional tests on her serum indicate that her serum does not contain antibodies to Rh-positive cells because no agglutination occurs. To perform the Coombs test, her serum is mixed with known Rh-positive cells and incubated to allow time for a reaction between antigen and antibody. At this point, in the case of nonagglutinating antibodies, the reaction shown in Fig. 4-7*a* has taken place. The red blood cells are centrifuged and washed 3 times in physiologic saline to remove all serum proteins free in the test. Washing does not remove antibody attached to the red blood cells. After washing the cells, anti-human globulin is added, which causes agglutination since antibodies are globulin (Fig. 4-7*b*). The anti-human-globulin serum is prepared by injecting human globulin into an experimental animal, e.g., rabbit or goat. The nonagglutinating antibody attached to the cells is human globulin and now acts as antigen in the reaction. The addition of antibody with specificity to human globulin causes agglutination. The reaction is diagrammed in Fig. 4-7*b* and is known as the *indirect Coombs*

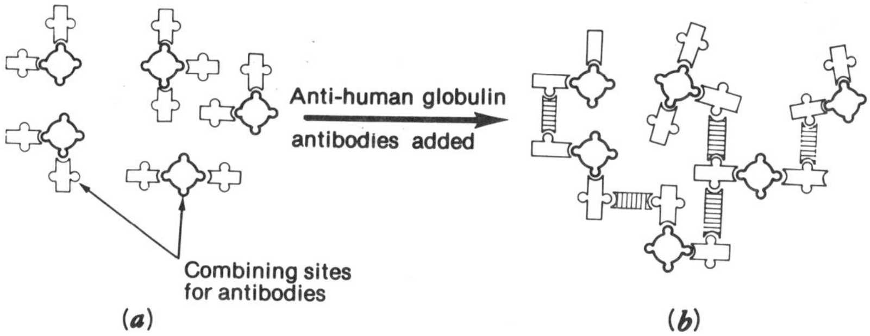

Figure 4-7 Indirect Coombs test employing anti-human-globulin antibodies to detect nonagglutinating antibodies combined with Rh-positive red blood cells. (*a*) Known Rh-positive rbc + patient's serum with anti-Rh nonagglutinating antibodies (hollow symbols). (*b*) Agglutination of red blood cells with attached human antibodies (nonagglutinating) by anti-human-globulin antibodies (hatched symbols).

test. The failure of IgG anti-Rh antibodies to cause agglutination and failure to fix complement (when complement is present) appear to be related not to any peculiarity in structure of the anti-Rh IgG antibodies but to the fact that Rh-antigen combining sites on the red blood cells are very sparsely distributed over the surface of the cell. The number of A and B antigen sites on red blood cells is at least 100 times greater. The strength of the antigen-antibody reaction with IgG anti-Rh antibodies appears to be insufficient to overcome the forces which cause red blood cells suspended in saline to repel each other. Repulsion is caused by the negative surface charge on red blood cells and by the cloud of positive ions (attracted by the negative surface charge) which surrounds the red blood cells (called the *zeta potential*). Antiglobulin antibodies are necessary for agglutination of red blood cells with IgG antibodies attached in order to bridge the zeta potential. In contrast, IgM anti-Rh antibodies can agglutinate Rh-positive red blood cells without the help of antiglobulin. Because of the pentamer structure of IgM, these anti-Rh antibodies are of sufficient size and combining strength to bridge or overcome the zeta potential. IgG anti-Rh antibodies can agglutinate trypsinized Rh-positive red blood cells or Rh-positive red blood cells suspended in albumin instead of saline. Enzyme treatment of red blood cells or suspension in albumin modifies the surface charges or repulsive forces and thereby facilitates agglutination by anti-Rh IgG antibodies.

4-15 In the direct Coombs test, the first step of the indirect test is omitted. For example, if red blood cells of an infant with erythroblastosis fetalis are suspected of having antibody attached to them, the cells should be washed 3 times in saline and then allowed to react with anti-human globulin. Erythroblastosis fetalis was discussed in Chap. 3. If an Rh-negative mother has been sensitized to Rh-positive cells and is carrying an Rh-positive fetus, her antibodies will go back to the fetus by way of the placenta, attach to red blood cells of the fetus and destroy them. Red blood cells with antibody attached are recognized as foreign by the body and are phagocytized. Removal by phagocytosis is enhanced because the attached anti-Rh antibodies are IgG, which are cytophilic for phagocytes and lead to opsonic adherence. As stated previously, these anti-Rh antibodies have been reported not to fix complement. At the time of birth, if erythroblastosis fetalis is expected, the direct Coombs test can be carried out. The antiglobulin test, sometimes called the development test for incomplete antibody, has found many applications besides testing for nonagglutinating antibodies. It is used to detect the attachment of small amounts of antibody to an antigen. For example, in acquired hemolytic anemia, an autoimmune disease, antibody is known to be formed to the patient's own red blood cells. Destruction occurs, with anemia resulting. To aid in diagnosis, a sample of the patient's blood is withdrawn and the red blood cells washed to remove free serum proteins. Anti-human globulin is added, which combines with human globulin attached to the red blood cells so that agglutination occurs. It has already been pointed out that antiglobulin antibodies are used to increase the sensitivity of a cross match for a blood transfusion (review Sec. 4-12).

Passive, or Indirect, Agglutination

4-16 The passive, or indirect, agglutination test is widely used. It is an extremely sensitive test because it will detect small amounts of antibody. The development of this test dates back many years, to a time when an attempt was made to coat collodion particles with a soluble antigen, e.g., an extract of heart tissue, and to test serum of rheumatic fever patients for antibodies to the adsorbed antigen. The technique was used for a number of years, usually unsuccessfully, because the collodion particles tended to aggregate nonspecifically. However, this technique paved the way for many similar passive agglutination tests in which various types of particles were used with specific antigens adhering to their surfaces. The two types of materials most frequently used as carrier particles for antigens are red blood cells and latex particles (polystyrene latex). The size of red blood cells is about 7μm; perfectly spherical latex particles can be obtained in different sizes and for this test are about 1 μm. To adsorb soluble antigens or antigens of small size onto large carrier particles such as red blood cells permits exploitation of the sensitivity of the agglutination reaction. The antibody is directed to the adsorbed material rather than to any antigens of the carrier particle, hence the terms passive or indirect agglutination. When red blood cells are used as carrier particles, the test is usually called passive or indirect hemagglutination. It has been shown that red blood cells adsorb polysaccharides but not protein antigens unless the red-blood-cell surface has been treated with a substance like tannic acid. Red blood cells treated with tannic acid are called *tanned cells.* Red blood cells are also treated with a preservative like formaldehyde to prevent deterioration or lysis.

4-17 Certain precautions must be observed when using red blood cells as carriers. The surface of red blood cells contains numerous antigens, and at least some of these antigens are the same as antigens of various animal and plant species. An antigen common to more than one species may be responsible for cross reactions in serologic tests. Common antigens occur not only in closely related species but also in unrelated ones. The term heterophile has been used to describe antibodies which cause cross reactions between antigens of distantly related or phylogenetically unrelated species. In carrying out the passive hemagglutination test, it is important to ascertain that the patient's serum does not contain heterophile antibodies to the red blood cells being used as carrier. Such antibodies must be removed or absorbed before the actual test is carried out. Latex particles as carriers have the advantage of having an antigenically inert surface. At present a variety of antigens coated on latex particles or preserved red blood cells are available commercially for rapid serologic testing. These include antigens from fungi such as *Coccidioides immitis* and nematodes such as *Trichinella spiralis.* Also tissue components, serum fractions, etc., associated with autoimmune diseases such as thyroglobulin, nucleoprotein, gamma globulin, etc., can be adsorbed onto carrier particles in order to test for antibodies to the adsorbed material. A specific test for syphilis has recently been introduced in which homogenized preparations of *T. pallidum* are adsorbed onto red blood cells (see Chap. 11). Latex particles are most frequently used in a slide test, and agglutination is observed within a few minutes after mixing of reagents. Tests with red blood cells as carriers for antigen are performed in tubes or U-shaped wells of plastic plates so that the pattern of settling can be observed. Results are read over a mirror. Nonagglutinated red blood cells settle into a compact button; agglutinated red blood cells settle into a diffuse pattern of agglutination on the bottom of the tubes or U-shaped wells (Fig. 4-8*a*). V-shaped wells, recently introduced, show a different settling pattern; agglutinated red

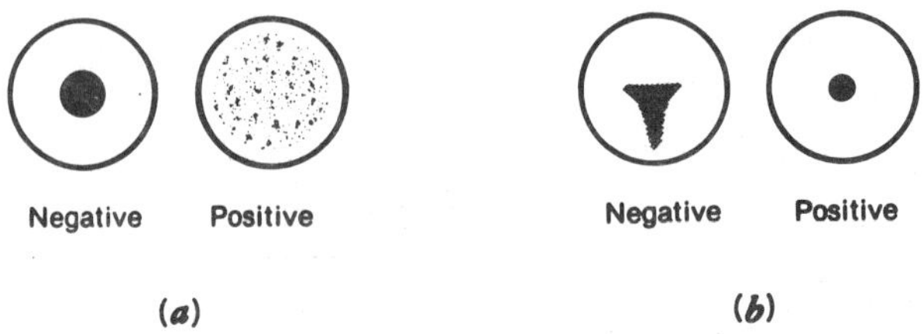

Figure 4-8 Patterns of settling of red blood cells in the passive, or indirect, hemagglutination test. Pattern shown for (*a*) U- and (*b*) V-shaped wells; negative = nonagglutinated and positive = agglutinated red blood cells.

blood cells appear as discrete dots while nonagglutinated red blood cells form a streak when the plate is incubated at a 45° angle (Fig. 4-8*b*).

4-18 The exquisite sensitivity of the passive agglutination reaction can be appreciated better if one considers the size of antibodies and soluble antigens. Some of the figures in this section showed antibody molecules drawn diagrammatically and about the same size as the antigen. Actually if the antigen in these figures had been sheep red blood cells and the antigen and antibody molecules had been drawn to scale, the antibody molecules in the drawing would have been so small they would have been no more than dots. Many of the soluble antigens used in the passive agglutination reaction are just as small and without adsorption onto a carrier particle would require many combinations of antigen with a very large amount of antibody in a precipitation reaction to give a positive visible result. In contrast, if the same soluble antigen is adsorbed onto a large carrier particle, a positive visible reaction is brought about by a much smaller amount of antibody. The lower limits of antibody nitrogen detectable by precipitation, complement fixation, agglutination, and passive hemagglutination are 5, 0.1, 0.05, and 0.005 μg/ml, respectively. Figure 4-9 attempts to show diagrammatically the difference in sensitivity between passive agglutination and precipitation.

Reversed Passive Agglutination, or Hemagglutination

4-19 Instead of coating the carrier particles with antigens, they can be coated with antibodies. This technique is sometimes referred to as *reversed passive agglutination* or *hemagglutination* (RPHA). For example, if latex particles are coated with antibodies to gamma globulin, they will be agglutinated by serum containing gamma globulin but not by the serum of a child with agammaglobulinemia. Recently the technique of RPHA has been used as a sensitive test for the detection of hepatitis B surface antigen. It is very important to determine whether a prospective blood donor has hepatitis virus in his blood. In the RPHA test, red blood cells are coated with antibodies to hepatitis B surface antigen and allowed to react with the serum to be tested for the presence of hepatitis B virus (see Fig. 4-10). After incubation, the pattern of settling of red blood cells is observed for agglutination. Appropriate controls must be used. Agglutination of the red blood cells coated with antibody will occur if the serum being tested contains hepatitis B virus. Other methods being used for the detection of hepatitis B virus include precipitation methods and radioimmunoassay, presented later in this chapter.

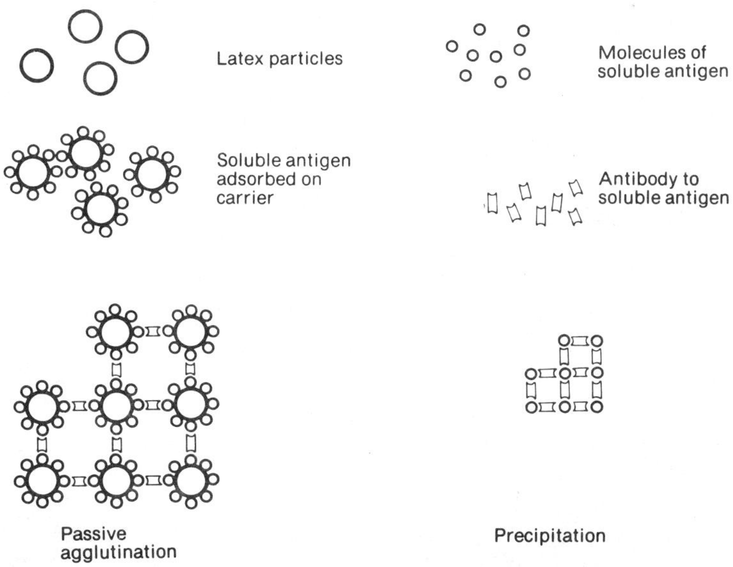

Figure 4-9 Manifestation of antibodies by passive agglutination and precipitation. Much fewer antibodies are required for a visible passive-agglutination reaction than for a visible precipitation reaction.

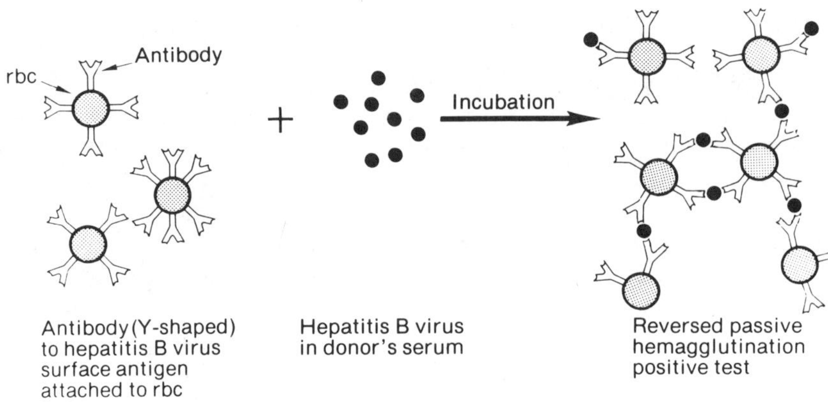

Figure 4-10 RPHA test for hepatitis B virus in the serum of a prospective donor.

Inhibition of Passive Agglutination, or Hemagglutination

4-20 Another modification of the passive, or indirect, agglutination test is one in which an antiserum known to have antibodies for the antigen adsorbed on the carrier particle and known to be capable of causing agglutination of these particles is allowed to react with a specimen suspected of containing the antigen. If the specimen contains the antigen, the antibodies in the diagnostic antiserum are saturated, so that when the carrier particles with the same antigen are added, agglutination does not occur. For example, a pregnancy test in current use employs latex particles coated with human chorionic gonadotropin (HCG) and an antiserum to HCG which agglutinates the HCG-coated particles. If the antiserum is incubated with the urine of a woman suspected of being pregnant (containing HCG in her urine) and then mixed with latex particles coated with HCG, the latex particles with HCG will not be agglutinated if the woman is pregnant.

Questions for Secs. 4-10 to 4-20

8. (*a*) What is the Widal test? (*b*) What is the flagella antigen called? (*c*) Is antibody to the flagella antigen associated with protection? (*d*) What two antigens are associated with virulence of *S. typhi*?

9. (*a*) When a transfusion reaction occurs due to Rh factor, what antigen is usually responsible? (*b*) What group of the ABO system contains naturally occurring antibodies in the serum to both A and B antigens? (*c*) Do the red blood cells of people in the blood group named in part (*b*) have A or B antigens? (*d*) What is the blood group of three patients with genotypes AO, OO, AB?

10. (*a*) Under what circumstances do minor blood groups cause transfusion reactions? (*b*) Which of the following combinations is the most important and is used for a cross match after donors of the same blood group have been obtained, the patient's cells and donor's serum or the patient's serum and donor's cells? (*c*) If the first step in a cross match shows no agglutination or hemolysis but agglutination occurs after addition of anti-human globulin to washed cells, can the blood be used? Explain your answer. (*d*) What effect would the antibodies in the serum of a group O individual have on the cells of a group AB patient if group O blood is used as a universal donor in an emergency?

11. (*a*) Do all four blood groups contain H substance? (*b*) In which blood group is H substance exposed so that it is recognized as a surface antigen? (*c*) What is the source of the letter H with regard to the H substance or antigen of red blood cells? (*d*) What is a Bombay-type individual?

12. (*a*) How is the indirect Coombs test used for detection of anti-Rh nonagglutinating antibodies in the serum of a Rh-negative person? (*b*) How does a person become sensitized to the Rh factor? (*c*) What are blocking antibodies? (*d*) Would anti-rabbit-globulin anti-

bodies cause agglutination of the red blood cells with human antibodies attached?

13. (*a*) How is the direct Coombs test used for detection of a mother's antibodies attached to the red blood cells of a newborn child with erythroblastosis fetalis? (*b*) To what immunoglobulin class do the mother's antibodies attached to the child's red blood cells belong? (*c*) If erythroblastosis fetalis was due to ABO system incompatibility rather than to Rh, would the addition of anti-human globulin to the red blood cells of the infant still cause agglutination? (*d*) Give another use besides diagnosis of erythroblastosis fetalis for the antiglobulin test.

14. (*a*) Must the antigens employed in the passive agglutination test be particulate, or cellular, in nature? (*b*) In the passive agglutination test, can haptens as well as antigens such as soluble antigens and virus particles be adsorbed onto carriers? (*c*) What is used as the carrier particle in passive hemagglutination? (*d*) Why is it necessary to treat red blood cells with tannic acid before adsorption of protein antigens? (*e*) Do the antibodies being assayed react with the carrier particle?

15. (*a*) Name one significant advantage of latex particles as carriers for antigens. (*b*) When red blood cells are used as carrier particles, why does the test serum need to be absorbed for heterophile antibodies? (*c*) Briefly describe the procedure for removal of antibodies in the patient's serum to carrier red blood cells before performing the passive hemagglutination test.

16. (*a*) Why can the passive, or indirect, agglutination test detect a much smaller amount of antibody to a soluble antigen than the precipitation reaction? (*b*) With regard to the smallest amount of antibody required for a positive reaction, list the following tests in order of their sensitivity; agglutination, complement fixation, passive hemagglutination, and precipitation.

17. (*a*) What is meant by reversed passive hemagglutination? (*b*) If latex particles coated with antibodies to human gamma globulin are allowed to react with the serum of a child suspected of having agammaglobulinemia or hypogammaglobulinemia and agglutination of the latex particles either fails to take place or gives a very weak reaction, does this indicate that the child's serum is deficient in gamma globulin?

18. In a test for pregnancy, the urine of a suspected pregnant woman is allowed to react with an antiserum to human chorionic gonadotropin (HCG), a hormone present in urine during pregnancy, and then latex particles coated with HCG are added. If agglutination does not occur, does this result indicate that the woman is pregnant? Explain your answer.

Answers

8. (*a*) A diagnostic agglutination test for typhoid fever. (*b*) H antigen. (*c*) No. (*d*) Vi and O antigens. (Sec. 4-10.)

9. Rh_0 (also called D). (*b*) Group O. (*c*) No, such a combination would be fatal. (*d*) A, O, and AB. (Sec. 4-11.)

10. (*a*) When a patient has to receive several transfusions containing the minor antigens with time in between transfusions to become sensitized. (*b*) The patient's serum and donor's cells. (*c*) No; agglutination after addition of anti-human globulin to the washed cells shows that antibodies of the patient were attached to the donor's cells and could cause transfusion reactions. (*d*) Probably no effect if they were present in O blood in amounts usually seen in O blood because they would be diluted with the patient's blood (about 7 liters); however, if they were present in high titer, they could cause a severe reaction. (Sec. 4-12.)

11. (*a*) Yes. (*b*) Group O. (*c*) H stands for heterogenetic antigen because it is also found in other animal species, not just in human beings. (*d*) A Bombay-type individual is one in whom the H gene is defective or absent, so that there is no H substance; since H substance is a building block for A and B antigens, they are also lacking. A Bombay-type individual may have in his serum anti-H, anti-A, and anti-B antibodies. (Sec. 4-13.)

12. (*a*) The serum of the patient is mixed with known Rh-positive red blood cells. The mixture is incubated and then the red blood cells are washed to remove all serum proteins except those which might be attached to the Rh-positive cells. Since antibodies are globulin, when anti-human globulin is added, any red blood cells with nonagglutinating antibodies attached are agglutinated. (*b*) By transfusion with improperly matched blood; an Rh-negative woman can be sensitized by an Rh-positive child, usually at parturition. (*c*) With regard to sensitization to Rh, blocking antibodies are nonagglutinating antibodies. (*d*) No, because the globulin nature of the antibodies is species-specific. (Secs. 4-14 and 4-15.)

13. (*a*) The red blood cells of the child are washed 3 times with physiological saline, the last supernatant fluid is removed, and anti-human-globulin antibodies are added to the red blood cells. Agglutination occurs if mother's antibodies are attached to the child's red blood cells. (*b*) IgG. (*c*) Yes. (*d*) For the detection of a small amount of antibody attached to red blood cells, as in acquired hemolytic anemia. (Sec. 4-15.)

14. (*a*) No. (*b*) Yes. (*c*) Red blood cell. (*d*) To modify the surface so that adsorption of protein antigens occurs. (*e*) No, they react with antigen adsorbed on the carrier. (Sec. 4-16.)

15. (*a*) Latex particles have an inert surface in that they contain no antigens as red blood cells do. (*b*) To remove antibodies to the carrier. (*c*) Mix patient's serum (inactivated at 56°C for 30 min) with a suspension of carrier red blood cells (without adsorbed antigen), incubate, centrifuge down the red blood cells or allow to settle, and use supernatant fluid. (Sec. 4-17.)

16. (*a*) In the passive-agglutination reaction, antigen is adsorbed onto a carrier which gives size to the antigen so that fewer antibodies are required for a visible reaction. (*b*) Passive hemagglutination, agglutination, complement fixation, and precipitation. (Sec. 4-18.)

17. (*a*) Antibody instead of antigen is adsorbed on a carrier. (*b*) Yes. (Sec. 4-19.)

18. Yes, because otherwise the antiserum would have agglutinated the latex particles with HCG adsorbed. (Sec. 4-20.)

Precipitation

4-21 The antigen in the precipitation reaction is very small and is referred to as *soluble* antigen. Examples of soluble antigens are pneumococcal polysaccharide and serum proteins. The basic mechanism of precipitation is believed to be the same as agglutination. Aggregation occurs as a result of lattice formation between multivalent soluble antigens and antibodies such as IgG or IgM which have a valence of two (IgG) or more (IgM). Antibodies which react with soluble antigens to cause precipitation have been termed *precipitins.* It is important to emphasize that unless precipitins and soluble antigens come together in the proper antigen-antibody ratios, i.e., *optimal proportions,* precipitation will not occur. Precipitation is inhibited by either an excess of antibody or an excess of antigen, as shown in Fig. 4-11. The *equivalence zone* is the zone in which antigen and antibody are present in optimal proportions to the extent that after the precipitate forms and settles out, there is neither ex-

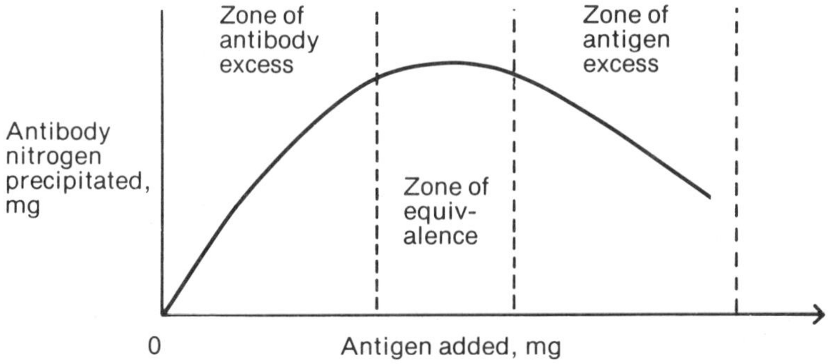

Figure 4-11 Effect of excess antibody or excess antigen on precipitation.

cess antibody nor antigen in the supernate. Diagnostic tests based on the precipitation reaction which are currently carried out in hospital laboratories are the ring test, agar-gel diffusion test including radial immunodiffusion, counterelectrophoresis, and immunoelectrophoresis.

Ring Test

4-22 The ring test is one of the earliest types of precipitation reactions used. It is very simple to perform but usually gives only a limited amount of information. It is called a ring test because in a positive reaction a ring of precipitation occurs at the antigen-antibody interphase. The test is carried out in tubes of very narrow diameter. The antiserum is delivered to the bottom of the tube to a depth of about 3/8 in. with a capillary pipet, and then a similar amount of antigen is layered (not mixed) onto the antiserum. The test results, along with controls, are read after an incubation period of about 30 min. Figure 4-12 shows positive and negative ring tests. In a positive test a turbid or white band of precipitation forms at the antigen-antibody interphase. In a negative test the antigen-antibody interphase does not change in appearance during the incubation period. The ring test has limited applications because it will not detect a multiplicity of antigen-antibody systems if more than one antigen-antibody system is present. The ring test is still used because it can be carried out easily and test results can be obtained in a short time. Examples of its use are grouping of streptococci using extracts of the organism and determination of species in forensic (legal) medicine using extracts of bloodstains, etc. With regard to technique, capillary tubing is often used in place of narrow-bore test tubes. After reagents are taken up into the capillary tubing, the tubing can be held upright with modeling clay for incubation.

Agar-Gel Diffusion (Ouchterlony Test)

4-23 The agar-gel diffusion method developed by Ouchterlony is often referred to as *double gel diffusion.* This test has many applications, e.g., determining the homogeneity of antigen-antibody systems and following the purification of antigens, but the method will not detect impurities which are not antigenic. In the agar-gel diffusion test, highly purified agar is used in a concentration of 1% in physiological saline; 0.01% merthiolate is added to prevent bacterial contamination during incubation. Agar is a mixture of two principal linear polysaccharides, agaropectin, the portion containing acid residues, and agarose, which is neutral. Agarose is frequently used now for immunodiffusion studies. Besides agar and agarose, other gels have been used for immunodiffusion but less often. Agar or agarose can be poured into petri dishes or layered on large glass slides. The reagents, solutions of antigen or antibody, are placed in wells cut in agar. Antigens and antibodies diffuse through the agar gel toward each other, and precipitation results where the optimal antigen and antibody ratios (optimal proportions) are reached; see Figure 4-13, which shows on the left side that a single antigen X diffusing from the antigen well (X) gives rise to a single line or precipitation with antibodies diffusing from the antiserum well (S). On the right side two antigens, Y and Z, are present; each antigen behaves independently of the other, so that two bands of precipitation can be seen between the antigen well and the antiserum well, which contains not only anti-X but also anti-Y and anti-Z. If several bands of precipitation had been evident, there would have been at least that many different antigen-antibody systems present.

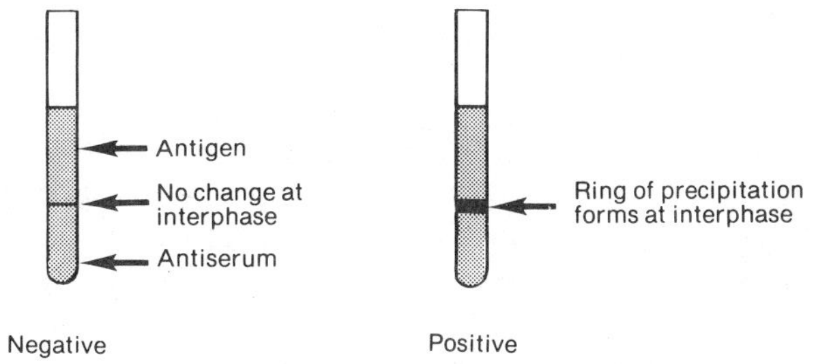

Figure 4-12 Ring-precipitation tests showing negative and positive results.

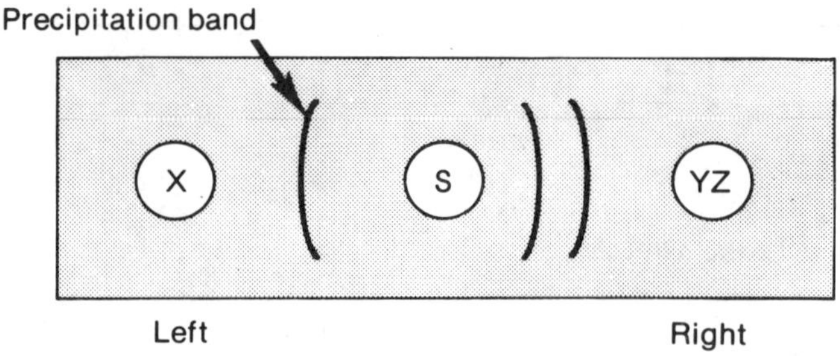

Figure 4-13 Agar-gel diffusion showing lines of precipitation with a single antigen-antibody system on the left and two independent antigen-antibody systems on the right. Each circle represents a well in agar, S = anti-X + anti-Y + anti-Z, X = antigen X, XY = antigens Y + Z.

4-24 One of the uses of the agar-gel diffusion test is to determine serological relationships between antigens. In Fig. 4-14*a* the precipitin band which forms between antiserum well S_1 and known antigen Z inclines toward S_1 and joins the precipitin band between S_2 and unknown antigen X. Joining of the two lines of precipitation indicates that the antigens are identical, or X = Z. In Fig. 4-14*b* the precipitin band which forms between antiserum S_1 and known antigen Z involves a component which gives a reaction of identity with a cross-reacting related antigen R and another component which does not, so that a spur is formed. In Fig. 4-14*c* different antigens, Y and Z, and antiserum S_2 to both Y and Z were placed in the wells as indicated. A double spur formed, which is interpreted to mean that the adjacent antigens, Y and Z, are unrelated. It is common practice to test a number of antigens against an antiserum at one time. For example, if antigens X, Y, Z, and R, described above, are tested against antiserum S_2 containing antibodies to Y and Z, the relationships shown in Fig. 4-15 would be observed.

4-25 In general, the technique of agar-gel diffusion employing 1% agar is not satisfactory for immunological studies on viruses unless soluble antigens of the viruses are being studied or the virus particles are very small. One of the requirements of the method of agar-gel diffusion is that the reactants be able to diffuse freely. Large viruses such as vaccinia do not diffuse well in 1% agar gel. The agar-gel diffusion test was the first test used for screening blood donors for hepatitis B virus before transfusion. Although this test has been largely replaced by more sensitive methods, it provided the first major breakthrough for such screening. Other tests for hepatitis B virus in serum are described in Secs. 4-19, 4-29, and 4-34.

4-26 The agar-gel diffusion technique was modified by Elek to test for toxigenic strains of *Corynebacterium diphtheriae,* the etiologic agent of diphtheria. Before this technique was developed by Elek,

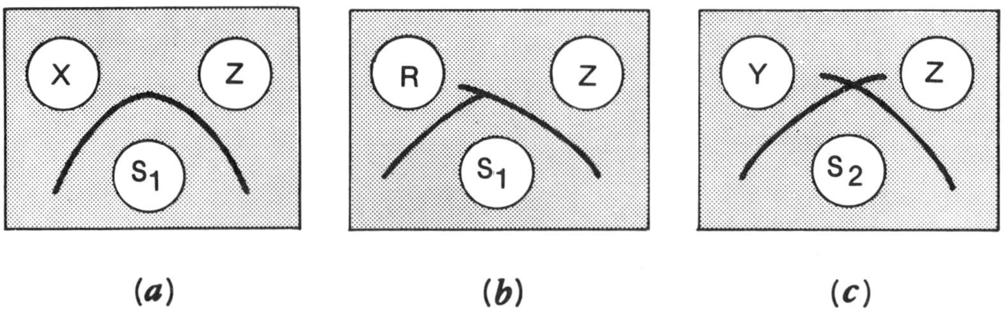

Figure 4-14 Agar-gel double-diffusion technique showing precipitation lines which correspond to the following reactions: (*a*) identity between antigens, S_1 = antiserum to Z, Z = known antigen, and X = unknown antigen; (*b*) partial identity between antigens, S_1 = antiserum to Z, Z = known antigen, R = related antigen; (*c*) nonidentity between antigens, S_2 = antiserum to Y and Z, Z = known antigen, and Y = unrelated antigen.

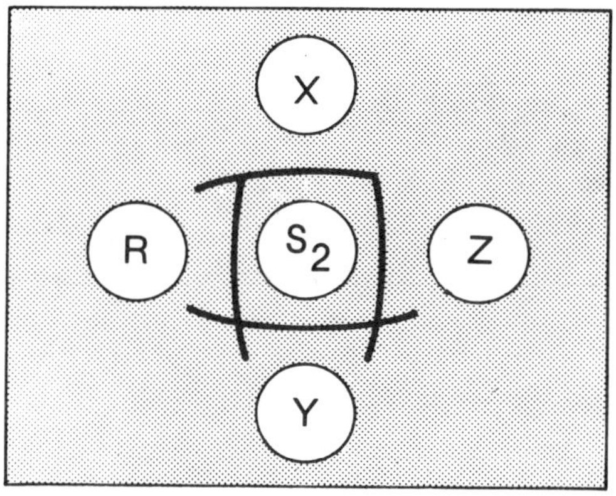

Figure 4-15 Use of agar-gel diffusion to show serological relationships between antigens; S_2 = anti-Y and anti-Z; antigens in outer well are X = Z, R (related to X and Z), and Y (not related to X, Z, or R).

tests for toxigenicity had to be carried out in laboratory animals. A 1% agar medium containing nutrients for growth of *C. diphtheriae* is prepared and poured into an agar plate. Before the agar hardens, a sterile strip of filter paper saturated with diphtheria antitoxin appropriately diluted is embedded in the center of the agar medium, as shown in Fig. 4-16. A single fairly wide streak of a known toxigenic culture of *C. diphtheriae* is streaked across the plate at right angles to the filter paper. The strain(s) being tested for exotoxin production are streaked across the plate in the same fashion. The plate is taped to prevent loss of moisture and is incubated for at least 48 h at 37°C. As shown in Fig. 4-16, a toxigenic strain of *C. diphtheriae* produces exotoxin, which diffuses out from the culture at right angles to the line of diffusion of the antitoxin from the filter paper. At points along the paths of their cross diffusion, antigen (toxin) and antibody (antitoxin) will be at optimal proportions, and a line of precipitation will form in the agar at these sites.

Radial Immunodiffusion

4-27 Radial immunodiffusion is a modification of the agar-gel diffusion technique; it is used for quantitation of immunoglobulins, complement components, etc. In radial immunodiffusion, monospecific antiserum is added to melted agar just before it is poured into plates or onto slides, so that antibodies are distributed throughout the medium. The specimens to be tested for antigen are placed in wells cut in the agar. For example, if one wants to assay for the C3 complement component (β_1C globulin), the antibodies in the agar will be to this component only. Antigen in the well diffuses radially, so that the greatest concentration of antigen is close to the well. At the point where antigen and

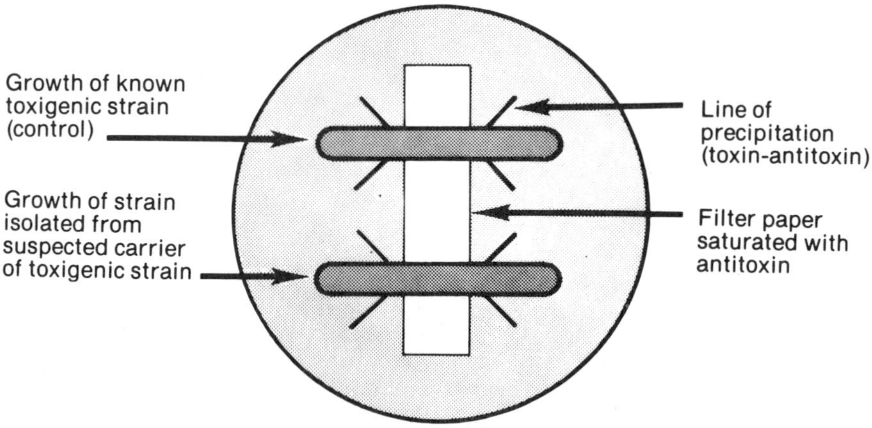

Figure 4-16 In vitro Elek test for toxin production by *C. diphtheriae* employing the technique of agar-gel diffusion.

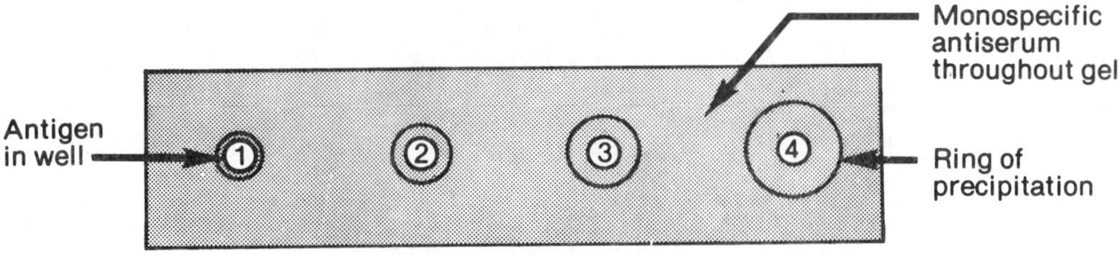

Figure 4-17 Radial-immunodiffusion technique for detection and quantitation of antigens. The concentration of antigen in wells 1 to 4 increases from left to right, as shown by the diameter of the ring of precipitation around the well.

antibody (which is constant) are in optimal proportions, a ring of precipitation is formed. The diameter of the ring is proportional to the antigen concentration (see Fig. 4-17). The quantity of antigen can be determined by comparing ring diameter to known standards. Tests are usually read at a stated time for the antigen being assayed because ring diameters can vary with time.

Immunoelectrophoresis

4-28 By combining the agar-gel double-diffusion method of Ouchterlony (1949) with electrophoretic separation on the same agar plate, Grabar and Williams (1953) developed a method whereby mixtures of proteins can be analyzed on the basis of both their antigenic and electrophoretic properties (review electrophoresis, Sec. 3-12). By using immunoelectrophoresis it is possible to detect more than 30 distinct antigenic proteins in normal human serum (see Fig. 4-18). Agarose gel has proved to be an excellent medium because it is transparent and neutrally charged and allows free diffusion of proteins. The test in Fig. 4-18 was carried out as follows. (1) Antigen was placed in the center wells, and an electric field was applied across the plate, causing the antigen (proteins) to migrate according to their intrinsic electrophoretic mobilities. At this point no visible change could be detected. (2) Antisera to the antigens were introduced into the narrow troughs *A* and *B*, in which the long axis is parallel to the axis of the antigen migration pattern. The separated components of the specimen and antibodies to them diffuse toward each other, and precipitation lines form at the optimal concentration zones after incubation. If permanent records are desired, the slide is dried and the precipitation lines are stained. Immunologic deficiency disorders such as agammaglobulinemia and the production of pathological immunoglobulins have been extensively studied by immunoelectrophoresis. For agammaglobulinemia it can be shown that an important serum component needed for protection is missing, while for the pathological immunoglobulins it can be shown that a certain immunoglobulin is present in an excessive amount. Figure 4-19 shows a serum specimen and control tested for IgG placed on each side of an antiserum trough containing anti-IgG. The specimen shows only a faint line of precipitation.

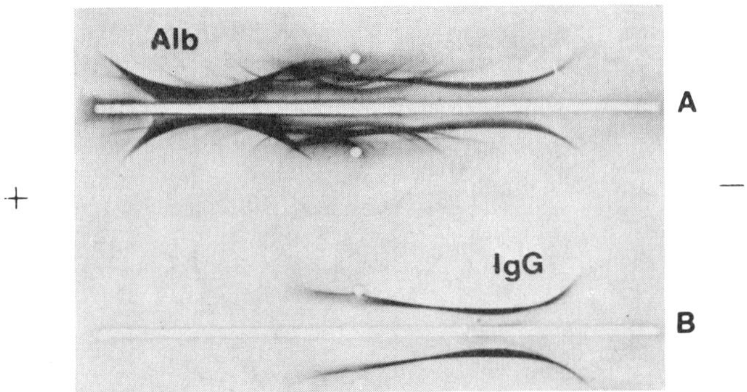

Figure 4-18 Immunoelectrophoresis of normal human serum. Normal human serum was placed in the center circular wells; after electrophoresis antiserum to human serum was placed in the trough labeled *A* and antiserum to IgG in the trough labeled *B*; Alb = albumin. (*Courtesy of B. P. Barton, Department of Pathology, Medical College of Georgia.*)

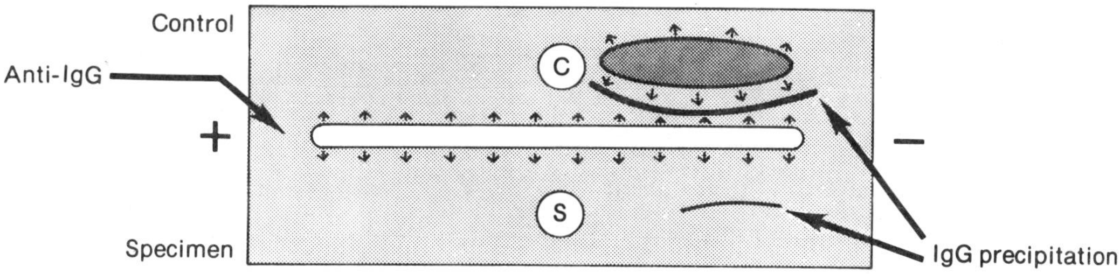

Figure 4-19 Immunoelectrophoresis on serum specimen of a child with hypogammaglobulinemia. Arrows indicate paths of diffusion after electrophoresis.

Rocket Electrophoresis and Counterelectrophoresis

4-29 In both rocket electrophoresis and counterelectrophoresis, reagents in the wells do not diffuse out from the wells in all directions; instead, they are drawn in one direction by electric current.
Rocket electrophoresis This is a procedure for quantitation of proteins. Like the procedure for radial immunodiffusion, monospecific antiserum is in the gel so that when an electric current is applied, antigen drawn to the anode forms a rocket- or flame-shaped precipitation arc with antibody in the gel (see Fig. 4-20). The antigen must have a greater mobility than antibody and a different isoelectric point. The length of the arc (rocket or flame) is related to antigen concentration and is compared with standards for quantitation of antigen (Ag).
Counterelectrophoresis This technique also employs diffusion of antigen from the well in one direction toward the anode. Antibody is placed in a well between antigen and the anode. This technique is not quantitative. Counterelectrophoresis makes use of endosomotic flow; during electrophoresis in a negatively charged gel this flow causes the slow-moving globulins, including antibody, to be displaced toward the cathode. Antigen and antibody are drawn together, so that precipitation occurs, giving a much more rapid and more sensitive method than simple gel diffusion (see Fig. 4-21). Other names by which the technique is known are immunoelectroosmophoresis, countercurrent electrophoresis, and crossover electrophoresis. One use of the technique has been to screen blood donors for hepatitis virus, but now federal regulations [Tests. . . (1975)] require more sensitive methods such as radioimmunoassay (Sec. 4-34) and reversed passive hemagglutination (Sec. 4-19). Counterelectrophoresis is used with a number of different kinds of soluble antigens such as α-fetoprotein (Chap. 10) and antigens extracted from bacteria and fungi. All tests based on precipitation in gels have a disadvantage in that reading lines of precipitation is subjective.

Questions for Secs. 4-21 to 4-29

19. (*a*) What kind of antigen is used in the precipitation reaction? (*b*) What are precipitins? (*c*) What is the effect of an excess of antibody or antigen on precipitation? (*d*) What

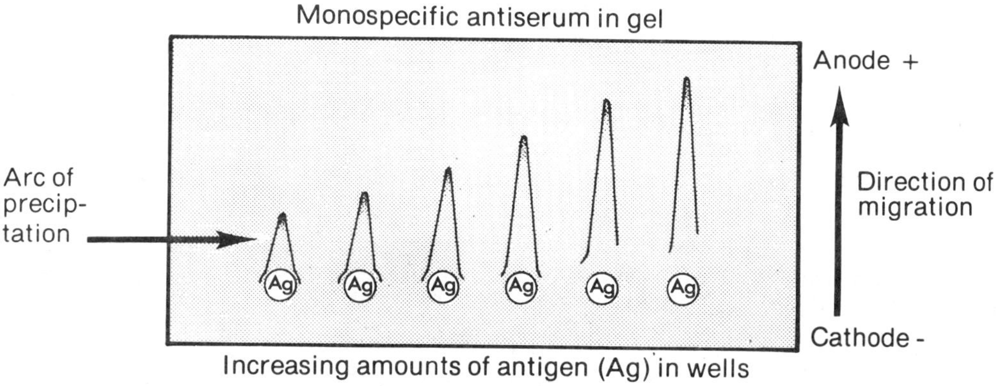

Figure 4-20 Rocket electrophoresis for quantitation of proteins by length of arc of precipitation.

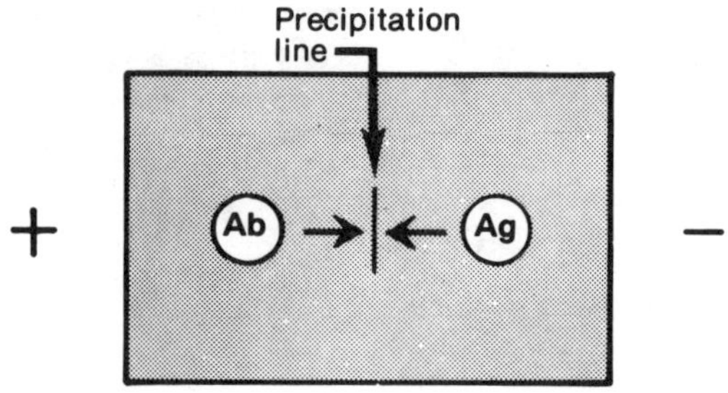

Figure 4-21 Counterelectrophoresis in which antigen (Ag) and antibody (Ab) are drawn together to form a visible line of precipitation.

happens to antibody and antigen in the equivalence zone of precipitation?

20. (*a*) If the reagents used in the ring test contained more than one antigen-antibody system, could the ring test differentiate between them? (*b*) Could the agar-gel diffusion method differentiate between them? (*c*) Why is merthiolate added to agar for the Ouchterlony test?

21. (*a*) Where do the lines of precipitation show up in an agar-gel diffusion test? (*b*) Sketch reactions of the agar-gel double-diffusion (Ouchterlony) test to show the following relationships between two adjacent antigens: (1) identity, (2) partial identity, and (3) nonidentity.

22. Can viruses or viral antigens be tested for by the agar-gel diffusion technique? Explain. (*b*) What organism was originally used in the Elek test for exotoxin production? (*c*) With regard to the Elek test for exotoxin production, why are nutrients added to the agar and merthiolate omitted? (*d*) Would a relatively small amount of antitoxin be more likely to precipitate with a small or large amount of exotoxin? (*e*) In the Elek test, why does the line of precipitation between exotoxin and antitoxin appear at approximately a 45° angle to the line of growth?

23. (*a*) In radial immunodiffusion, where are the reagents placed? (*b*) How can this test be used to determine whether or not a certain complement component is present in a patient's serum and if present what the quantity of it is?

24. (*a*) What two tests are the basis of immunoelectrophoresis? (*b*) How are the components of human serum separated? (*c*) After the components of human serum are separated, what reagent is used to make the components visible? (*d*) Can slides showing results of agar-gel diffusion be kept for a permanent record? Explain.

25. (*a*) What are some other names used to refer to immunoelectroosmophoresis? (*b*) On what principle is counterelectrophoresis based? (*c*) What are the main advantages of counterelectrophoresis over agar-gel diffusion as a diagnostic test?

Answers

19. (*a*) Soluble antigen. (*b*) Antibodies capable of precipitating with antigen. (*c*) An excess of antibody or antigen can either completely inhibit or reduce the amount of precipitation. (*d*) They are completely precipitated so that there is neither excess antigen nor antibody in the supernatant fluid after the precipitate settles. (Sec. 4-21.)

20. (*a*) No. (*b*) Yes. (*c*) To prevent growth of microbial air contaminants. The agar has no nutritive value, but the antiserum and antigen being tested do contain nutrients for bacterial growth. (Secs. 4-22 and 4-23.)

21. (*a*) Where diffusion of antigen molecules and antibodies takes place so that they are present in optimal proportions. (*b*) Precipitation lines are shown below for (1) identity, (2) partial identity and (3) nonidentity of antigens after reaction with antibodies diffusing from antiserum in bottom wells. (Sec. 4-24.)

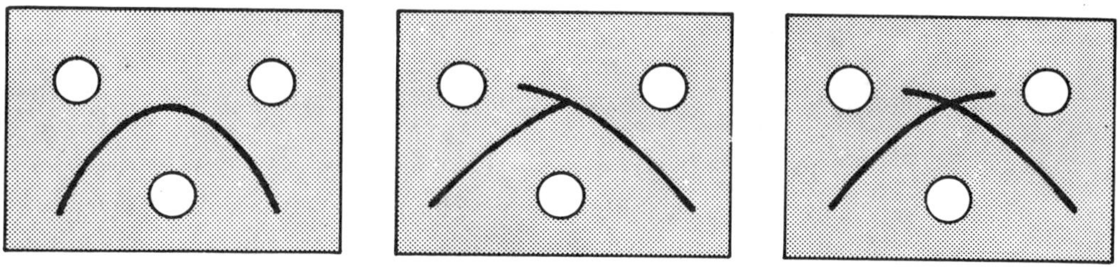

(1) Lines join (2) Spur appears (3) Lines cross

22. (*a*) Small viruses or soluble antigens of viruses can be tested for by agar-gel diffusion. The method is not suitable for any particles which are not freely diffusible in the agar medium used. (*b*) *Corynebacterium diphtheriae.* (*c*) For the Elek test, nutrients are added so that toxigenic strains of *C. diphtheriae* can grow and produce exotoxin; merthiolate is not added because it would prevent growth of *C. diphtheriae* and the test would be worthless, because if the organism does not grow, toxin will not be produced. (*d*) Small. (*e*) Because of the direction of diffusion of toxin and antitoxin as shown below and the fact that visible lines of precipitation occur in zones of optimal proportions. (Secs. 4-25 and 4-26.)

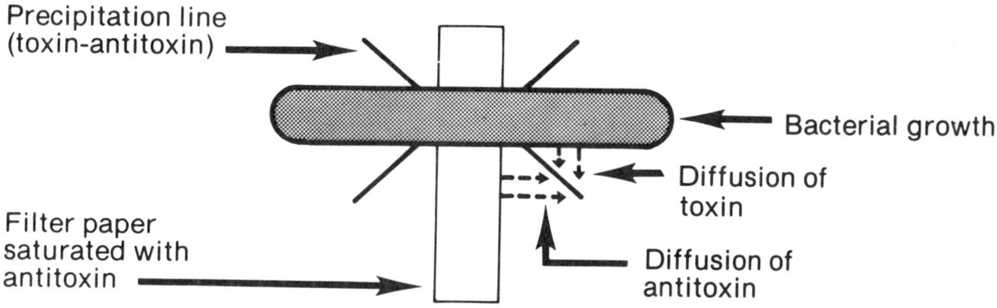

23. (*a*) Antiserum is incorporated into melted agar at 45 to 50°C so that after the gel solidifies, antibodies are distributed throughout the gel. The antibodies in the gel must be specific for a single antigen. The specimen to be tested for antigen is placed in a well cut in the gel. (*b*) Antigen in the well diffuses in all directions and forms a ring of precipitation with antibodies in the gel where antigen and antibody are in optimal proportions. The diameter of the ring is proportional to the amount of antigen present. The amount of antigen can be determined by comparison of the diameter of the ring with a standard curve. (Sec. 4-27.)

24. (*a*) Agar-gel diffusion and electrophoresis. (*b*) By electrophoresis in agar gel. (*c*) Antiserum containing antibodies to human serum. Such an antiserum could be prepared by injection of rabbits or other animals with human serum. (*d*) Yes, the slides can be dried, stained, and filed for reference. (Sec. 4-28.)

25. (*a*) Counterelectrophoresis, countercurrent electrophoresis, and crossover electrophoresis. (*b*) Counterelectrophoresis, or immunoelectroosmophoresis, is based on the principle of endosmotic flow. During electrophoresis in a negatively charged gel, the slower-moving globulins, especially gamma globulins, are displaced to the cathode, in a direction opposite to the movement of the antigen. (*c*) In counterelectrophoresis, the antigen and antibody molecules are drawn together by electrophoresis so that a line of precipitation forms much sooner than with agar-gel diffusion. It is a more sensitive test than agar-gel diffusion. (Sec. 4-29.)

Radioimmunoassay

4-30 Radioimmunoassays generally use radioactive-labeled antigens or haptens, but in some procedures, e.g., the method to be described later for detection of hepatitis B virus, antibodies are labeled with radioactivity. Proteins are commonly labeled with ^{125}I or ^{131}I. Three main advantages of radioiodine as a trace label are (1) that the labeling can be performed in vitro to obtain labeled proteins of very high specific activity, (2) that the label is covalently linked firmly to the protein molecule, so that there is no exchange with other protein molecules, and (3) that many proteins can be labeled so that the native protein is indistinguishable from the labeled protein. ^{125}I, which is probably used more often than ^{131}I, has a half-life of 57 days with low-energy gamma emission. ^{131}I is a beta- and gamma-ray emitter with a half-life of 8 days. Many modifications can be made in the radioimmunoassay procedure to suit the substance being assayed. In general, radioimmunoassay is very sensitive and quite versatile. Rosalyn S. Yalow was one of the 1977 recipients of the Nobel prize for her work on radioimmunoassay. Two general methods of procedure will be described, competitive and direct radioimmunoassay.

Competitive Radioimmunoassay

4-31 The basic underlying mechanism of the test is that a standardized amount of radioactive-labeled antigen will compete with unlabeled antigen of the same specificity for antibody sites during an antigen-antibody reaction. Although in some modifications of radioimmunoassay, soluble complexes may form, precipitation does not occur in the initial reaction between antibody and labeled and unlabeled antigens because only very small amounts of known antibody and labeled antigen are added. It was pointed out earlier that the precipitation reaction is a rather insensitive method for detection of antigen and antibody. The endpoint which is read in radioimmunoassay is not precipitation but the amount of radioactivity present, which is determined by using isotope-counting equipment. Since visible precipitation does not occur during the initial reaction between known antibody and labeled and unlabeled antigens, some procedure has to be employed to separate antigen bound to antibody from unbound antigen. Figure 4-22 shows the use of specific antiglobulin to separate out antibody-bound antigen, one of several procedures that have been used. The higher the concentration of antigen (unlabeled) in the specimen, the less labeled antigen bound to antibody there will be, as a result of competition between unlabeled and labeled antigen. The effect of the competition of known amounts of unlabeled antigen on the percent of radioactive antigen which is bound by antibody is shown in the standard curve in Fig. 4-23. From this curve the unknown amount of antigen in the specimen can be determined.

4-32 Since radioimmunoassay has been used extensively in research, numerous modifications in technique have been made by various investigators. Farr used radioimmunoassay to measure antibody concentration after mixing serum with a standard amount of radioactive ligand. He used a high concentration of ammonium sulfate to bring down, or salt out, antibody-bound ligand. It is necessary for unbound ligand to be soluble in the concentration of ammonium sulfate used. Still another method is the use of *insoluble supports,* or *immunoadsorbants,* which can be centrifuged down to

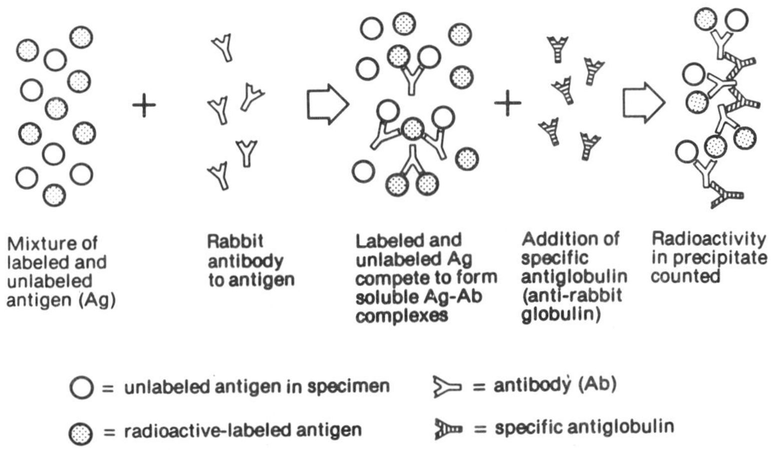

Figure 4-22 Competitive radioimmunoassay employing isotope-labeled antigen and specific antiglobulin to precipitate antibody-bound antigen.

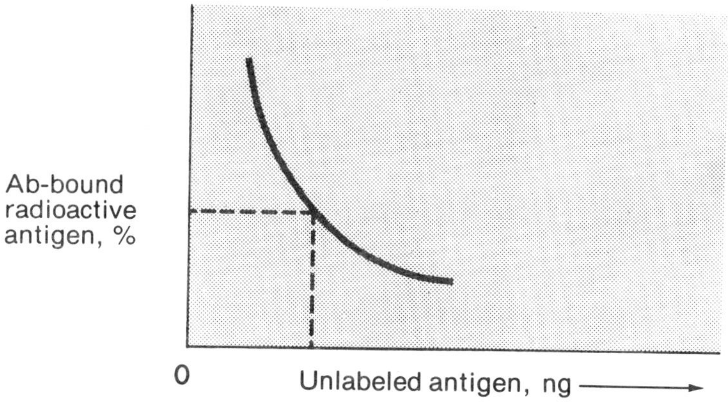

Figure 4-23 Standard curve to determine the effect of known amounts of unlabeled antigen on the percentage of antibody-bound radioactive antigen.

determine radioactivity. For example, radioimmunoassays for IgE have been devised using Sephadex beads as immunoadsorbants for antigen or antibody, as the case warrants. Techniques for assay of IgE are described in Chap. 5 in connection with atopy. One technique for IgE is called the *radioimmunosorbent test* (RIST); the other technique is called the *radioallergosorbent test* (RAST). Both competitive and direct RIST assays have been described. The RAST technique is a direct one and also identifies the specificity of IgE.

4-33 A technique used in hospital laboratories is based in part on the observation that test tubes made out of some unsubstituted polymers, e.g., polystyrene and polypropylene, can adsorb antibody. If an antiserum is delivered to the lower part of the tube, there will be a uniform coat of antibody on the lower inside surface of the tube. One test for human growth hormone (HGH) in serum is based on the observation that in a radioimmunoassay, antibody bound to the wall of a polystyrene or polypropylene tube will react specifically and bind labeled and unlabeled antigen in proportion to their concentration in the tube. HGH is labeled with radioactive iodine, ^{125}I. If one wishes to assay for HGH in a patient's serum, tubes are coated with antibody to HGH, the patient's serum is added, followed by the addition of ^{125}I-labeled HGH. After suitable incubation, the sample is counted, and then unbound antigen (labeled and unlabeled) is removed by washing. The tube is then counted again in order to determine the amount of bound labeled antigen, which is inversely proportional to the amount of unlabeled antigen or HGH in the patient's serum. In other words, the higher the count after washing, the less HGH in the patient's serum.

Direct Radioimmunoassay

4-34 One test currently used to detect hepatitis B virus (HB_V) or hepatitis B surface antigen (HB_SAg) in donor serum employs large plastic beads coated with antibody to the surface antigen of the virus. Antiserum (anti-HB_SAg) is prepared by injecting guinea pigs with HB_V or HB_SAg. The donor's serum suspected of containing hepatitis B virus is added to the test tubes or U-shaped wells in plastic trays. Each tube or well contains a large antibody-coated bead. After a suitable incubation period, the tube is aspirated and the bead washed. ^{125}I-labeled anti-HB_SAg is added. If the donor's serum contained HB_V, the virus would have been bound to unlabeled antibody adhering to the surface of the bead and now the bound HB_V would combine with labeled antibody to HB_SAg. The technique employed here is sometimes referred to as a *sandwich technique*. In the last step, the bead is washed to remove free labeled antibody. The radioactivity on the bead is counted in a gamma scintillation detector. A negative control which has been carried through the same procedure is assayed. The amount of virus or viral antigen in the serum of the donor is determined by referring to a standard curve. In this direct radioimmunoassay, the more radioactivity at the end of the test, the more HB_V or HB_SAg in the prospective donor's serum (see Fig. 4-24).

4-35 The procedure just described can be modified to test for antibodies to hepatitis B virus (or its surface antigen) in the serum of a prospective blood donor or in the serum of a patient believed to

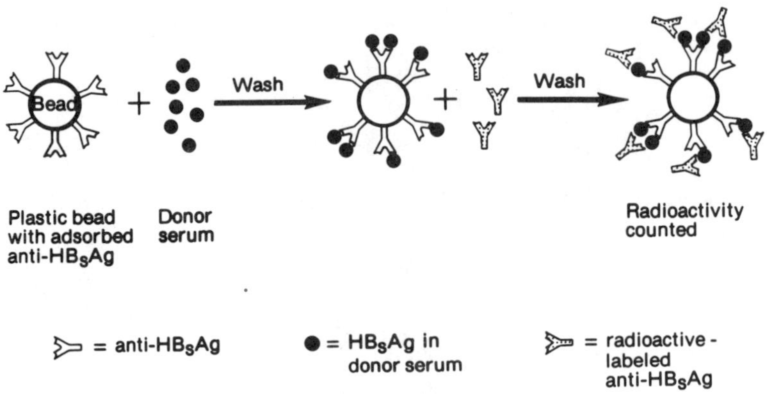

Figure 4-24 Direct radioimmunoassay for hepatitis B virus or hepatitis B surface antigen (HB_sAg) in serum of a prospective blood donor.

have hepatitis. Hepatitis B surface antigen (HB_SAg) is adsorbed onto the surface of large plastic beads. A single bead is placed in a tube or well and a donor's or patient's serum is added. After incubation, the bead is washed, and ^{125}I-labeled antigen is added. After the second incubation period, the bead is again washed and radioactivity counted. The sandwich technique is also employed here. If the donor or patient had serum antibodies, they would react with antigen adsorbed on the bead and would not be removed by washing. When radioactive antigen (HB_SAG) is added, it would combine with the antibodies which had reacted with unlabeled antigen adsorbed on the bead. If the serum being tested contained no antibodies, there would be nothing present in the test system with which labeled antigen could react and it would all be removed by washing (see Fig. 4-25).

Hepatitis B Virus: Comparison of Diagnostic Serologic Tests for HB_SAg

4-36 Hepatitis B surface antigen (HB_SAg) has also been called serum hepatitis or SH antigen, hepatitis-associated antigen (HAA), and Australia antigen. In Sec. 1-28 it was mentioned that hepatitis with a very long incubation period and caused by an agent present in serum was recognized for the first time during World War II. This agent, now known to be a virus, has proved very difficult to cultivate and study. Blumberg (1964) and his associates discovered Australia antigen when they found that an antibody in the blood of a transfused hemophiliac patient from New York reacted with an antigen which had been found in the serum of an Australian aborigine. In 1976, Blumberg shared the Nobel prize in medicine for his work on Australia antigen. Work with Australia antigen provided the first method for testing for hepatitis B virus in the blood of prospective donors. Although HB_SAg or Australia antigen is not considered to be the virus particle itself, it is believed to be an antigen associated with the virus. Presumably antibodies to HB_SAg would react not only with the surface antigen but also with the virus particle. It is important to detect hepatitis B viral infection in the blood of a prospective donor because this virus causes a very serious disease. Since there is a long incubation period, the prospective donor may have the virus in his blood without showing any

Figure 4-25 Direct radioimmunoassay for serum antibodies to hepatitis B surface antigen (HB_sAg).

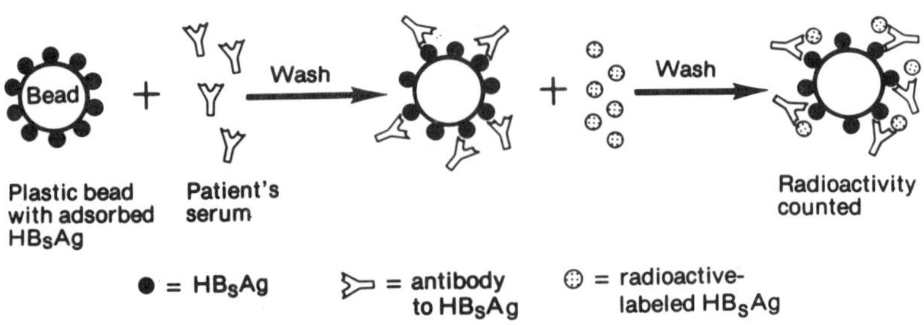

symptoms at the time of blood donation. The agar-gel diffusion method is not sufficiently sensitive for small amounts of HB_SAg. Counterelectrophoresis (Sec. 4-29) is more sensitive than agar-gel diffusion but not as sensitive as reversed passive hemagglutination (Sec. 4-19) or radioimmunoassay (Sec. 4-34).

Questions for Secs. 4-30 to 4-36

26. (*a*) With what radioactive substance(s) is antigen often labeled? (*b*) What is the half-life of the labeled material? (*c*) Can labeling take place in vitro? (*d*) Are labeled and unlabeled antigens sufficiently similar in structure to react with specific antibody to unlabeled antigen?

27. (*a*) What is the mechanism of competitive radioimmunoassay (RIA) when used to determine the amount of antigen in a specimen? (*b*) In the above test, what reagents are present in standardized amounts? (*c*) What effect would a large amount of antigen in a specimen have on the amount of bound labeled antigen?

28. (*a*) Give three ways in which soluble complexes can be separated from unbound ligand (labeled or unlabeled) in order to determine the amount of bound labeled ligand? (*b*) What is the RAST test?

29. (*a*) Briefly describe a radioimmunoassay (RIA) currently used to screen blood donors for hepatitis B virus. (*b*) How is antiserum for the test prepared? (*c*) Why is the technique called a sandwich technique? (*d*) Is the technique based on competitive or direct RIA?

30. (*a*) What is the relationship between serum hepatitis or SH antigen, Australia antigen, hepatitis-associated antigen (HAA), and hepatitis B surface antigen (HB_SAg)? (*b*) Which of the above terms is preferred at present? (*c*) Why is it important to test a blood donor for HB_SAg?

31. (*a*) What tests have been used to detect HB_SAg in the serum of a prospective donor? (*b*) What test(s) are not sufficiently sensitive to detect a very small amount of HB_SAg? (*c*) Which test is probably the most sensitive but requires very expensive equipment? (*d*) Which test is very sensitive and requires inexpensive equipment to perform? (*e*) Are reagents for the above diagnostic tests available commercially? (*f*) How is radioactivity counted in RIA?

Answers

26. (*a*) ^{125}I or ^{131}I. (*b*) 57 days for ^{125}I and 8 days for ^{131}I. (*c*) Yes. (*d*) Yes. (Sec. 4-30.)

27. (*a*) Competitive radioimmunoassay is based on the fact that labeled and unlabeled antigen are the same structurally and therefore compete for specific antibodies. The amount of labeled antigen which is bound is inversely proportional to the amount of unlabeled antigen present in the specimen. (*b*) Antibody and labeled antigen are present in standardized amounts. (*c*) Less labeled antigen would be bound. (Sec. 4-31.)

28. (*a*) Three ways in which soluble complexes can be separated from unbound ligand (antigen or hapten) are (1) specific precipitation with the appropriate antiglobulin, (2) nonspecific precipitation, or salting out, of antibody-bound ligand with a high concentration of ammonium sulfate in which the ligand is soluble, (3) adsorption of antibody on insoluble supports. (*b*) The RAST test is frequently used in clinical laboratories to test for IgE. RAST stands for radioallergosorbent test. (Secs. 4-32 and 4-33.)

29. (*a*) Specific antibodies to HB_SAg are adsorbed onto large plastic beads. A bead is placed in a tube, and the donor's serum is added. If hepatitis B virus or particles of HB_SAg are present in donor serum, they will form a link between unlabeled antibodies and labeled antibodies which are subsequently added after washing the bead. (*b*) By injecting guinea pigs with viral particles or antigens obtained by high-speed centrifugation. (*c*) Because anti-

gen is between two antibody molecules (unlabeled and labeled). (*d*) Direct RIA. (Sec. 4-34.)

30. (*a*) Different names for the same antigen. (*b*) Hepatitis B surface antigen (HB_SAg). (*c*) The incubation period is long, and donor could have virus in blood without showing symptoms of the disease. (Sec. 4-36.)

31. (*a*) Agar-gel diffusion; counterelectrophoresis; reversed passive hemagglutination, and radioimmunoassay. (*b*) Agar-gel diffusion and counterelectrophoresis. (*c*) Radioimmunoassay. (*d*) Reversed passive hemagglutination. (*e*) Yes. (*f*) In a gamma scintillation counter. (Secs. 4-34 and 4-36.)

Complement-Fixation Test

4-37 The observation that complement enters into reactions between antigens and specific antibodies was used in 1901 by Bordet for the development of a very sensitive serologic test called the complement-fixation (CF) test. Complement-fixation tests are frequently used to diagnose viral, rickettsial, and fungal infections; however, the technique of complement fixation can be used with a wide variety of antigens. The sensitivity of CF tests was compared with that of other serologic tests in Sec. 4-18. The CF test is more sensitive than precipitation tests but less sensitive than agglutination; however, unlike both these tests, the CF test can be used with either soluble or particulate antigens. Complement is not fixed by antigen or antibody alone but by the specific combination of the two. In order to understand this test, one should know a few basic facts about the nature of complement (review complement in Chap. 3). Complement is a humoral factor which, in addition to antibodies, is important in immune reactions. Complement (C′) is composed of nine separate components designated C1, C2, ... C1 consists of three subcomponents, bringing the total number of complement proteins to 11. All components of complement are required for specific lysis of bacteria (bacteriolysis), for specific lysis of red blood cells (hemolysis), and for specific destruction of other cells (cytotoxic reactions). Complement is present in the serum of all warm-blooded animals, and the content of complement in the serum is not increased by immunization. Guinea pig serum is usually employed as a source of complement for CF tests carried out in the laboratory because of the relatively high amount of complement components in serum of this species. Complement is present in serum separated from freshly drawn blood; it is unstable in the refrigerator at 5 to 10°C but is preserved by freezing or (better) lyophilization. Since complement is heat-labile, it can be inactivated by heating serum. The standard procedure for inactivation of complement (or decomplementation of serum) is by heating serum at 56°C for 30 min.

Mechanism of the CF Test

4-38 If antigen and antibody combine in the presence of complement, complement is fixed in the reaction. The antigen can be either particulate or soluble. The only antibodies known to fix complement are those belonging to classes IgG and IgM, the latter being the more efficient. Microorganisms such as fungi, which are not suitable for either agglutination or precipitation tests, can be employed as antigen in the CF test. The CF test combines two distinct reactions, both of which utilize complement. Figure 4-26 gives an outline of the test. The first reaction or main test system does not give a visible reaction; the second reaction, which constitutes the indicator system, does give a visible reaction and indicates whether or not complement was fixed in the first reaction. In the indicator system, when specific antibodies to sheep red blood cells react with sheep red blood cells in the presence of all of the components of complement, small holes are formed in the red-blood-cell membrane, so that hemoglobin leaks out into the surrounding fluid phase to cause a clear red solution. If lysis does not occur, the turbid suspension of cells settles on standing to show a colorless supernate. The CF test is based on the addition of just enough complement (pretitrated) to be completely fixed in one system of the test but not both. Any complement present in the patient's serum is inactivated by heating the serum at 56°C for 30 min. The main test system may consist either of the patient's serum tested for antibody by using a known antigen, as shown in Fig. 4-26, or of a specimen suspected of contain-

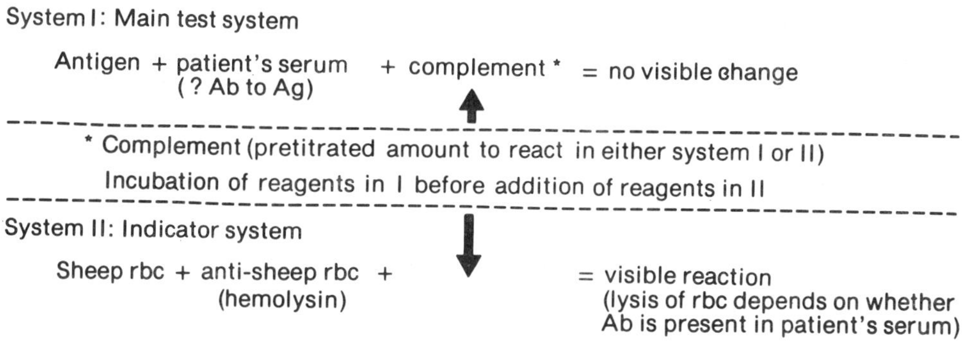

Figure 4-26 Mechanism of CF test, which consists of two different antigen-antibody systems. Complement is fixed in the first system if an antigen-antibody reaction occurs.

ing a certain antigen tested with an antiserum known to contain antibody for that antigen. The CF test is usually carried out with the patient's serum and a known antigen.

4-39 In performing the CF test, a serum control must be run on each patient's serum to show the absence of anticomplementary substances, i.e., those which nonspecifically bind complement. The serum control is set up at the same time as the main test system and contains the same reagents except for antigen. If the serum control binds complement in the absence of antigen, the CF test is not readable. Figure 4-27 represents diagrammatically what happens to complement in positive and negative results of the CF test on sera of patients 1 and 2. For patient 3 the figure shows only the result obtained with the serum control. Since patient 3 has an anticomplementary serum, the test on his serum is not readable because it fixes complement nonspecifically. Anticomplementary activity is not a permanent quality of a patient's serum but may be due to contamination of serum, etc. It is important to collect blood aseptically and to ship it under proper conditions to the laboratory. If the serum is anticomplementary, the laboratory may be able to remove this undesirable activity by various methods, e.g., passage through a Sephadex column. It may be necessary to supply another blood specimen.

Titration of Reagents, Performance of the Test, and Reading Test Results

4-40 The CF test is not difficult to carry out after all the reagents have been titrated. Table 4-2 gives a test procedure. Since all reagents must be titrated with respect to each other, titration can be tedious and time-consuming. It is essential to use the proper amount of antigen if the antibody content of an unknown serum is to be determined. Some antigens are anticomplementary, a fact which must also be determined in advance of the test. The amount of antigen used in the test must meet several criteria: it must be in a sensitive range which can detect minute amounts of antibodies; it should not be anticomplementary or hemolytic; and it should be able to bind all complement in the system if sufficient specific antibodies are present. In Fig. 4-27 the reagents for the indicator system

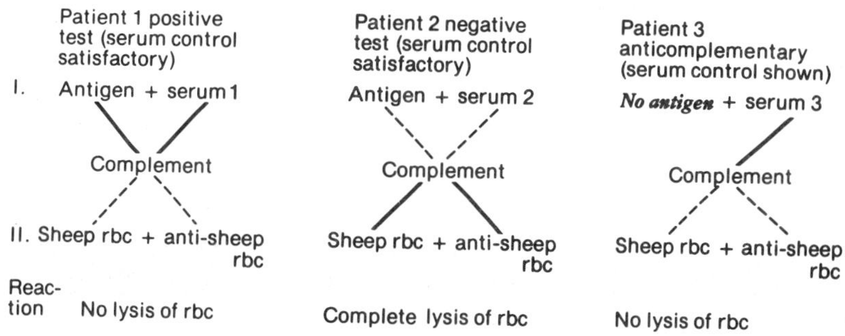

Figure 4-27 Results which may be obtained in a CF test. Solid lines show binding of complement; broken lines indicate combination with complement which might theoretically occur but does not with result obtained.

Table 4-2 Procedure for a CF Test

Tube no.	Patient's serum no.	Amount of serum, ml	Antigen, ml	Complement (2 units), ml	Saline, ml	Anti-sheep rbc, ml	Sheep rbc, ml	Results	Interpretation
1	1	0.2	0.5	1.0	–	0.5	0.5		
1C*	1	0.2	–	1.0	0.5	0.5	0.5		
2	2	0.2	0.5	1.0	–	0.5	0.5		
2C*	2	0.2	–	1.0	0.5	0.5	0.5		
3	3	0.2	0.5	1.0	–	0.5	0.5		
3C*	3	0.2	–	1.0	0.5	0.5	0.5		
	Controls†								
4	Positive serum	0.2	0.5	1.0	–	0.5	0.5		
4C*	Positive serum	0.2	–	1.0	0.5	0.5	0.5		
5	Negative serum	0.2	0.5	1.0	–	0.5	0.5		
5C*	Negative serum	0.2	–	1.0	0.5	0.5	0.5		
6	Antigen	–	0.5	1.0	0.2	0.5	0.5		
7	Hemolytic system	–	–	1.0	0.7	0.5	0.5		
8	Complement	–	–	1.0	1.2	–	0.5		
9	Hemolysin‡	–	–	–	1.7	0.5	0.5		
10	Sheep rbc	–	–	–	2.2	–	0.5		

Incubation (between Saline and Anti-sheep rbc; between Sheep rbc and Results)

Arrangement of tubes in racks with serum control (C) directly behind test

Row	Tests			Controls						
Back	1C	2C	3C	4C	5C					
Front	1	2	3	4	5	6	7	8	9	10

*C = Serum control.

†Antigen control (tube 6) should show that the antigen is not anticomplementary; tube 7 should show that the indicator system is working properly; complement (tube 8) and hemolysin (tube 9) controls should show that these reagents alone are not hemolytic; sheep rbc control (tube 10) should show that the cells are not fragile or lysing spontaneously.

‡Hemolysin = anti-sheep rbc.

were titrated so that complete lysis of the sheep red blood cells was used as the endpoint of the test. Frequently, 50 percent lysis determined photometrically is taken as the endpoint, so that anything less than 50 percent lysis of a standardized amount of red blood cells constitutes a positive reaction. The volume of reagents used for CF tests varies; some tests use only 2 units of complement while others use 3, but the principle of the test remains the same. In the past few years, disposable molded plastic plates (with round-bottom wells) have become commercially available for microtechniques, which have the advantage of conserving reagents and equipment.

Questions for Secs. 4-37 to 4-40

32. (*a*) Is antigen in the CF test soluble or particulate? (*b*) What is complement? (*c*)

How many components of complement are there? (*d*) Are all components of complement required for lysis of red blood cells? (*e*) Name a good source of complement. (*f*) Is complement stable at refrigeration temperature? (*g*) How is complement best preserved? (*h*) What is the procedure for routine inactivation of complement?

33. (*a*) What is the principle of the CF test? (*b*) What are the components of the indicator system? (*c*) What is a specific hemolysin? (*d*) Why are sheep red blood cells used for the indicator system in most CF tests? (*e*) Is the principle of the CF test the same for the wide variety of diseases for which it is used? (*f*) Do all antibodies fix complement? Explain.

34. (*a*) What is an anticomplementary serum? (*b*) Can the CF test be carried out on a patient's serum if the serum is anticomplementary? (*c*) Is it possible to remove the substance(s) causing the serum to be anticomplementary? If so, how?

35. (*a*) What is read as an endpoint for the CF test? (*b*) Why is the CF test a more satisfactory test for fungal infection than precipitation and agglutination? (*c*) Why is the CF test difficult to perform?

36. Table 4-2 shows the procedure for a CF test. (*a*) Assume that the results on patients 1, 2, and 3, respectively, were positive, negative, and anticomplementary. Record the reactions with regard to lysis you would expect to observe for each of these patients if the test had been standardized for complete lysis to represent the test endpoint. (*b*) Assume that all controls were satisfactory and record the results you would expect in tubes 4 to 10.
4 to 10.

Answers

32. (*a*) Antigen may be either soluble or particulate. (*b*) Complement is present in normal serum of warm-blooded animals and takes part in reactions between certain antibodies (IgG and IgM) and the corresponding antigens. (*c*) Nine (C1 to C9), but since C1 has three subcomponents, there are eleven complement proteins. (*d*) Yes. (*e*) Normal guinea pig serum. (*f*) No. (*g*) By lyophilization. (*h*) Heating serum at 56°C for 30 min. (Sec. 4-37.)

33. (*a*) If complement is present when specific antibodies, IgG or IgM, react with antigen, complement will be fixed. Since no visible change occurs, an indicator system is added. Complement must be carefully titrated so that there is only enough present to react in one system, not both. (*b*) Sheep red blood cells and antibodies to sheep red blood cells and complement if it is not fixed in the main test system. (*c*) A specific hemolysin is a specific antibody to red blood cells which causes their lysis in the presence of complement. (*d*) No one is sure why sheep red blood cells were used so extensively by early investigators for the CF test. Since sheep are large animals, they offer a relatively inexpensive source of red blood cells. The system of sheep red blood cells and specific hemolysin has been used for over 50 years, so that it has been well studied and characterized. (*e*) The principle of the CF test is the same regardless of what antigens are being used or diseases diagnosed. (*f*) No, only IgG and IgM. Since IgM structurally is a pentamer, a small amount of IgM is more efficient in binding complement than a small amount of IgG. (Sec. 4-38.)

34. (*a*) A serum which nonspecifically fixes complement in the absence of antigen. (*b*) No. (*c*) In some cases such as by filtration through a Sephadex column. In many cases it is necessary to request another serum specimen. The anticomplementary state is not a permanent quality of a patient's serum but is due to contamination or other substances in the serum. (Sec. 4-39.)

35. (*a*) Lysis, complete or 50 percent (*b*) It is difficult to obtain suitable fungal antigens in a soluble form for precipitation. In the particulate state, they tend to settle out in the absence of specific antibodies. (*c*) All the reagents must be carefully titrated with regard to each other. (Sec. 4-40.)

36. The appropriate reactions for Table 4-2 are as follows:

(*a*) Patient	Lysis	Interpretation	(*b*) Control	Lysis	Interpretation
1	None or partial	Positive	4	None or partial	Positive
1C	Complete		4C	Complete	
2	Complete	Negative	5	Complete	Negative
2C	Complete		5C	Complete	
3	None or partial	Anticomplementary	6	Complete	Satisfactory control
3C	None or partial		7	Complete	Satisfactory control
			8	None	Satisfactory control
			9	None	Satisfactory control
			10	None	Satisfactory control

(Sec. 4-40.)

Immunomicroscopic Tests; Fluorescent-Antibody (FA) Tests

4-41 The technique of *immunofluorescence*, in which antibody molecules are labeled or tagged with a fluorescent dye, was first described by Coons et al, (1942). This technique now is used extensively both for research and diagnosis. A number of fluorescent dyes have been employed, but the most common is fluorescein isothiocyanate (FITC). This dye is used for both the direct and indirect methods. The conjugation of antibodies with dye is a chemical reaction. FITC fluoresces in the ultraviolet wavelength of 550 to 640 nm to give a yellow-green color. Specimens are observed with an ultraviolet-light microscope with a dark-field condenser. For the preparation of labeled antibody, antiserum is obtained by immunization of animals in the usual way. The gamma-globulin fraction of the antiserum is separated by precipitation with ammonium sulfate. After sufficient purification, the gamma-globulin fraction containing antibodies to be labeled is incubated with FITC. Any dye which fails to become conjugated with antibodies is removed. The preparation of labeled antibodies or conjugate is titrated and standardized with the antigen it is supposed to detect and identify.

Direct FA Technique

4-42 The direct FA technique is widely used for the diagnosis of bacterial and fungal infections, autoimmune diseases, etc. Although the indirect method is more frequently used with viral infections (Sec. 4-46), the direct method has been used for a long time for the diagnosis of rabies in animals by examination of impression smears of their brain tissue. The main steps in the direct FA test are as follows: (1) the specimen containing the antigen to be identified is fixed to a slide; (2) antibodies labeled with FITC are added to the slide and allowed to react specifically with antigen; (3) the slide is washed to remove antibodies and serum components not bound to antigen on the slide; and (4) the slide is dried and examined with an ultraviolet-light microscope for yellow-green fluorescence.

4-43 One of the most frequently used direct FA techniques is that for rapid recognition of group A streptococci. Group A streptococci (beta-hemolytic) cause a very severe form of pharyngitis and less frequently other conditions such as scarlet fever and impetigo. Infection with group A streptococci may lead to serious sequelae, e.g., rheumatic fever and glomerulonephritis. It is important for infection with group A streptococci to be recognized as soon as possible and to be properly treated in order to prevent these sequelae. A person with a sore throat can be tested for group A streptococcal infection by making a throat culture and placing the throat swab in broth for growth at 37°C for 2 to 5 h. After incubation, the broth is centrifuged to sediment bacterial cells, and the cells are washed twice in buffered saline. The sediment of cells from the last washing is used to prepare smears of the culture (see Fig. 4-28). The smears are fixed by 95% ethanol. Next FITC-labeled antibodies to group A streptococci are added to the smear and incubated. After incubation, the slide is washed to remove antibodies which did not react with bacteria on the slide. The slide is examined with the ultraviolet-light microscope for fluorescence of streptococci. If streptococci are present which do not belong to group A, they will not show fluorescence. One of the advantages of the FA technique in the diag-

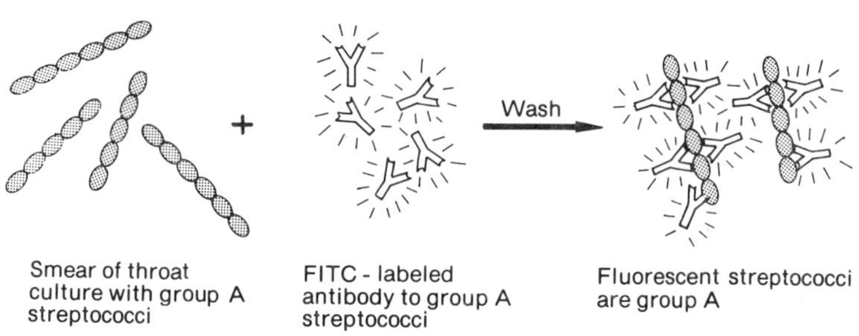

Figure 4-28 Direct FA technique for detection and identification of group A streptococci in patient's throat culture; FITC = fluorescein isothiocyanate.

nosis of bacterial infections is that a report usually can be made much sooner with FA than with the usual culture identification methods.

4-44 For the diagnosis of most viral infections, the indirect method is used; however, with regard to the diagnosis of rabies, the direct FA method has been used successfully for many years to detect foci of rabies-virus infection in animal brain tissue. The direct method can be modified so that inhibition of fluorescence is used as an endpoint rather than fluorescence in a test known as the *rabies fluorescent-focus-inhibition test.* This modification has been used to determine whether or not a patient receiving immunization against rabies has developed a sufficiently high level of protective antibodies. Antibodies in the patient's serum (serially diluted) would combine with rabies virus in brain tissue on a slide and saturate the viral antigens for antibody so that when serum conjugate with labeled antibodies to rabies virus is added, fluorescence is inhibited.

Indirect FA Technique

4-45 The indirect technique is especially useful when patients' sera need to be examined for antibody. It would be very difficult to try to label each patient's serum, as there would probably be insufficient serum for the process; even if there were enough serum, the procedure for conjugating antibodies with dye and appropriately standardizing the conjugate would be tedious. Figure 4-29 illustrates the steps in an indirect FA test; the example used is the *fluorescent Treponema antibody* (FTA) *test* for syphilis. In the indirect method, patient's serum is allowed to react on a slide with the specimen containing antigen; the slide containing the specimen and patient's serum is then thoroughly washed to remove all serum components except antibody bound to antigen. In order to detect antibody bound to antigen, anti-human globulin labeled with FITC is added, incubated, and then washed from the slide. The slide is examined with the ultraviolet-light microscope for yellow-green fluorescence.

4-46 In most cases of examination of tissue for virus, the indirect FA method is considered the more sensitive method, especially if only a small amount of virus is present in the tissue. Most viruses are quite small, so that only a limited number of antibodies can attach to their surface in tissue. The attachment of unlabeled antibodies to virus surface gives a greater surface area for attachment of labeled antibodies (antiglobulin) and therefore a better chance that a small focus of virus infection

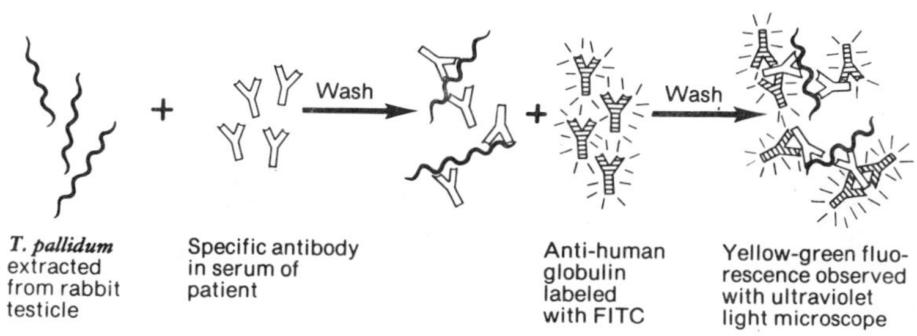

Figure 4-29 FTA test to illustrate the indirect FA technique, in which antiglobulin is labeled with FITC.

will be detected. The indirect FA method is sometimes called a *sandwich technique* (see figure 4-30). Protein molecules such as exotoxin are smaller than the smallest viruses. When exotoxin is produced, it diffuses into the surrounding tissue and does not remain localized, as viruses do, in an area of virus infection in tissue. Although attempts to modify the FA technique so that it can be used for detection and identification of exotoxins in tissue are continuing, technically it has been difficult to get enough labeled antibody on toxin molecules, even by the sandwich technique, to make them visible.

4-47 The FA method is also used in the study of autoimmune diseases and immune-complex diseases to detect antibodies bound to tissue components or the deposition of immune complexes (antigen-antibody aggregates) in tissue. FITC-labeled anti-human globulin is used in a direct FA method for these studies. For example, in Goodpasture's syndrome, antibodies bound to tissue (lung and kidney) show a smooth linear pattern of fluorescence (Chap. 6). In immune-complex diseases, e.g., systemic lupus erythematosus, immune complexes in kidney tissue show an irregular pattern of fluorescence often described as "lumpy bumpy." In addition to labeling antibodies to human globulin, antibodies to human-complement components have been produced, labeled with fluorescent dye, and used to show that complement is bound to tissue in immune reactions.

Immunoenzyme Tests

4-48 Tests have been developed recently in which antibody molecules are labeled with enzymes, e.g., horseradish peroxidase. The immunoperoxidase technique has the advantage that peroxidase-labeled antibodies can be visualized with the light microscope and the preparations are permanent. With some enzyme substrates, electron-dense molecules are produced, so that the technique can also be used with the electron microscope. Enzyme-labeled antibodies can be employed in direct and indirect methods in the same way that fluorescein-labeled antibodies are used with FA tests. Since horseradish peroxidase has a molecular weight of 40,000, there is no problem of penetration within tissues for this enzyme. After reaction of enzyme-labeled antibodies with antigen in tissue, enzyme substrate is added to the tissue. Peroxidase activity can be detected with a number of substrates which yield different colored reaction products. For example a blue reaction product is obtained with benzidine as substrate; brown with 3,3-diaminobenzidine; brown with *o*-dianisidine, and red with α-naphthol. The fine brown precipitate formed by the reaction of enzyme with 3,3-diaminobenzidine is electron-dense and can be used for localization of antigen with both light and electron microscopy. Since benzidine and naphthol are potential carcinogens, their use as enzyme substrates must conform to federal safety regulations. The immunoenzyme test can be applied to the diagnosis of a number of disease states. This technique has been used for the diagnosis of viral infections, e.g., those caused by the herpes group.

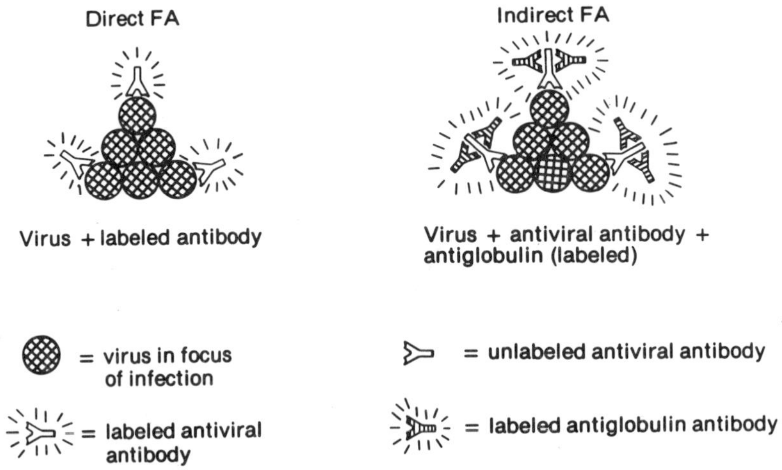

Figure 4-30 Comparison of the direct and indirect FA techniques for detection of a small focus of viral infection in tissue.

Immunoelectronmicroscopy

4-49 An immunoenzyme test which can be used with the electron microscope was described in Sec. 4-48. In another frequently used method antibodies are labeled with ferritin, an electron-dense material. Structures which have reacted with ferritin-labeled antibodies can easily be recognized when sections are viewed with the transmission electron microscope. Recently, antibodies labeled with latex particles have been used in scanning electron microscopy to study surface antigens.

Questions for Secs. 4-41 to 4-49

37. (*a*) Who first described the FA technique? (*b*) What dye is most frequently used to label antibody for diagnostic tests? (*c*) Why must specimens be examined with an ultraviolet-light microscope?

38. (*a*) Is the morphology of bacilli, spirochetes, and streptococci apparent with the direct FA test? (*b*) What test can be used to determine the antibody titer of a person exposed to, and immunized against, rabies?

39. (*a*) Name the main difference or differences between the direct and indirect FA techniques. (*b*) Explain the mechanism of the indirect FTA test for syphilis. (*c*) With regard to the labeling of reagents, what is the advantage of the indirect method?

40. (*a*) Can anything be determined about the morphology of viruses with the FA technique? (*b*) Why is the indirect FA method considered more sensitive for the detection of a small amount of virus in tissue? (*c*) If you are trying to detect the presence of a virus antigen in tissue and you use unlabeled antibody or antiserum prepared in guinea pigs, what kind of antibody do you have to use next in order to determine whether or not the virus is present in the tissue specimen?

41. (*a*) Can the FA test be used to demonstrate the reaction of antibody with tissue in autoimmune diseases? (*b*) What term has been used to describe the appearance of immune complexes in tissue as shown by the FA test? (*c*) How can the fixation of complement to tissue be demonstrated in autoimmune reactions?

42. (*a*) What is the principle of immunomicroscopic enzyme tests used for diagnosis? (*b*) What enzyme is frequently used to label antibodies for these tests? (*c*) What label is electron-dense and is used to label antibodies for electron-microscopy studies?

Answers

37. (*a*) Coons. The test is infrequently called Coons test and should not be confused with the Coombs test. (*b*) Fluorescein isothiocyanate (FITC). (*c*) FITC and other dyes used in the FA test fluoresce in the ultraviolet wavelength. (Sec. 4-41.)

38. (*a*) Yes. (*b*) The rabies fluorescent-focus-inhibition test. (Secs. 4-43 and 4-44.)

39. (*a*) In the direct FA test, antibody to antigen being tested for is labeled; in the indirect test instead of this antibody an antiglobulin antibody which combines with the antibody to antigen is labeled. (*b*) *T. pallidum* spirochetes are fixed on the slide, and the patient's serum is allowed to react with them. The slide is washed, and labeled anti-human globulin is added. If the patient had antibodies to the spirochetes, the antibodies attached to the spirochetes would react with labeled anti-human globulin antibodies. (*c*) It would be very difficult to label each patient's serum, and with the indirect method it is not necessary. When diagnostic sera to many different antigens are used, they need not be labeled if labeled antiglobulin serum to the appropriate animal species is available. (Secs. 4-43 and 4-45.)

40. (*a*) No. The ultraviolet-light microscope can detect areas of virus infection, but the individual virus particles are too small for this microscope to reveal anything about the structure of the virus particle. (*b*) Because with labeled antiglobulin antibodies attached to antibodies which have reacted with virus particles there is a greater area of fluorescence than by the direct method. (*c*) Labeled anti-guinea pig globulin. (Secs. 4-44 and 4-46.)

41. (*a*) Yes. (*b*) Antibodies to tissue such as antibodies to basement membrane cause a fairly smooth pattern of immunofluorescence, but when immune complexes (antigen-antibody aggregates) are deposited in tissue, there is an irregular, or lumpy-bumpy, pattern of fluorescence. (*c*) By using labeled antiserum prepared against complement. (Sec. 4-47.)

42. (*a*) Antibody is labeled with an enzyme which reacts with its substrate added to tissue to give colored reaction products. Thus with the light microscope one can recognize the site where labeled antibody has reacted with antigen. Some reaction products are electron-dense, so that the technique can also be used with the electron microscope. (*b*) Horseradish peroxidase. (*c*) Ferritin. (Secs. 4-48 and 4-49.)

Neutralization

4-50 Neutralization tests include tests for neutralization of bacterial exotoxins and neutralization of viruses. The need to carry out neutralization tests for bacterial exotoxins seldom arises. The Elek test (Sec. 4-26) was designed to detect toxigenic strains of *C. diphtheriae* by in vitro precipitation methods and is usually carried out now for study of toxigenic strains of this organism instead of neutralization tests, such as animal protection tests. In botulism food poisoning, if some of the contaminated food is obtained and an extract of it made, the antigenic type of exotoxin can be determined by neutralization tests in mice with known antitoxin. There are six distinct types of *Clostridium botulinum*, A to F. Since each type produces an antigenically different exotoxin, antitoxin must be prepared against each kind of exotoxin. Polyvalent antiserum or a mixture of antitoxins to different types is available for emergency use. Types A, B, and E are the ones usually associated with human cases. The radioimmunoassay test is also being used now for the detection of *C. botulinum* exotoxin and the determination of antigenic type. In addition to use with toxins, neutralization tests are used for the diagnosis of virus infections. The principle of virus neutralization tests is that specific protective or virus-neutralizing antibodies can be measured by adding serum containing these antibodies to a suspension of virus; after incubation the antibody-virus mixture is inoculated into susceptible experimental animals, embryonated eggs, or tissue-cultured cells, depending on the virus.

Neutralization of Cytopathic Effect in Tissue Culture

4-51 The use of tissue-culture cells in neutralization tests is based on neutralization of cytopathic effect (CPE) caused by the virus and is one of the most frequently used techniques in the diagnosis of viral infections. Cultured cells attach to glass or plastic and then continue to grow, spreading out to form a single layer of cells called a *monolayer*. One kind of CPE on the monolayer is destruction of cells by virus, so that holes appear in the monolayer of cells. Viral antibody specifically neutralizes the virus and prevents CPE. The type of tissue cells used depends on the virus being studied. Not all viruses show a CPE in tissue culture, but many do. Primary cultures of monkey kidney tissue are usually suitable for the study of most human viruses. The amount of virus used is standardized and recorded as $TCID_{50}$ (tissue culture infectious dose). Table 4-3 shows the results of a neutralization test on the paired sera of a patient tested against three known viruses. Since many viruses infect human beings, it is helpful for the physician to give the laboratory some idea what viral infections are suspected from the history of the patient. For paired sera, a specimen is collected when the physician first sees the patient and again about 2 weeks later to allow time for a rise in antibody titer. The neutralization test with paired sera is incubated at 35°C for 4 to 7 days, during which time each tube is examined microscopically for CPE. The controls and each serum dilution should consist of at least four tubes. Table 4-3 shows a significant rise in antobidy titer with virus A. A patient suspected of having poliomyelitis virus would have had to be tested against all three types of poliomyelitis virus. If viruses A, B, and C had been types 1, 2, and 3 poliomyelitis virus, the patient would have type 1 infection. Neutralization tests carried out in tissue culture may be used to diagnose a viral infection either by determination of antibody titers on paired sera using known virus or by specific identification of a virus isolated from the patient using known antisera.

Viruses (virus inoculum = 100 $TCID_{50}$)	Paired sera, days after onset of symptoms	CPE observed with mixtures of virus and patient's serum			
		Dilution of patient's serum			
		1:5	1:25	1:125	1:625
Virus A	1	0000	++++	++++	++++
	15	0000	0000	0000	++++
Virus B	1	++++	++++	++++	++++
	15	00++	++++	++++	++++
Virus C	1	++++	++++	++++	++++
	15	++++	++++	++++	++++
Control (no virus)	1	0000	Not done	Not done	Not done
	15	0000			

Key: TCID = tissue-culture infectious dose; + = CPE; 0 = no CPE; 00++ = two tubes without CPE and two tubes with CPE.

Table 4-3 Principle of Tissue-Culture Neutralization Test for Diagnosis of Viral Infection Using Paired Sera of Patient Tested against Known Viruses

Serologic Tests Frequently Used for Diagnosis of Viral Infections

4-5 Serologic methods which are frequently used in the diagnosis of viral infections are as follows:

Complement-fixation tests, Secs. 4-37 to 4-40

Immunomicroscopic tests:

- Fluorescent antibody tests, Secs. 4-41 to 4-47
- Immunoenzyme tests, Sec. 4-48

Neutralization tests, Sec. 4-51

Passive hemagglutination tests, Secs. 4-16 to 4-19

Radioimmunoassays, Secs. 4-30 to 4-36

Viral hemagglutination-inhibition tests, Secs. 4-53 to 4-55

Viral hemadsorption-inhibition tests, Secs. 4-56

Viral Hemagglutination-Inhibition Test

4-53 The term hemagglutination means agglutination of red blood cells; it is frequently used to refer to passive (indirect) hemagglutination and to viral hemagglutination. Often it is left to the reader to discern which type of hemagglutination is meant. Since passive hemagglutination involves a reaction between antigens (or haptens) and antibodies, it is a serologic test. In contrast, viral hemagglutination is not a serologic test because it involves a reaction only between viruses and red blood cells. Not all viruses will cause hemagglutination. Some viruses, e.g., influenza, find receptors on the surface of the red blood cells similar to tissue receptors and attach to the red blood cells, causing hemagglutination. In this case the virus particle is the hemagglutinin. Other viruses, e.g., vaccinia, produce a soluble substance separable from the virus particle which is responsible for hemagglutination. The virus used in the test determines the species and age of red blood cells to be used. The *hemagglutination-inhibition test,* developed for viruses which cause hemagglutination, is based on the observation that antibody to the virus will inhibit hemagglutination. This test is easy to perform and provides a method of both identifying and titrating antibodies to the virus.

4-54 In order to titrate antibodies to viruses by the hemagglutination-inhibition test, one must have a preparation of the virus and know the amount of virus hemagglutinin present. The hemagglutinin is titrated by making serial dilutions of the virus in phosphate-buffered saline (PBS) and then adding a constant amount of a light suspension of suitable red blood cells (see Fig. 4-31). In viral hemagglutination, the agglutination reaction is often very weak and can best be determined by observing the pattern formed by red blood cells after settling. The pattern on the bottom of the tubes is viewed in a mirror. A positive reaction (tubes 1 to 6) shows diffuse settling of the agglutinated cells on the bottom of the tube, while a negative reaction (tubes 7 to 10) shows the nonagglutinated cells settling in a compact button. Between the two patterns, intermediate stages of partial agglutination can be recognized. Tube 6 contains the highest dilution of virus which causes hemagglutination. This dilution (1:320) contains 1 hemagglutinating (HA) unit of virus. Four HA units, or a dilution of 1:80, of the above virus preparation would be used in the hemagglutination-inhibition test (provided the volume is the same).

4-55 For the hemagglutination-inhibition (HI) test the serum is diluted in PBS from 1:10 to 1:640, and a constant amount of the virus preparation containing 4 HA units is added to each serum dilution. Next a constant amount of a light suspension of suitable red blood cells washed 3 times is added to each tube (see Fig. 4-32). The cells are allowed to settle, and the pattern of sedimented cells is read. The endpoint is the highest dilution of serum inhibiting hemagglutination by the virus. The virus control, tube 8, which contained no serum, showed hemagglutination, as it should have; while the serum control, tube 9, contained no virus and showed that the lowest dilution of serum used (1:10) had no antibodies to red blood cells. The red-blood-cell control, tube 10, contained only red blood cells in PBS and showed no spontaneous hemagglutination. All the controls were satisfactory. The endpoint of the test was read as the highest dilution of the serum which inhibited viral hemagglutination, and this was 1:160 in tube 5. In other words, the antibody titer to the virus was

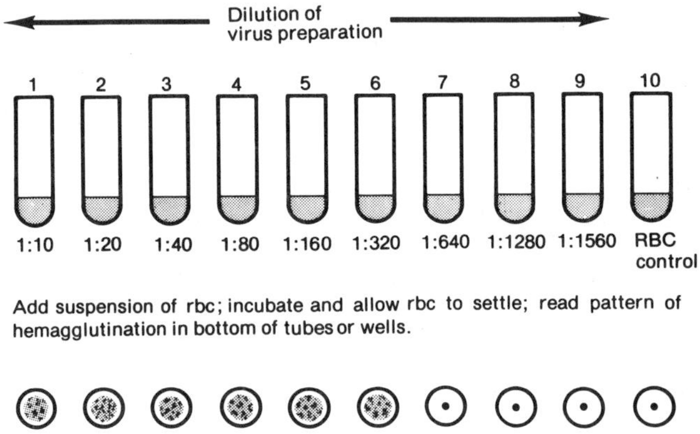

Figure 4-31 Titration of viral hemagglutinins. Results of the titration show that the 1:320 virus dilution contains 1 HA unit of virus.

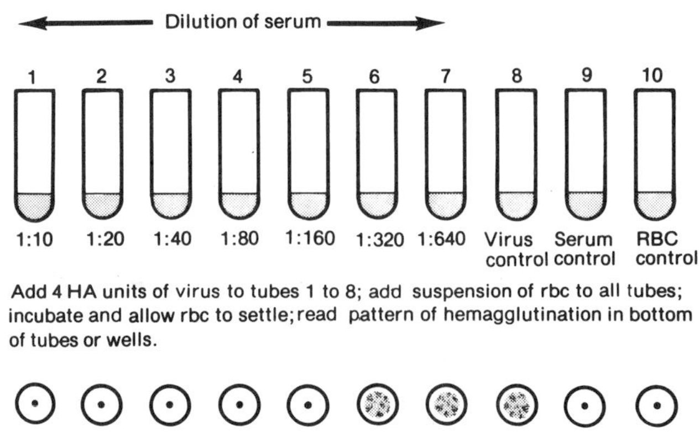

Figure 4-32 Hemagglutination-inhibition test. Results of test show that antibody titer is 1:160.

1:160. The hemagglutination-inhibition test is very valuable because of its high specificity; i.e., it is possible to distinguish antibodies to various substrains or variants of viruses such as the Asian and Victoria variants of type A_2 influenza virus.

Viral Hemadsorption-Inhibition Test

4-56 Some viruses grow in tissue culture but show no CPE such as the destruction of tissue cells. For example, influenza virus grows in monolayers of chicken fibroblasts without showing any characteristic CPE. Influenza viruses "bud," or are shed from the cell membrane, while the tissue-cultured monolayer remains intact. It was pointed out in Sec. 4-53 that certain red blood cells have receptors for virus which are responsible for hemagglutination. These same receptors are responsible for hemadsorption in tissue culture. When a washed light suspension of red blood cells is added to a monolayer infected with influenza virus, the red blood cells adhere to areas of virus infection. The adsorbed red blood cells are not removed by washing and can be observed with the light microscope. The specificity of this reaction can be determined by hemadsorption inhibition. If specific antiserum to the virus is added first to the infected monolayer, virus at the surface of the cells is neutralized so that hemadsorption does not occur on addition of red blood cells.

Miscellaneous Serologic Diagnostic Tests

4-57 A serologic test known as the *enzyme linked immunosorbent assay* (ELISA) was developed in 1972 and is now being applied to the diagnosis of many different disease states. Like many other tests presented in this chapter, this test can be carried out in wells of microtiter plastic trays. The principle of the test is shown diagrammatically in Fig. 4-33. Alkaline phosphatase is one of the enzymes which has been used to label antibodies directed to globulin. The enzyme is bound to antibody in such a way that enzymic activity is not affected. The enzyme substrate is *p*-nitrophenylphosphate. Results of enzymic hydrolysis are read in a spectrophotometer. The amount of antibody present in the patient's serum is directly proportional to the amount of substrate hydrolyzed by enzyme.

4-58 The *antistreptolysin O* (ASO) titration has been frequently used to diagnose conditions associated with such group A beta-hemolytic streptococci infections as rheumatic fever and glomerulonephritis. Streptolysin is a protein metabolic product excreted by beta-hemolytic streptococci. Since streptolysin is antigenic, patients develop antibodies to it. Streptolysin is a nonspecific hemolysin in that it is not an antibody and causes lysis of many different kinds of red blood cells. A suspension of 5 percent rabbit cells is used in this test. Suitable dilutions of the patient's serum are made and added to a commercial preparation of streptolysin O. After incubation, the suspension of red blood cells is added. If a patient has antibodies to streptolysin, the hemolytic property is neutralized and lysis of red blood cells does not occur. The endpoint, or antibody titer, is read as the highest dilution of patient's serum causing complete inhibition of lysis of red blood cells.

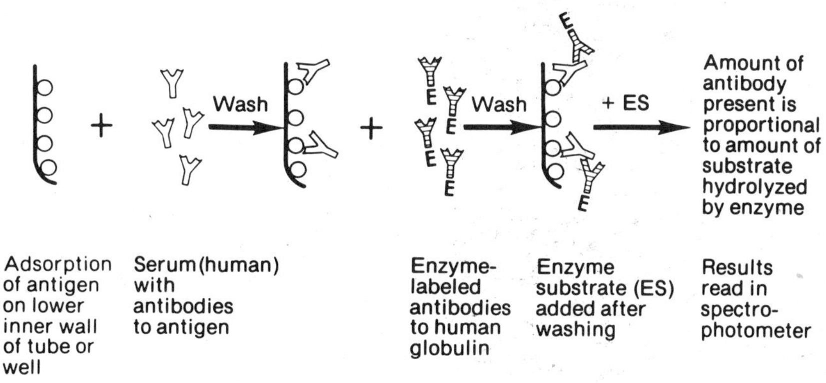

Figure 4-33 Principle of ELISA assay.

4-59 The *Quellung reaction*, or test, for capsular swelling is based on the observation that after reaction with specific antibodies, the capsule of encapsulated organisms such as pneumococci and meningococci appears enlarged compared with that of controls. This test is of historical interest because before the discovery of antibiotics, it was used to type pneumococci for administration of pneumococal antisera. This test is still used in laboratory diagnosis, e.g., to determine the antigenic types of certain encapsulated organisms like those mentioned above and also *Hemophilus influenzae.* Meningitis caused by *H. influenzae* is most frequently caused by the type b strain. The determination of serologic type is of epidemiological importance and helps confirm identification of the organism.
4-60 *Cytotoxic tests* used for tissue typing are described in Chap. 9. In one kind of cytotoxic test, the *dye-exclusion test,* when a suspension of intact viable cells is exposed to vital dyes, such as trypan blue or eosin Y, these dyes are excluded from the cells. In contrast, the dyes are taken up by dead or damaged cells which have previously reacted with specific antibodies and complement.

Skin Tests

4-61 Skin tests are useful diagnostic aids. Unlike most other tests described in this section, skin tests are carried out in vivo. The three main types of skin tests employed today are (1) those based on neutralization of exotoxin, (2) those based on immediate-type hypersensitivity skin reactions, and (3) those based on delayed-type hypersensitivity skin reactions. The basic immune mechanism underlying each type of test will be described with some examples indicating the use of each type. Regardless of the type of test carried out, antigen is usually injected intradermally (intracutaneously) in order to hold the antigen in a circumscribed area. The formation of a bleb at the injection site indicates that the test was carried out properly. A skin-test needle (3/8 in. case, 26 guage) is used, and generally no more than an 0.1 ml is injected (see Fig. 4-34). There are two other methods for skin testing. In the *scratch test*, antigen is placed on the skin, and then the antigen is scratched into the skin. In the *patch test*, a piece of material containing antigen is taped to the skin.
4-62 Neutralization of exotoxin Examples of skin tests based on neutralization of exotoxin are the *Schick test,* for susceptibility to diphtheria, and the *Dick test,* for susceptibility to scarlet fever. The Dick test is seldom used. For immunized children to be resistant to diphtheria, they must have a certain level of antitoxin to neutralize diphtheria exotoxin. To carry out the Schick test, exotoxin is injected in an amount equal to 1/50 MLD (minimum lethal dose) for 250-g guinea pigs. Diphtheria toxin is a dermonecrotic toxin; if unneutralized, it causes reddening of the skin followed by a brownish desquamation. The effect of the toxin does not become apparent for several hours, and then the reaction develops in intensity over a period of several days. This type of reaction is read as positive and indicates that antibody (antitoxin) was not present to neutralize the toxin. If no reaction is observed, the test is read as negative, indicating that the toxin injected was neutralized by antibody.
4-63 Immediate-type hypersensitivity (allergic) reaction This type of skin test is used to test for hypersensitivity to foreign protein in biological preparations of antibodies (other than human antitoxin or human antiserum), e.g., foreign antiserum to rabies virus for passive immunization. This type of skin test is also used to determine what allergens are responsible for atopy. A positive reaction, characterized by the *wheal-and-flare* (erythema) *reaction,* shows a small area of circumscribed edema (the wheal) surrounded by spreading erythema (the flare). A positive reaction appears in 15 to 30 min and disappears in a few hours. A positive immediate allergic skin test is due to a reaction between antigen and antibody (IgE attached to tissue), in which histamine or substances similar in action

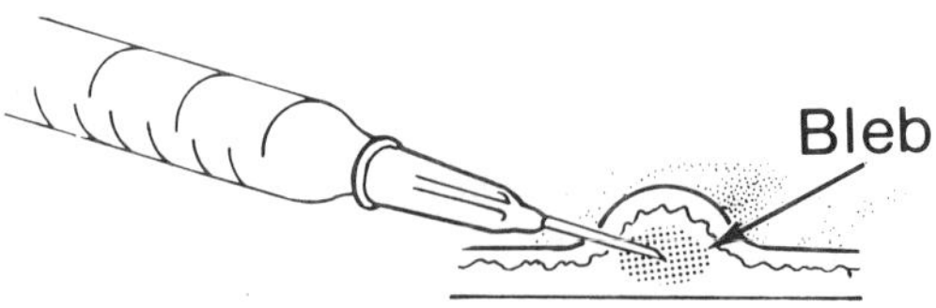

Figure 4-34 Intracutaneous injection of skin-test antigen should show a bleb at the injection site.

are released. If no reaction is observed, the test is read as negative, indicating that antibody is absent and the person is not sensitive to the skin-test material. The immediate-type hypersensitivity (allergic) skin reaction is also called *cutaneous anaphylaxis.* The Prausnitz-Küstner (PK) test is based on the same mechanism, but in this test the serum of the patient is transferred to the skin of a nonallergic individual, time is allowed for IgE to attach to mast cells, and then antigen is injected. This test is seldom performed now because of the danger of transferring hepatitis viruses.

4-64 Delayed-type hypersensitivity (allergic) reaction Skin tests for infectious diseases (bacterial, viral, or fungal) are of this type. The reaction is read in 48 h. A positive reaction shows erythema, induration, and sometimes necrosis. A positive reaction is brought on by sensitized lymphocytes and indicates previous or present infection. Examples of frequently used skin tests are the tuberculin test and the skin test for exposure to histoplasmosis. The skin-test material may be a suspension of the microorganism (usually inactivated) or an extract or metabolic product of the organism.

4-65 In some skin tests a combination of immediate and delayed types of sensitivity reactions may be observed. In addition to the three basic immune mechanisms underlying skin tests cited in Sec. 4-61, another mechanism which may be involved is the *Arthus reaction* (Chap. 5), which is caused by the formation of immune complexes in the presence of complement. Skin-test reactions due to the Arthus reaction develop in 7 to 8 h and become resolved in about 36 to 48 h. The Arthus type of skin reaction is usually large, erythematous, soft, and edematous with an ill-defined margin. In some cases there may be central induration with limited evidence of hemorrhage. Antigens which may give this type of skin reaction are heterologous serum proteins, extracts of tissue, extracts of helminths such as ascaris, and extracts of microorganisms such as fungi.

Questions for Secs. 4-50 to 4-65

43. Do specific antibodies effectively neutralize (*a*) exotoxins, (*b*) endotoxins, (*c*) viruses?

44. Besides neutralization tests, what serologic tests are currently used for detection of (*a*) production of exotoxin by a strain of *C. diphtheriae,* (*b*) presence of botulism toxin in food?

45. Viruses are propagated only in living cells; name three cell systems which are used for virus-neutralization tests.

46. (*a*) To what does cytopathic effect (CPE) in tissue culture refer? (*b*) How is neutralization in tissue culture carried out? (*c*) Why is tissue culture used so extensively now for neutralization tests instead of experimental animals or embryonated eggs?

47. (*a*) Do all viruses cause hemagglutination? (*b*) If a virus does not cause hemagglutination, can it be used in the viral hemagglutination-inhibition test? (*c*) Do viruses which cause hemagglutination agglutinate red blood cells of any animal species and of any age? (*d*) Is viral hemagglutination caused by a reaction with antibody? (*e*) What is the hemagglutinin which holds the red blood cells together in this test?

48. (*a*) How is 1 HA (hemagglutinating) unit of virus determined? (*b*) Is it possible by the viral hemagglutination-inhibition test to determine the specificity of the antibody to the virus and also to titrate the amount of antibody in the serum?

49. (*a*) If a virus does not cause hemagglutination, can the passive hemagglutination test be used to identify and titrate antibodies to the virus? (*b*) What are some other serologic tests used for diagnosis of viral infections?

50. (*a*) If a virus such as influenza does not cause a cytopathic effect in tissue culture, how can the area of viral infection be detected? (*b*) Could the method just cited be used with virus which does not cause hemagglutination? (*c*) How can the specificity of the reaction be determined?

51. (*a*) What is the ELISA test? (*b*) How is this test read? (*c*) Does the linking of enzyme to antibody affect enzyme activity?

52. (*a*) What test is used to determine whether or not infection has recently occurred with group A beta-hemolytic streptococci? (*b*) What test can be used to determine the

serologic type of an organism which is encapsulated? (*c*) In the dye-exclusion test, is trypan blue excluded by living or dead cells?

53. (*a*) What substance is used as antigen for the Schick test? (*b*) If a child has a positive Schick test, does this indicate that the child, if exposed, would be resistant or susceptible to diphtheria?

54. (*a*) A child who has diphtheria is being skin-tested before administration of diphtheria antitoxin produced in horses to see whether or not she is sensitive to horse protein. Human diphtheria antitoxin was not available at the time. She shows a positive skin reaction with horse serum diluted 1:100. Does this mean that she is sensitive to a component of the antitoxin? (*b*) What chemical substance is released and is responsible for a positive reaction? (*c*) What is the basis of the PK test? (*d*) What risk is associated with performance of the PK test?

55. (*a*) A person has a positive tuberculin reaction. Does this mean that he has tuberculosis? (*b*) What mechanism is responsible for a positive delayed allergic reaction?

Answers

43. (*a*) Yes. (*b*) No. (*c*) Yes. (Sec. 4-50.)

44. (*a*) Elek test (agar-gel diffusion precipitation test). (*b*) Radioimmunoassay. (Sec. 4-50.)

45. Intact animals, embryonated eggs, and tissue culture. (Sec. 4-50.)

46. (*a*) CPE refers to damage to cells in tissue culture. CPE caused by some viruses is characteristic for the virus. (*b*) If virus is mixed with antibody, the mixture incubated, and then inoculated into test tubes or bottles containing tissue-cultured cells, CPE does not occur if the virus has been neutralized. Control tubes of cells containing only virus show CPE. Control tubes of cells with no virus show no CPE. (*c*) It is easier and more economical because each tube or bottle of cultured cells is equivalent to an experimental animal or embryonated egg. Although not all viruses grow in all tissue cells, most viruses grow in tissue culture provided the appropriate tissue is used. (Sec. 4-51.)

47. (*a*) No. (*b*) No. (*c*) No, both species and age are important. For example, only 1-day-old chicken cells are used in the viral hemagglutination-inhibition test for German measles virus (rubella). (*d*) No. (*e*) Virus or soluble antigen of virus. Viral hemagglutination is used to titrate virus but is not a serologic test. Viral hemagglutination-inhibition is a serologic test. (Sec. 4-53.)

48. (*a*) 1 HA unit is the highest dilution of virus which agglutinates a standard amount of red blood cells. The virus preparation is titrated by making serial twofold dilutions of virus and then adding red blood cells. (*b*) Yes. (Secs. 4-54 and 4-55.)

49. (*a*) Yes, with many viruses. (*b*) In addition to passive hemagglutination and hemagglutination inhibition, other tests which may be used are complement fixation, fluorescent-antibody tests (direct and indirect), immunoenzyme tests, neutralization, radioimmunoassay, and viral hemadsorption inhibition. (Sec. 4-52.)

50. (*a*) By hemadsorption of the appropriate red blood cells. (*b*) No. (*c*) By hemadsorption inhibition. (Sec. 4-56.)

51. (*a*) ELISA stands for enzyme-linked immunosorbent assay. Antigen is adsorbed onto the lower inner wall of a test tube or well in a plastic tray. Combination of specific antibody with antigen is determined after washing by the addition of enzyme-linked antiglobulin. (*b*) Enzyme substrate is added, and the amount of substrate hydrolyzed by enzyme is read in a spectrophotometer. (*c*) No. (Sec. 4-57.)

52. (*a*) Antistreptolysin O (ASO) titration. (*b*) Quellung reaction, or swelling of the capsule in specific antiserum. (*c*) Living cells. (Secs. 4-58 to 4-60.)

53. (*a*) Toxin, not toxoid, is used for antigen. (*b*) A positive test indicates that the action of the toxin was not neutralized and the child would be susceptible. (Sec. 4-62.)

54. (*a*) Yes, she is sensitive to horse protein in the antitoxin. (*b*) Histamine is released when IgE bound to tissue mast cells reacts with antigen. (*c*) The PK (Prausnitz-Küstner test) is an immediate-type allergic reaction; serum of the patient is passively transferred to the skin of a nonallergic donor. After allowing time for IgE to become attached to donor skin, antigen is injected at the same site. (*d*) One of the hepatitis viruses may be transferred with the patient's serum. (Sec. 4-63.)

55. (*a*) A positive tuberculin reaction indicates either disease or previous exposure without disease. (*b*) Reaction of sensitized lymphocytes with skin-test antigen is responsible for a positive test. (Sec. 4-64.)

REFERENCES

Ackroyd, J. F. (1964): "Immunological Methods," Blackwell, Oxford.

Addison, G. M., and C. N. Hales (1975): Radioactive Immunoassay, pp. 259-281 in P. H. Gell, R. R. A. Coombs, and P. J. Lackmann (eds.), "Clinical Aspects of Immunology," 3d ed., Blackwell, Oxford.

Backhausz, R., and K. Merētey (1974): Antigen-Antibody Reactions *in Vitro*, pp. 439-537 in E. Rajka and S. Korossy (eds.), "Immunological Aspects of Allergy and Allergic Diseases," vol. 2, "Methods in Experimental Immunology," Plenum, London.

Benjamin, D. R. (1975): Use of Immunoperoxidase for Rapid Viral Diagnosis, pp. 89-96 in D. Schlessinger (ed.), "Microbiology: 1975," American Society for Microbiology, Washington, D.C.

Blumberg, B. S. (1964): Polymorphisms of the Serum Proteins and the Development of Isoprecipitins in Transfused Patients, *Bull. N. Y. Acad. Med.*, **40**:377-386.

Boyden, S. V. (1951): The Adsorption of Proteins on Erythrocytes Treated with Tannic Acid and Subsequent Hemagglutination by Antiprotein Sera, *J. Exp. Med.*, **93**:107-120.

Bussard, A. (1959): Descriptions d'une technique combinant simultanēment l'elēctrophorēse et la precipitation immunologique dans un gel: l'ēlectrosynērēse, *Biochim. Biophys. Acta*, **34**: 258-260.

Campbell, D. H., J. S. Garvey, M. E. Cremer, and D. H. Sussdorf (1970): "Methods in Immunology," 2d ed., Benjamin, New York.

Carpenter, P. L. (1975): "Immunology and Serology," 3d ed., Saunders, Philadelphia.

Cherry, W. B., and M. D. Moody (1965): Fluorescent-Antibody Techniques in Diagnostic Bacteriology, *Bacteriol. Rev.*, **29**:222-250.

Coombs, R. R. A., A. E. Mourant, and R. R. Race (1945): Detection of Weak and "Incomplete" Rh Agglutinins: A New Test, *Lancet*, **1945**(2):15-16.

Coons, A. H., H. J. Creech, and R. N. Jones (1941): Immunological Properties of an Antibody Containing a Fluorescent Group, *Proc. Soc. Exp. Biol. Med.*, **47**:200-202.

——, ——, ——, and E. Berliner (1942): The Demonstration of Pneumococcal Antigen in Tissues by the Use of Fluorescent Antibody, *J. Immunol.*, **45**:159-170.

Davidson, I., and J. B. Henry (1974): "Todd-Sanford Clinical Diagnosis by Laboratory Methods," 15th ed., Saunders, Philadelphia.

Elek, S. D. (1948): The Recognition of Toxigenic Strains *in Vitro*, *Br. Med. J.*, **1**:493-496.

Engvall, E., and P. Perlmann (1972): Enzyme-linked Immunosorbent Assay (ELISA): Quantitation of Specific Antibodies by Enzyme-labeled Anti-immunoglobulin in Antigen Coated Tubes, *J. Immunol.*, **109**:129-135.

Freifelder, D. (1976): "Physical Biochemistry: Application to Biochemistry and Molecular Biology," Freeman, San Francisco.

Gocke, D. J., and C. Howe. (1970): Rapid Detection of Australia Antigen by Counterimmunoelectrophoresis, *J. Immunol.*, **104**:1031-1032.

Grabar, P., and C. A. Williams, Jr. (1953): Mēthodes permettant l'ētude conjugēe des propriētēs ēlectrophorētiques et immunochimiques d'une mēlange de protēines: application au serum sanguin, *Biophys. Acta*, **10**:193-194.

Kabat, E. A., and M. M. Mayer (1961): "Experimental Immunochemistry," 2d ed., Thomas, Springfield, Ill.

Kofman, S. (1971): "Radioimmunoassays: Abbott Programmed Learning Course," Abbott Laboratories, North Chicago, Ill.

Kwapinski, J. B. G. (1972): "Methodology of Immunochemical and Immunological Research," Wiley-Interscience, New York.

Laurell, C. B. (1966): Quantitative Estimation of Proteins by Electrophoresis in Agarose Gel Containing Antibodies, *Anal. Biochem.*, **15**:45-52.

Lewis, J. H., and J. E. Coram (1972): Australia Antigen Detection: Comparison of Results Obtained with Five CEP and One RIA Test Systems, *Transfusion*, **12**:301-305.
Mancini, G., A. O. Carbonara, and J. F. Heremans (1965): Immunochemical Quantitation of Antigens by Single Radial Immunodiffusion, *Immunochemistry*, **2**:235-254.
Miller, W. V. (ed.) (1974): "Technical Methods and Procedures of the American Association of Blood Banks," American Association of Blood Banks, Washington, D.C.
Nakamura, R. M. (ed.) (1974): "Immunopathology, Clinical Laboratory Concepts and Methods," Little, Brown, Boston.
Nakamura, S. (1966): "Crossed Electrophoresis: Its Principles and Applications," Elsevier, New York.
Ouchterlony, Ö (1949): Antigen-Antibody Reactions in Gels, *Acta Path. Microbiol. Scand.*, **26**: 507-515.
——(1958): Diffusion-in-Gel Methods for Immunological Analysis, *Progr. Allergy*, **5**:1-78.
Pepys, J. (1975): Skin Tests in Diagnosis, pp. 55-80 in P. H. Gell, R. R. A. Coombs, and P. J. Lackmann (eds.), "Clinical Aspects of Immunology," 3d ed., Blackwell, Oxford.
Ritzmann, S. E., and J. C. Daniels (1975): "Serum Protein Abnormalities, Diagnostic and Clinical Aspects," Little, Brown, Boston.
Rose, N. R., and H. Friedman (1976): "Manual of Clinical Immunology," American Society for Microbiology, Washington, D.C.
Shulman, N. R. (1970): Hepatitis-associated Antigen, *Am. J. Med.*, **49**:669-692.
Singer, S. J., and A. F. Schick (1961). The Properties of Specific Stains for Electron Microscopy Prepared by the Conjugation of Antibody Molecules with Ferritin, *J. Biophys. Biochem. Cytol.*, **9**:519-537.
Sutnick, A. I. (1973): Australia Antigen: Progress Report, *Med. Clin. North Am.*, **57**:1029-1043.
Tests for Hepatitis B Surface Antigens (1975): *Fed. Regist.*, **40**(136):29706-29710.
Thompson, R. A. (ed.) (1977): "Techniques in Clinical Immunology," Blackwell, Oxford.
Voller, A., C. C. Drapes, D. E. Bidwell, and A. Barttlett (1975): Microplate Enzyme-linked Immunosorbent Assay for Chagas Disease, *Lancet*, **1975**(1):426-429.
Weir, D. M. (ed.) (1977): "Handbook of Experimental Immunology," 3d ed., Blackwell, Oxford.
Wilson, G. S., and A. Miles (eds.) (1975): "Topley and Wilson's Principles of Bacteriology and Immunology," vol. 1, Williams & Wilkins, Baltimore.
Yalow, R. S., and S. A. Berson (1973): Big, Big Insulin, *Metabolism*, **22**:703-713.

5

Hypersensitivity: Immediate and Delayed Types

HYPERSENSITIVITY AND ALLERGY

Explanation of Terms

5-1 For many years after the discovery by Jenner in 1798 and Pasteur in 1881 that immunization can confer protection on the host, the immune response was viewed as an entirely favorable event for the host. When it was later shown by a number of investigators that the injection of foreign proteins (usually soluble proteins) can elicit a very unfavorable response in the host and even cause death, the term *allergy* was introduced. The word is derived from two Greek words, *allos*, which means "other" or "altered," and *ergon*, which means "work" or "effect." The antigen responsible for initiating an allergic response is often referred to as an *allergen*. Although the word allergy was originally introduced to refer to altered reactivity on the part of the host, it is often used now as if it were synonymous with hypersensitivity. *Hypersensitivity* is a state of increased reactivity. The process by which an individual becomes hypersensitive is usually called sensitization in preference to immunization, since the latter term has the connotation of resistance. *Hyposensitivity* is a state of decreased reactivity, and *anergy* is a state in which a previously sensitized host shows no kind of allergic response on exposure to the allergen.

5-2 The terms immediate and delayed were originally used to differentiate between allergies in which the onset of symptoms appeared within a short time, say minutes, after exposure to antigen and those in which onset was delayed by several hours or even days. It was found that the time of onset can be misleading. Now the terms immediate and delayed are used to refer mainly to different mechanisms; the immediate type is caused by reactions between antigens and antibodies, so that immediate hypersensitivity is transferable to an appropriate host by injection of serum containing the antibodies. The delayed type is cell-mediated, is caused by a reaction of sensitized lymphocytes with antigen, and is not transferable by injection of serum. Other differences between immediate and delayed types of hypersensitivity reactions were discussed in Chap. 2 and will be discussed again later in this chapter. Although anaphylactic shock, atopy, and the Arthus reaction are all examples of antibody-mediated reactions, anaphylactic shock and atopy are caused by IgE attached to tissue mast cells in the affected organ while the Arthus reaction is caused by the formation of immune complexes or precipitates of IgG or IgM and antigen. IgE antibodies are often referred to as reagins (IgE reagins should not be confused with Wassermann antibodies of syphilis, also called reagins, see Chap. 11).

Types I to IV: Classification of Immune Reactions Which Produce Tissue Damage

5-3 In 1963 Coombs and Gell proposed a classification of what they considered to be the four main types of reactions by which an animal or individual sensitized by a previous exposure to an antigen or allergen may react and show symptoms of clinical hypersensitivity. Types I, II, and III are antibody-mediated, and type IV is cell-mediated by activated or sensitized lymphocytes or by lymphokines produced by them. In cases of clinical hypersensitivity, one or more types of reactions may be responsible for the condition of the patient. The classification of Coombs and Gell is primarily a classification of initiating mechanisms and not a classification of diseases.

5-4 *Type I reactions* (*IgE-dependent*) are brought on when antigen reacts with IgE bound to tissue mast cells or blood basophils, to cause degranulation of these cells and release of vasoactive amines such as histamine. Examples are atopy and both systemic and cutaneous anaphylaxis.

5-5 *Type II reactions* (*cytotoxic or cell-stimulating*) are brought about when IgG or IgM antibody reacts with antigenic components of a cell or with antigens and haptens bound to a cell. Cell damage usually occurs in the presence of complement but in some cases may occur in the absence of complement due to the action of K cells (non-T lymphocytes), which react with IgG antibody bound to target cells to bring about cytolysis [called antibody-dependent cytolysis (ADC)] (see Chaps. 9 and 10). K cells, which are found in peripheral blood, have Fc receptors for IgG. Transfusion reactions to ABO and Rh incompatibility are examples of cytotoxic reactions. Cell lysis due to ABO incompatibility occurs in the presence of complement. Sensitized Rh-positive cells appear not to undergo lysis in the presence of complement but are destroyed after phagocytosis. In still other cases, antibodies may react with cells and cause their stimulation. For example, a protein called *long-acting thyroid stimulator* (LATS) is thought to be an autoantibody which reacts with cells of the thyroid gland and leads to excessive hormone excretion.

5-6 *Type III reactions* (*damage by immune complexes*) are brought about when there is a sufficient amount of circulating precipitating antibodies to cause the formation of aggregates with antigen, usually in the zone of antigen excess. Tissue damage is caused when these aggregates or complexes are formed in the presence of complement and leukocytes and the complexes are deposited in blood-vessel walls or in the basement membrane of tissue. Host reaction, ranging from transient infiltration of polymorphonuclear leukocytes to extensive vascular thrombosis and local necrosis, is related to the extent of formation of soluble complexes. Anaphylatoxins and other substances are released which cause injury to bystander cells. Examples of allergic conditions brought on by in vivo formation of immune complexes are the Arthus reaction and serum sickness. When complexes of any antigen-antibody ratio lodge in biological filtration membranes, e.g., glomerular basement membrane of the kidney, function is affected.

5-7 *Type IV reactions (delayed-type hypersensitivity, cellular hypersensitivity, or cell-mediated allergy)* are brought on by reaction of activated or sensitized lymphocytes with antigen. Many different kinds of substances known as *lymphokines* may be released, so that these reactions can also be described as lymphokine-mediated. Mechanisms associated with delayed-type hypersensitivity were discussed in Chap. 2. Histologically type IV reactions show infiltration of predominantly mononuclear cells although even in mild reactions, polymorphonuclear leukocytes may also be present. Examples of type IV reactions are the Koch phenomenon, the positive tuberculin skin-test reaction, rejection of tissue transplants, some kinds of autoimmune diseases, and immune surveillance against cancer (Sec. 10-1).

5-8 Some immunologists feel that the four types of reactions described by Coombs and Gell do not completely cover the mechanisms responsible for tissue damage. In an article by Myrvik et al. (1975) objections were raised to the classification of Coombs and Gell because although it differentiates between bystander- (type III) and target-cell injury (type II) mediated by humoral antibody reactions, it fails to make this distinction in cell-mediated hypersensitivity reactions (type IV). Myrvik et al. propose the classification below, which adds three more types of reactions to give a total of seven. The seventh type had been proposed before by Riott (as type V) and was included by Coombs and Gell in their type II mechanism.

1. Immediate hypersensitivity (anaphylactic, PK, atopic)
2. Target-cell injuries by immunoglobulins (antigen intrinsic to target cell)
3. Immune-complex injury (injury to bystander cells)
4. Cell-mediated hypersensitivity (target-cell injury; antigen intrinsic to target cell)
5. Cell-mediated hypersensitivity (bystander-cell injury)
6. Blocking or neutralization of a critical hormone or metabolite
7. Stimulation of cell

Target cells are cells which react directly with antibodies or sensitized T lymphocytes. *Bystander cells* do not act directly with antibodies or sensitized T lymphocytes but are injured or destroyed by products released as a result of immune reactions.

Questions for Secs. 5-1 to 5-8

1. (*a*) By derivation, what does allergy mean? (*b*) By derivation, is allergy synonymous with hypersensitivity? (*c*) By usage, is allergy often used synonymously with hypersensitivity? (*d*) What is anergy?

2. (*a*) Is the main difference between immediate and delayed types of hypersensitivity in the time of appearance of the reactions? (*b*) If your answer to part (*a*) is no, name the main difference(s). (*c*) Anaphylactic shock and the Arthus reaction are antibody-mediated, but the underlying mechanisms are different. What mechanisms are involved?

3. (*a*) What reactions concerned with cell damage are classified as type II by Coombs and Gell? (*b*) Do these reactions require complement?

4. (*a*) What is the type III reaction described by Coombs and Gell? Does this reaction require complement?

5. (*a*) What are target cells? (*b*) What are bystander cells?

Answers

1. (*a*) Altered reactivity. (*b*) No. (*c*) Yes. (*d*) Anergy is the lack of any kind of allergic response in a previously sensitized individual. (Sec 5-1.)

2. (*a*) No. (*b*) In the basic mechanisms responsible for the reactions; immediate-type hypersensitivity is antibody-mediated; delayed-type hypersensitivity is cell-mediated or mediated by release of lymphokines. (*c*) Anaphylactic shock is brought on by reaction of antigen with IgE antibodies bound to tissue mast cells and blood basophils to release vasoactive amines such as histamine; the Arthus reaction is caused by the formation of immune complexes in the presence of complement and neutrophils. (Secs. 5-2, 5-4, and 5-6.)

3. (*a*) Antibody-mediated cytotoxic reactions. (*b*) Many but not all type II reactions require complement. (Sec. 5-5.)

4. (*a*) Tissue damage due to the formation of immune complexes. (*b*) Yes, complement is bound in the immune complexes. During activation of complement, anaphylatoxins are released. Complement also has chemotactic properties which attract neutrophils. The accumulation of neutrophils can cause tissue damage. (Sec. 5-6.)

5. (*a*) Target cells are cells which react directly with antibodies or sensitized lymphocytes. (*b*) Bystander cells are cells which do not act directly with antibodies or sensitized lymphocytes but which are nearby and may be injured or destroyed by products released as a result of immune reactions. (Sec. 5-8.)

ANTIBODY-MEDIATED AND IMMEDIATE-TYPE HYPERSENSITIVITY REACTIONS

Anaphylactic Shock (Systemic Anaphylaxis)

5-9 By derivation *anaphylaxis* means "against protection" (*ana-* means "against" and *phylaxis* means "protection"). Anaphylactic shock is commonly demonstrated for a student experiment by the injection of horse serum into guinea pigs. When horse serum is injected into a guinea pig, the first injection appears harmless to the animal; in contrast, a second injection made intravenously 14 days later will kill the guinea pig. This simple experiment illustrates the elements necessary for anaphylactic shock, which are (1) sensitizing exposure, (2) period during which antibodies are formed and attach to tissue mast cells, and (3) a challenging injection made in such a way that antigen enters the circulation and there is a rapid reaction between antigen and antibody attached to tissue cells. The guinea pig shows extreme difficulty in breathing and dies within a few minutes. If this animal is autopsied, the lungs are found to be greatly distended with air because the animal was able to suck in air but was not able to expel it due to contraction of smooth muscles in the bronchioles. Manifestations of anaphylactic shock vary with different animal species, depending on the principal site of reaction or shock organ.

5-10 Antibodies attached to tissue cells are called *cytotropic antibodies*. They bind to mast cells in tissue and to basophils in the blood. Mast cells are widely distributed throughout the body but are especially numerous in connective tissue, in lung and uterus, and around blood vessels. They are abundant in liver, kidney, spleen, heart, and other organs. The cytoplasm of mast cells is filled with granules. Tissue mast cells are similar in appearance to basophilic leukocytes. When cytotropic antibodies attached to mast cells combine with antigen, degranulation occurs, with the release of histamine. Lysis of mast cells is not necessary for degranulation to occur. When lysis of mast cells does not occur, the granules are "spit out" of the cells and extracellular dissolution of granules with release of histamine occurs. Histamine causes contraction of smooth muscle, dilatation of blood capillaries, increased capillary permeability, and a fall in blood pressure. Failure of the blood to coagulate properly is caused by the release of heparin in addition to histamine from the mast cells. Other chemical mediators of anaphylaxis are serotonin, bradykinin, slow-reacting substances of anaphylaxis (SRS-A), and eosinophil chemotactic factor of anaphylaxis (EFC-A). The Schultz-Dale reaction, known as in vitro anaphylaxis, demonstrates clearly that cell-bound or cytotropic antibodies are responsible for anaphylactic shock. When uterus or a segment of ileum from a sensitized guinea pig is washed free of circulating antibodies and then exposed in a water bath to the antigen used for sensitization, contraction of the tissue occurs.

5-11 IgE has been identified as the cytotropic antibody responsible for anaphylactic shock in human beings. IgE attached to mast cells or basophils combines with antigen to cause degranulation of the cells with release of histamine. Although anaphylactic shock is rare in human beings, it has been observed following the injection of certain biologic preparations or soluble antigens such as antitoxin prepared in a foreign species. The number of cases of anaphylactic shock following injection of antitoxin has been greatly reduced because antitoxin is now refined to eliminate almost all foreign protein except antibody; also antitoxin prepared in human beings is used whenever it is available. Anaphylactic shock has been reported to occur as a result of transfusion with blood containing IgA allotype to which the patient has been previously sensitized (review Chap. 3). Immunoglobulin allotypes are immunoglobulins with structural differences common to some members of a species but not all. Allotypes of IgA (subclass IgA_2) designated Am have been associated with transfusion reactions. Anaphylactic shock may also occur after an insect bite such as a bee sting. Bee venom is a soluble antigen. It is fortunate that insulin, which is a soluble protein, is a very poor antigen, but some people still become sensitized to it. IgE antibodies to insulin can be demonstrated. Insulin has a low molecular weight of about 6000; it has 51 amino acids, 48 of the sequence being identical in different animal species with only the 3 terminal amino acids showing a sequential variation, responsible for differences in antigenicity. Foreign protein from the insulin donor may also cause sensitization. Anaphylactic shock and even death may occur following injection of drugs such as penicillin into a sensitized individual. Sensitization of an individual following the injection of penicillin (a hapten) is due to the ease with which metabolic degradation products of penicillin combine with tissue proteins to form complete antigens such as penicilloyl proteins.

5-12 Antitoxins and other substances which cause anaphylactic shock are multivalent ligands (more than one combining site for antibody). Additional information concerning anaphylactic shock and some other forms of hypersensitivity has been obtained by injection of monovalent ligands. Since the injection of monovalent ligands seems to interfere specifically with anaphylaxis, it was deduced that multivalent ligands probably initiate shock by aggregation or cross linking of IgE molecules already bound to the mast-cell surface (see Fig. 5-1). The mechanism of degranulation of mast cells seems to be brought on by physical distortion of cell-bound antibody molecules after reaction with antigen. This reaction activates serine esterase enzymes in a pathway similar to the classical complement cascade (Chap. 3). Activation of the enzyme cascade causes dissolution or expulsion of mast-cell granules so that histamine and so forth are released. The speed and completeness of activation of the enzyme cascade in mast cells are modulated by the balance between cyclic adenosine monophosphate (cAMP) and cyclic guanosine monophosphate in the cytoplasm of target cells. A rise in intracellular cAMP causes a decrease in release of histamine and similar mediators of anaphylaxis. Most of the experimental work on anaphylactic shock has been carried out in guinea pigs. IgE immunoglobulins do not occur in guinea pigs, but a homocytotropic IgG antibody does. Homocytotropic antibody is antibody which attaches to cells of the same animal species. Human IgE is homocytotropic, while IgG is heterocytotropic (attachment of antibody to cells of a different animal species).

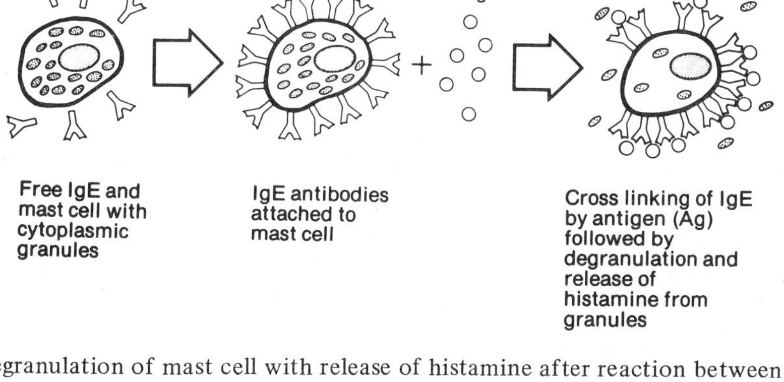

Figure 5-1 Degranulation of mast cell with release of histamine after reaction between antigen and IgE attached to the mast cell. Note cross linking of IgE molecules by antigen.

Skin Tests for Hypersensitivity (Immediate-Type)

5-13 Because of the rapidity and seriousness of anaphylactic shock, every precaution should be taken to prevent its occurrence. When antiserum containing foreign protein has to be used, the patient must be skin-tested first (see the description of the immediate allergic skin reaction in Sec. 4-63). The immediate allergic skin reaction is sometimes referred to as local or cutaneous anaphylaxis, in contrast to systemic or generalized anaphylaxis (anaphylactic shock). A patient should not be injected with any substance for which he has shown a positive skin-test reaction unless it is possible to desensitize the patient first. It is safer to do prick skin tests first and if these are negative to do intradermal tests, especially when testing for sensitivity to penicillin. Skin tests for sensitivity to penicillin have proved unsatisfactory; some severe reactions have occurred during skin testing. The basophil-degranulation test is an in vitro test developed to test for sensitivity to penicillin. A similar test measures histamine release from a suspension of the patient's blood leukocytes (basophils with IgE) after mixing with antigen. The amount of histamine released can be measured spectrofluorometrically.

Desensitization (Acute) against Anaphylaxis

5-14 If diphtheria antitoxin of human origin is not available and a patient with diptheria is found to be sensitive to the protein of the animal species in which antitoxin was produced, the patient must be desensitized to the foreign protein. This type of desensitization can be accomplished by giving the antitoxin (foreign protein) in small divided doses at approximately 15-min intervals. Injections should not be made intravenously. It may take several hours to administer the therapeutic dose. Although the mechanism of this type of desensitization is not well understood, it is thought that by this procedure all bound antibody is gradually exhausted by reaction with small amounts of antigen so that the chemical mediators of anaphylaxis are not released in a sufficient amount at any time to bring on shock. Desensitization of this kind should be carried out only when there is no substitute for the material to which the patient is sensitive. For example, only a specific antitoxin will neutralize exotoxins such as those of diphtheria, botulism, etc. During the entire desensitization process, epinephrine, which will counteract anaphylactic shock, should be on hand in a syringe ready for injection in case shock occurs. This type of desensitization lasts only about 2 weeks. Desensitization to penicillin is dangerous and should not be attempted if the microorganism is susceptible to another antibiotic.

Aggregate Anaphylaxis

5-15 *Soluble complexes* are formed when the antigen-antibody reaction takes place in the region of antigen excess. Aggregate anaphylaxis refers to the intravenous injection of preformed soluble antigen-antibody complexes (aggregates) into unsensitized experimental animals. In the guinea pigs, it has been reported that symptoms very similar to those of classical anaphylaxis are induced. There is considerable evidence that in aggregate anaphylaxis, soluble antigen-antibody complexes act on the same mediator cells; however, there are conflicting reports concerning mast-cell degranulation and release of histamine. Absence of degranulation and failure to release histamine have also been reported for aggregate anaphylaxis in some other experimental animals; therefore, the mechanisms involved in aggregate anaphylaxis require clarification. It has been reported with some experiments on the guinea pig that the soluble complexes or aggregates must be of an antigen (Ag) and antibody (Ab) composition which will fix complement, such as Ag_3Ab_2. Binding of complement by the complexes causes its activation and release of anaphylatoxins, C3a and C5a, which act on tissue to cause release of histamine. Injection of soluble aggregates formed in the region of extreme antigen excess Ag_3Ab_1 did not induce shock. Complexes formed in zones of antibody excess were not highly effective in triggering anaphylactic shock but did cause mild shock.

Anaphylactoid Shock

X **5-16** *Anaphylactoid shock* displays the same symptoms as anaphylactic shock but is not brought on by the injection of antigen into a sensitized animal. Anaphylactoid shock occurs when such substances as peptone, precipitates of barium sulfate, and heat-aggregated globulins are injected into a nonsensitized animal. In Sec. 1-31 the danger of intravenous injection of immune gamma globulin was pointed out; small aggregates of globulin may be present and cause anaphylactoid shock. Gamma globulin for passive immunization should be injected intramuscularly and never intravenously.

Questions for Secs. 5-9 to 5-16

6. (*a*) What events lead to anaphylactic shock? (*b*) Why does a guinea pig which has died in anaphylactic shock show lungs distended with air at autopsy?

7. (*a*) What type of cells are mainly involved in initiation of anaphylaxis? (*b*) What are the chemical mediators of anaphylactic shock? (*c*) What reactions in the host follow the liberation of histamine? (*d*) Is histamine responsible for incoagulability of the blood? (*e*) If your answer to part (*d*) was no, what substance is responsible? (*f*) What is the Schultz-Dale reaction?

8. (*a*) What class of immunoglobulins is responsible for anaphylactic shock in human beings? (*b*) Why might the injection of antitoxin lead to anaphylactic shock? (*c*) Would antitoxin of human origin be expected to cause an allergic reaction? (*d*) Why do some people treated with penicillin become sensitized? (*e*) Are patients sensitized to penicillin or to metabolic degradation products of penicillin? (*f*) Has the injection of penicillin into a patient ever caused anaphylactic shock and death?

9. (*a*) If monovalent ligands combine with antibody attached to tissue, is anaphylactic shock likely to occur? Explain your answer. (*b*) What are homocytotropic antibodies? (*c*) Is IgE homocytotropic for human tissue?

10. (*a*) How can you determine whether or not a person is allergic to a foreign protein? (*b*) What sensitivity tests are carried out with basophils?

11. (*a*) How can a person be desensitized to foreign protein in antiserum in order to prevent anaphylactic shock? (*b*) What is the mechanism of this type of desensitization?

12. (*a*) What is meant by aggregate anaphylaxis? (*b*) What is the antigen and antibody composition of aggregates which cause shock? (*c*) Will Ag_2Ab_1 cause shock?

13. (*a*) How does the mechanism of anaphylactoid shock differ from that of anaphylaxis? (*b*) Give examples of substances which cause anaphylactoid shock.

Answers

6. (*a*) Exposure to allergen, usually by injection; formation of IgE immunoglobulins and attachment to mast cells of affected tissue and also to blood basophils; reexposure to allergen in such a way that there is rapid reaction between antigen and antibody attached to tissue mast cells. Entrance of allergen into bloodstream is more likely to cause anaphylactic shock. (*b*) Anaphylactic shock in guinea pigs causes contraction of smooth muscle of bronchioles; air is sucked in but cannot be forced out. (Sec. 5-9.)

7. (*a*) Tissue mast cells and blood basophils. (*b*) Histamine; serotonin; bradykinin, slow-reacting substances of anaphylaxis (SRS-A), and eosinophil chemotactic factor of anaphylaxis (ECF-A). (*c*) Contraction of smooth muscles; dilatation of blood capillaries; increased capillary permeability and fall in blood pressure. (*d*) No. (*e*) Heparin (*f*) In vitro demonstration of mechanism of anaphylactic shock with contraction of washed smooth muscle from sensitized animal after exposure to antigen. (Sec. 5-10.)

8. (*a*) IgE. (*b*) If antitoxin is prepared in a different species, it is foreign and antigenic. Also it is a soluble antigen. (*c*) No. (*d*) Because metabolic degradation products of penicillin such as penicilloyl readily combine with tissue proteins to form complete antigens and become antigenic. (*e*) Metabolic degradation products of penicillin. (*f*) Yes. (Sec. 5-11.)

9. (*a*) No, because they cannot cross-link receptors of IgE attached to mast cells. (*b*) Antibodies which bind to cells of the same animal species. (*c*) Yes. (Sec. 5-12.)

10. (*a*) By skin testing and performing in vitro tests for IgE. (*b*) In vitro tests in which

a suspension of blood leukocytes mixed with antigen are tested for basophil degranulation or histamine release. (Sec. 5-13.)

11. (*a*) By injection of antiserum (containing foreign protein) in small divided doses at intervals of 15 to 30 min. Start with very small dose and increase amount at next injection provided no reaction has occurred. (*b*) Supposedly, bound IgE is gradually exhausted by reaction with small amounts of antigen so that the chemical mediators of anaphylaxis are not released in a sufficient amount at any time to induce shock. (Sec. 5-14.)

12. (*a*) Shock due to injection of soluble antigen and antibody complexes (aggregates). (*b*) Ag_3Ab_2. (*c*) No. (Sec. 5-15.)

13. (*a*) Anaphylactoid shock is not brought on by an immediate-type hypersensitivity reaction, i.e., a reaction between antigen and antibody. (*b*) Intravenous injection of peptones, aggregated globulins, etc. (Sec. 5-16.)

Atopy

5-17 *Atopy* means "strangeness" and was originally used to describe allergic illnesses in which the nature of the antigenic exposure and the production of antibody were not clear. It is now known that about 10 percent of the population in the United States may be sensitized through natural exposure to substances in the environment. Atopic illnesses were among the first antibody-associated diseases noted to have a strong familial or hereditary tendency. The mechanism of atopy is similar to that of anaphylactic shock except that the rate of the reaction in atopy is much slower. Atopy is caused by reaction of allergens with IgE bound to tissue mast cells in the affected organ followed by the degranulation of mast cells and release of histamine and other vasoactive amines (see Fig 5-1). Almost everyone has a small amount of IgE in his serum. An atopic individual appears to produce IgE readily and in elevated amounts to one or more allergens.

Allergens of Atopy

5-18 Sensitization in atopy is usually through inhalation or ingestion. Hay fever, a common form of atopy, is characterized by sneezing, watery reddened eyes, running nose, and respiratory distress. Pollens of plants may sensitize a person through contact with the mucous membranes of eyes, nose, and throat. After sensitization, reexposure of these surfaces during a following pollen season may cause recurrence of symptoms. Another common cause of inhalant allergy is house dust. The demonstration that mites in house dust often contain the major antigenic components to which a patient is sensitive was a significant advance in understanding this type of allergy. Other common causes of allergy by inhalation are molds (fungi) and animal danders. Some of the molds associated with atopy are *Alternaria* and *Aspergillus*. Animal danders are epithelial scales or dandruff shed by the skin of various animals such as horses etc. A person may become sensitized to danders of pets such as cats, dogs, parrots, parakeets, and canaries; to laboratory animals such as rabbits, guinea pigs, rats, and mice; and to farm animals such as sheep, goats, cows, and hogs. It is not always necessary to come in contact with the animal in order to become sensitized. For example, a person may become sensitized to feathers in pillows (goose, duck, or chicken).

IgE (Reagin) in Atopy

5-19 Long before the different classes of antibodies were described, it was recognized that the antibody responsible for atopy is different from classical antibody. IgE is heat-labile and nonprecipitating. The attachment of IgE to tissue mast cells with degranulation and release of histamine after reaction with antigen has been described (Sec. 5-10). IgE is sometimes called reagin, a use which has led to confusion since the term reagin also refers to the antibody detected in tests for syphilis employing a nonspecific cardiolipin hapten. IgE is also called *homocytotropic* and *anaphylactic antibody*. IgE binds to tissue cells by the Fc portion of the antibody molecule (review Sec. 5-12). Patients with atopy have elevated levels of IgE in their serum. Patients with parasitic diseases also have high IgE levels, but their significance is not yet understood. There is recent evidence that serum IgE is elevated in venereal diseases (gonorrhea and syphilis) and in vaginitis caused by *Trichomonas*.

Anaphylaxis versus Atopy

5-20 Since the mechanism of anaphylactic shock is essentially the same as that of atopy, anaphylaxis is considered by many to be a manifestation of atopy or vice versa. Historically anaphylactic shock is a rapid, often fatal reaction which may follow injection of a soluble antigen into a sensitized individual whereas atopy is an allergic disorder with hereditary tendency caused by natural exposure to an allergen, e.g., by inhalation or ingestion. Anaphylactic shock was discussed separately in this chapter because of its importance. It rarely occurs in human beings, but when it does, it is often fatal. Atopy (excluding anaphylactic shock) occurs in about 10 percent of the population and although atopy causes much discomfort, it is rarely fatal.

Clinical Manifestations of Atopy

5-21 If IgE is fixed to tissue in the respiratory tract, exposure to the specific allergen may cause symptoms of asthma, allergic rhinitis, and sinusitis. Ingestion may cause gastrointestinal allergy with symptoms of vomiting, diarrhea, bloating, etc. Ingestion of an allergen more frequently causes atopic skin disorders, e.g., urticaria, or hives, when IgE is present in the skin. Urticaria, or hives, may also be brought on by injections of an allergen. An allergic reaction in atopy usually is not brought on by contact because the epithelium serves as a barrier. Contact dermatitis is a delayed-type hypersensitivity reaction. Clinical symptoms of atopy can be relieved by treatment with antihistamine or adrenergic drugs.

Prolonged Desensitization to Prevent Symptoms of Atopy

5-22 Desensitization can be carried out by injections of the allergen (antigen) to which the patient is sensitive; e.g., before the pollen season, a person may receive a series of injections of the allergen. The rationale of immunization as a desensitizing procedure for atopy is based on the formation of a high titer of circulating antibodies. The circulating antibodies are IgG and act as blocking antibodies to combine with antigen before antigen has a chance to react with IgE attached to the cells. Desensitization for atopy is carried out over several weeks. The underlying mechanism of desensitization to prevent symptoms of atopy is different from that to prevent anaphylactic shock. There is some evidence that the formation of a high level of IgG to allergen during desensitization depresses the formation of IgE and is antigen-specific.

Tests for Sensitization with IgE

5-23 *Skin tests* based on the immediate-type hypersensitivity reaction or cutaneous anaphylaxis described in Sec. 4-63 can be carried out. The scratch (or prick) method is frequently used for the inoculation of allergen into the skin of a patient with atopy in order to determine the allergen(s) responsible. Some allergists feel that the scratch method is safer than the intracutaneous skin-test method. Others feel that the intracutaneous method is safe and more accurate and therefore preferable. There are cases on record where extremely hypersensitive patients have gone into anaphylactic shock and died during skin testing. Presumably the allergen was injected in such a way that it entered a blood capillary and caused a rapid systemic reaction rather than a local cutaneous reaction.

5-24 The *Prausnitz-Küstner* (PK) test is a skin test used in the past to demonstrate IgE in the serum of a patient with atopy. In this test, the patient's serum is injected intradermally into the skin of a nonsensitive individual. After allowing time (24 to 48 h) for IgE to attach to tissue mast cells and for other antibodies in serum to diffuse away, antigen is injected intradermally at the same site. Specific antigen causes a positive immediate allergic reaction characterized by the wheal-and-flare reaction. It has been shown that IgE remains fixed to tissue fairly long. The PK test is seldom used now. It has two disadvantages: (1) a skin donor must be obtained and (2) there is the danger of transferring hepatitis virus to the donor by injection of human serum. In human beings the PK test is comparable to passive cutaneous anaphylaxis test in guinea pigs. A blue dye, Evans blue, is used in the guinea pig test for better visualization of increased tissue permeability due to release of histamine. It has been found that the Fc fragment of IgE obtained by proteolysis with papain can inhibit the PK test in human beings. This finding may have future clinical application.

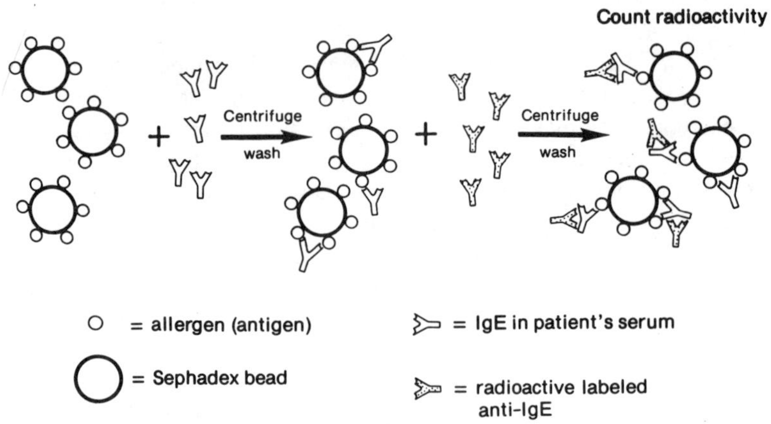

Figure 5-2 Radioallergosorbent test (RAST) for IgE.

5-25 The *radioallergosorbent test* (RAST) is an in vitro test frequently used to assay for antigen-specific IgE in the serum of a patient. The suspected allergen is adsorbed on, or coupled to, Sephadex beads and then allowed to react with the patient's serum. This "insoluble" allergen is washed and tested for IgE by adding anti-IgE radiolabeled with ^{125}I. The RAST test is a direct radioimmunoassay test. The procedure is outlined in Fig. 5-2. The *radioimmunosorbent test* (RIST) is a quantitative test for IgE but is not antigen-specific. It is similar to RAST but uses anti-IgE coupled to an insoluble support such as Sephadex or paper. Reaction of IgE in patient's serum with anti-IgE is detected by the addition (after washing) of ^{125}I-labeled anti-IgE. Other in vitro tests include the *leukocyte histamine-release test.* Leukocytes (white blood cells containing basophils) are separated from the red blood cells of the patient's blood. These leukocytes are mixed with antigen, and the amount of histamine released is measured fluorometrically.

5-26 The *provocative test*, sometimes used in the diagnosis of atopy, consists of exposing the patient to the suspected allergen and observing for symptoms of atopy. Exposure may take place by inhalation or ingestion.

Questions for Secs. 5-17 to 5-26

14. (*a*) How was the term atopy originally used? (*b*) Is there a hereditary tendency to atopy? (*c*) How does the mechanism of anaphylactic shock differ from that of atopy?

15. (*a*) What is one of the main antigenic substances in most samples of house dust? (*b*) What are some other allergens (antigens) which frequently cause allergies by inhalation?

16. (*a*) What terms are used to refer to IgE? (*b*) Does serum IgE show an increase in atopy? (*c*) What part of IgE attaches to tissue?

17. What are some of the clinical manifestations of atopy?

18. (*a*) Why are IgG antibodies produced during desensitization for atopy called blocking antibodies? (*b*) Is the mechanism of desensitization for anaphylactic shock the same as that for atopy? Explain.

19. (*a*) How is the Prausnitz-Küstner (PK) skin test carried out? (*b*) Why is it seldom used now? (*c*) What test carried out in guinea pigs is similar to the PK test?

20. (*a*) Briefly outline the mechanism of the radioallergosorbent test (RAST). (*b*) How does the RIST test differ from the RAST test?

Answers

14. (*a*) Atopy means "strangeness," so that the term was originally used to describe allergic illnesses following natural exposure, e.g., to pollens, in which the nature of both the antigen and antibody produced to antigen was not clear. (*b*) Yes. (*c*) The mechanism is the same, but it occurs more slowly in atopy. (Sec. 5-17.)

15. (*a*) Mites. (*b*) Plant pollens, molds (fungi), animal danders (dandruff). (Sec. 5-18.)

16. (*a*) Reagin, homocytotropic and anaphylactic antibody. (*b*) Yes. (*c*) Fc. (Sec. 5-19.)

17. Respiratory symptoms such as asthma, rhinitis, and sinusitis; skin reactions such as urticaria (hives); gastrointestinal symptoms such as vomiting, diarrhea, and bloating. (Sec. 5-21.)

18. (*a*) IgG antibodies are produced during a series of injections with the allergen, e.g., before the hay fever season. Later when exposure to allergen occurs, these antibodies are available to react with allergen, with luck before allergen has the chance to react with IgE antibodies fixed to tissue. In other words they tend to block reaction of allergen with IgE and therefore are called blocking antibodies. (*b*) No. Desensitization against anaphylactic shock must take place over a short time (no longer than a few hours), for example, if antitoxin needs to be given. Desensitization for anaphylactic shock allows only a small amount of antigen and IgE on mast cells to react at any time until the desired dose of antiserum has been injected. (Sec. 5-22.)

19. (*a*) First a skin donor is obtained. The patient's serum is injected intradermally into sites on the donor's back; 24 to 48 h later, after time has been allowed for fixation of IgE to tissue and for other antibodies to diffuse away, the antigens to be tested are injected into these sites. (*b*) Because of the possibility of transferring hepatitis viruses. (*c*) Passive cutaneous anaphylaxis. (Sec. 5-24.)

20. The suspected allergen is coupled onto an insoluble support such as Sephadex beads or paper so that washing can be accomplished easily when necessary. This "insoluble" allergen is mixed with patient's serum, allowed to react, washed, and then mixed with anti-IgE labeled with ^{125}I. After another incubation period and washing, the insoluble allergen is tested for radioactivity. (*b*) The RIST test is a quantitative radioimmunoassay for IgE but does not identify the specificity of IgE. (Sec. 5-25.)

Serum Sickness and Serum-Sickness Syndrome

5-27 Before the discovery of antibiotics, serum therapy was used not only to treat diseases, like diphtheria and tetanus, caused by exotoxins but also such diseases as pneumococcal pneumonia and meningococcus meningitis. Most bacterial diseases are now treated with antibiotics although a few are still treated with antitoxin since antibiotics will not neutralize exotoxins. The injection of antitoxin causes fewer cases of serum sickness than formerly because either human antitoxin is employed or the preparation of antitoxin is refined to the extent that most of the foreign protein is removed except the specific antibodies (antitoxin molecules). How serum sickness is brought on by the injection of antitoxin prepared in horses (or other antisera such as antilymphocyte serum) can be outlined as follows:

1. Injection of antitoxin (antibody molecule has antigenicity of horse protein); with regard to the production of serum sickness, the antitoxin acts as an antigen.
2. Patient begins to form antibody to antigen (in this case horse protein); see curve *A*, Fig. 5-3, for rise in antibody titer.
3. Antigen is gradually eliminated from body; see Fig. 5-3, curve *B*, for antigen decline.
4. Before antigen is eliminated, antibody production occurs and antigen and antibody react to cause symptoms of serum sickness.

5-28 The only really unusual thing about serum sickness as a form of antibody-mediated allergy is the fact that the sensitizing dose and the dose of antigen which brings on symptoms may be one and the same. Symptoms of serum sickness usually appear within 7 to 14 days after injection of serum; however, if a patient has been previously sensitized, an anamnestic response occurs and symptoms develop in 3 to 5 days. The form brought on by the anamnestic response, or rapid production of antibody, has been called *accelerated serum sickness.* Serum sickness is an allergic reaction characterized by hives, extensive edema (especially about the face, neck, and joints), joint pain, malaise, and

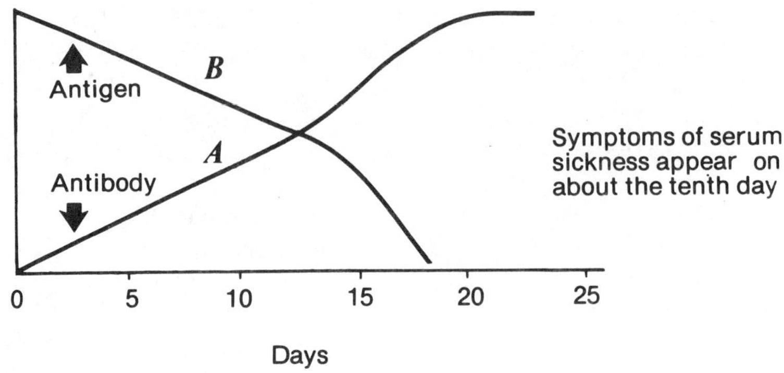

Figure 5-3 Production of serum sickness after injection of foreign serum into a patient not previously sensitized; curve A = production of antibody; curve B = elimination of antigen.

fever. It appears that two mechanisms may contribute to the symptoms of serum sickness. (1) Soluble complexes formed between antibody (IgG) and antigen in the region of antigen excess bind and activate complement. Through the formation of anaphylatoxins, C3a and C5a (Chap. 3), histamine and other chemical mediators are released. In addition to the symptoms mentioned above, transitory eosinophilia, albuminuria, and decrease in complement may occur. Serum sickness may have serious consequences especially when soluble immune complexes are filtered through the kidneys and cause severe kidney damage or glomerulonephritis. (2) IgE also appears to be formed. Immediate-type allergic skin tests are positive. IgE antibodies attach to tissue mast cells, react with antigen, and cause release of histamine. Whatever the mechanism of serum sickness, the reactions between antigen and antibody occur as the antibody is produced, so that a sudden release of histamine does not occur to cause shock. Symptoms of serum sickness occur following the injection of other substances besides serum; e.g., penicillin has been one of the most common causes of the syndrome known as serum sickness.

Arthus Reaction

5-29 In 1903 Arthus reported his observation that when rabbits were injected subcutaneously each week with horse serum, no reaction appeared at the site of injection until several weeks later, when localized inflammatory reactions began to appear. The lesion, which was at first hemorrhagic and edematous, eventually became necrotic. Similar reactions were soon described in human beings and were called *Arthus reactions.* The Arthus reaction, sometimes called the Arthus phenomenon, is initiated by the formation of precipitates in small blood vessels. Precipitates form in the region of antibody excess so that a high level of circulating antibody favors the development of the Arthus reaction when antigen is injected. Complement and neutrophils are also required for the development of the Arthus reaction. Necrosis is not due to the liberation of histamine or other vasoactive amines but to the activation of complement, the release of chemotactic factors, and the accumulation of neutrophils and their products. The stages in the development of the Arthus reaction can be outlined as follows:

1. Circulating antibody meets soluble antigen in blood vessels, where precipitation occurs.
2. Complement is fixed and anaphylatoxins (C3a and C5a) are released, which cause increase in vascular permeability and deposition of the precipitates.
3. Infiltration of neutrophils occurs due to the chemotactic properties of C3a and C5a. Neutrophils adhere to precipitates and subsequently phagocytize them. Lysosomal materials are released extracellularly during phagocytosis.
4. Proteolytic enzymes released by the phagocytic cells contribute to tissue damage (hemorrhage and necrosis).
5. Precipitates may bind to platelets, causing platelet aggregation and release of stored vasoactive

amines. This reaction appears to occur more readily with complexes formed in antibody excess.

The Arthus reaction requires 6 to 12 h or longer to develop. Since the reaction is caused by formation of precipitates with IgG (or IgM) and is not dependent upon fixation of IgE to mast cells and their degranulation, antihistamines and adrenergic drugs are ineffective in preventing or ameliorating the Arthus reaction. Skin tests which are positive as a result of the Arthus reaction were considered in Sec. 4-65.

5-30 The Arthus reaction may occur in ways other than injection. For example, a pulmonary condition known as *farmer's lung* is considered to result from an Arthus reaction in the lungs when spores from moldy hay are inhaled. Symptoms appear in 6 to 8 h after exposure of a sensitized individual. A thermophilic strain of *Actinomycetes* capable of propagating in hay at high temperatures is one of the microorganisms which has been shown to cause this condition. Extracts of the organism precipitate with antibodies in the patient's serum. Aslo IgG precipitates can be demonstrated in biopsies of lung tissue. Farmer's lung belongs to a group of diseases known as *extrinsic allergic alveolitis* or *pneumonitis.* Others include cheese-worker's lung (spores of moldy cheese), mushroom-worker's lung (spores), and bird-fancier's lung (organic dust of excreta).

5-31 Tissue changes brought on by the Arthus reaction are similar to those seen in the Shwartzman phenomenon, although the latter is not considered to result from an immune reaction. In 1927 Shwartzman showed that when a filtrate of *Salmonella typhi* was injected into the skin of rabbits and followed 24 h later by an intravenous injection of the same material, hemorrhagic necrosis developed at the site of the first injection. The filtrate contained endotoxin. Endotoxin from many different gram-negative organisms will bring on this reaction, and the endotoxins for the two injections may be different. Sanarelli previously had made the observation (in 1916) that an intraperitoneal injection of nonlethal dose of *Vibrio cholera* followed by an intravenous injection of a small quantity of *Escherichia coli* caused death of the animals. This generalized, or systemic, type of Shwartzman reaction is often called the *Sanarelli-Shwartzman phenomenon.* A few investigators feel that the Shwartzman reaction may be a form of hypersensitivity; however, the mechanism of this reaction is still not clear. In general, it is not viewed as antibody-mediated. Clinical conditions which have been associated with a Shwartzman reaction are toxemia in pregnancy and the Waterhouse-Friderichsen syndrome (acute adrenal insufficiency) seen with gram-negative endotoxin-containing diplococci *Neisseria meningitidis.*

Immune-Complex Disorders

5-32 There are many diseases which are associated with the formation and deposit of immune complexes in tissue. Two of them, serum sickness and the Arthus reaction were discussed above. Immune complexes may be formed as a result of infections (bacterial, viral, and parasitic), autoimmune disorders such as systemic lupus erythematosus, disseminated malignancy, cryoglobulinemia, and drug reactions. Immune complexes may be formed with antigen and either IgG or IgM antibodies, but those formed with IgG usually cause the most trouble. The size of the complex is very significant. Large complexes like those which would be formed with IgM are readily phagocytized. Complexes formed in extreme antigen excess do not fix complement and are unlikely to cause immune-complex disorders. Complexes of antigen and IgG having the molecular formula Ag_3Ab_2 have been shown experimentally to cause immune-complex disorders. The importance of complement and polymorphonuclear leukocytes has already been discussed. Immune complexes may also bind to platelet membranes, causing the release of vasoactive amines stored in platelets. Immune complexes formed in antigen excess appear to be less active in binding platelets than complexes formed in antibody excess, like those found in the Arthus reaction.

Questions for Secs. 5-27 to 5-32

21. (*a*) Why does serum sickness rarely occur now? (*b*) What kind of antisera are still used that might cause serum sickness? (*c*) Do antibodies or antigen(s) in the antisera cause serum sickness? (*d*) Do symptoms of serum sickness occur after the injection of antigens

(or haptens) other than serum? Give an example.

22. (*a*) Can a person who has not been previously sensitized develop serum sickness? (*b*) Is serum sickness an immediate-type hypersensitivity reaction with regard to appearance of symptoms? (*c*) Name several factors which would not favor the production of serum sickness. (*d*) What is accelerated serum sickness? (*e*) Name the underlying mechanism(s) of serum sickness. (*f*) Why doesn't shock occur when antigen and antibody react? (*g*) What are the symptoms of serum sickness? (*h*) What might be a serious complication of serum sickness?

23. (*a*) Is the Arthus reaction an immediate-type hypersensitivity reaction with regard to time of appearance of symptoms? (*b*) Why is the Arthus reaction classified as an immediate-type hypersensitivity reaction? (*c*) What factors are responsible for the Arthus reaction? (*d*) Does a high level of precipitating antibodies favor or hinder the Arthus reaction? (*e*) Is the Arthus reaction brought on by the release of histamine? (*f*) Would antihistamine drugs counteract the Arthus reaction?

24. (*a*) Give several examples of allergic alveolitis. (*b*) What reaction is believed to be responsible? (*c*) How does exposure of the patient take place?

25. (*a*) With regard to pathological tissue changes, what reaction does the Shwartzman reaction resemble? (*b*) Is the Shwartzman reaction brought on by an immune reaction? (*c*) What substance characterizes the material used to induce a Shwartzman reaction?

26. (*a*) What class of immunoglobulins is usually associated with immune-complex disease? (*b*) Are the soluble complexes formed in the region of antibody or antigen excess? (*c*) Why is serum complement less at the height of the illness? (*d*) Do immune-complex disorders occur with viruses?

Answers

21. (*a*) Since the introduction of antibiotics, antiserum therapy is not used for treatment of bacterial infections except some of those caused by bacteria which excrete an exotoxin, for example, *C. diphtheriae.* Antitoxin used is highly refined to remove as much foreign protein as possible and whenever possible, human antitoxin (gamma globulin) is used. (*b*) Antitoxin, antirabies serum, antilymphocyte serum. (*c*) Antigens. (*d*) Yes; penicillin. (Sec. 5-27.)

22. (*a*) Yes. Antibody may be produced to the injected antigen and react with antigen before antigen is eliminated from the body. (*b*) No, but it is still classified as immediate-type hypersensitivity because it is antibody-mediated. (*c*) Serum sickness may not occur if a small amount of antigen (serum, drug, etc.) is injected, if antigen is eliminated before antibody is formed, or if a person is a poor producer of antibody. (*d*) Symptoms occur earlier in a previously sensitized person because there is an anamnestic response with sufficient antibody formed in 3 to 5 days to cause symptoms. Of course, a previously sensitized person could show anaphylactic shock instead of accelerated serum sickness. (*e*) Immune-complex formation (with IgG) and possibly also production of IgE, with attachment to tissue and with liberation of histamine when bound IgE subsequently reacts with antigen. (*f*) Because there is a slow or gradual combination between antigen and antibody when antibody is produced. (*g*) Hives, edema, joint pain, malaise, and fever. (*h*) Glomerulonephritis. (Secs. 5-27 and 5-28.)

23. (*a*) No. (*b*) It is antibody-mediated. (*c*) Complex formation in blood vessels with complement fixation, activation, and release of anaphylatoxins C3a and C5a from complement, attraction of neutrophils into area, and phagocytosis of complexes with release of lysosomal enzymes. (*d*) Favor. (*e*) No. (*f*) No. (Sec. 5-29.)

24. (*a*) Farmer's lung, cheese-worker's lung, mushroom-worker's lung, bird-fancier's lung. (*b*) Arthus. (*c*) By inhalation. (Sec. 5-30.)

25. (*a*) Arthus reaction. (*b*) In general, no. (*c*) Endotoxin. (Sec. 5-31.)

26. (*a*) IgG (*b*) Antigen (*c*) Because it is fixed to the complexes. (*d*) Yes (Sec. 5-32.)

CELL-MEDIATED AND DELAYED-TYPE HYPERSENSITIVITY REACTIONS

Delayed-Type Hypersensitivity (Cell-mediated)

X **5-33** Delayed-type hypersensitivity is cell-mediated and is caused by reaction of sensitized T lymphocytes with antigen. The basic underlying mechanisms of delayed-type hypersensitivity and cell-mediated immunity are essentially the same, but the latter term has the connotation of a beneficial event. The terms are often used interchangeably by many investigators. Some examples of delayed-type hypersensitivity or cell-mediated immunity are

- The Koch phenomenon (of historical interest)
- Positive tuberculin skin reaction
- Resistance to certain microorganisms, e.g., those causing tuberculosis and fungal infections
- Resistance to many intracellular parasites, e.g., viruses
- Rejection of allografts
- Graft-versus-host reaction
- Tumor immunity
- Contact dermatitis
- Some autoimmune diseases

The underlying mechanisms of cell-mediated reactions were discussed in Chap. 2. Cell-mediated reactions are brought about by thymus-dependent lymphocytes (T cells) and not by antibodies derived from plasma cells of B-lymphocyte origin (review Chap. 2).

X **5-34** Delayed-type hypersensitivity reactions were classified as type IV reactions by Coombs and Gell (Sec. 5-7). The nature of the receptors on T lymphocytes which are responsible for recognition of antigen is not clear at present. After T lymphocytes encounter the specific antigen, the T lymphocytes are triggered to divide and produce a clone of many daughter cells, which in turn contribute to the release of an increased amount of lymphokines on reencounter of this cell line with specific antigen. See Sec. 2-27 for a list of some of the lymphokines which have been recognized. Lymphokines such as macrophage chemotactic factor (MCF), migration-inhibition factor (MIF), and macrophage-activating factor are responsible for the accumulation of macrophages and their destructive activity at a particular site, e.g., invasion of living tissue by tubercle bacilli. In some cases different lymphokine activity is caused by the same substance; MIF and macrophage-activating factor appear to be the same, for example. With regard to chemical composition, lymphokines have been reported to be proteins or glycoproteins. Cell-mediated immunity or delayed-type hypersensitivity cannot be transferred to another person with serum but can be transferred with sensitized T lymphocytes. The latter process, called *adoptive immunization*, is dangerous because it can cause the graft-versus-host reaction and even death. Transfer factor prepared as an extract of T lymphocytes can transfer cell-mediated immunity provided the person whose lymphocytes were extracted had the desired immunity. Transfer factor is now being used experimentally in T-cell immunologic deficiency disorders (Chap. 7). Figure 5-4 summarizes stages in the development of immediate-type (antibody-mediated) and delayed-type (cell-mediated) hypersensitivities.

Koch Phenomenon

5-35 Delayed-type allergy of infection was first described by Koch in 1890 with tubercle bacilli and is now known as the Koch phenomenon. Subcutaneous injection of a normal guinea pig with tubercle bacilli caused the development of a nodule at the injection site after 10 to 15 days. Tubercle bacilli spread to the regional lymph nodes and then to many other tissues, such as the lungs; death of the

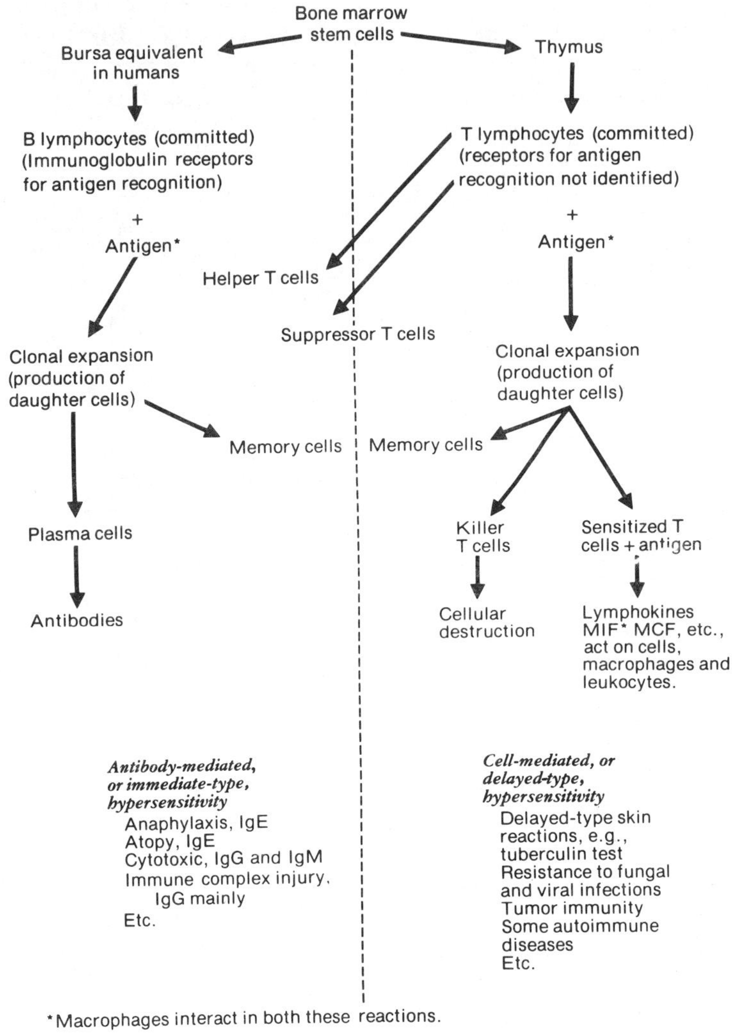

Figure 5-4 Summary of development of hypersensitivity in human beings.

pig followed in about 10 weeks. When the same amount of virulent tubercle bacilli was injected subcutaneously into a guinea pig which had been infected at least a week earlier, a local erythematous tissue reaction developed within 24 to 48 h. This reaction showed a shallow type of ulceration, resulting in sloughing off of tissue with subsequent healing; the tubercle bacilli in this injection did not spread to the lymph nodes.

Tuberculin Skin Test

5-36 Koch believed that the sloughing-tissue reaction in a sensitized animal described above was a favorable one since tubercle bacilli were eliminated and the lesion healed rapidly. He tried to duplicate this reaction with a culture filtrate of tubercle bacilli. The preparation by Koch is now known as *old tuberculin* (OT). The active principle in old tuberculin was purified by Seibert in 1934 and called *purified protein derivative* (PPD); it has a molecular weight of only 10,500 and cannot sensitize or immunize a person. Koch did not succeed in developing a substance which could be used for immunization against tuberculosis, but he did prepare one which has been used extensively in screening populations for exposure to, or infection with, tubercle bacilli. At present PPD is more commonly used. A positive tuberculin test shows a delayed allergic skin reaction. A positive test begins to appear in about 6 h; it should be read between 48 and 72 h. Induration, characteristic of the tuberculin reaction, is caused by the accumulation of mononuclear cells. The average diameter of induration (not just erythema) is measured; a reaction 10 mm in diameter is definitely positive.

the tuberculin reaction, is caused by the accumulation of mononuclear cells. The average diameter of induration (not just erythema) is measured; a reaction 10 mm in diameter is definitely positive.

5-37 Skin testing for tuberculosis must be performed with care. If too large a dose of tuberculin or PPD is injected into a highly sensitized individual, there may occur not only a local skin-test reaction but also a focal reaction at the site of infection, e.g., in the lungs. A focal reaction could cause breakdown of a healed lesion or walled-off focus of infection with spread of tubercle bacilli to other areas. Also too large an injection of tuberculin into a sensitized individual could cause a generalized systemic reaction. Both OT and PPD are standardized in terms of their biologic activity as *tuberculin units* (TU). First-strength tuberculin has 1 TU; intermediate strength, 5 TU; and second strength, 100 to 250 TU. Intermediate strength (5 TU) is chosen for routine use. In children suspected of having tuberculosis, 1 TU may be used to avoid a focal reaction; if there is no response, the test is repeated with intermediate-strength tuberculin. On the other hand, patients who have shown a negative or doubtful reaction with 5 TU but are suspected of being infected with tubercle bacilli or cross-reacting atypical mycobacteria may be tested with second-strength tuberculin.

5-38 The tuberculin test has been carried out by the patch-test and scratch-test methods, but the Mantoux test is usually preferred. In it 0.1 ml of PPD is injected intracutaneously. In a method designed to provide a rapid and easy procedure for tuberculin testing large population groups, called the *tine test*, a mechanical device containing several small tines is used, so that tuberculin on the points of the tines is introduced by puncture into the skin. Other mechanical devices for inoculation have also been developed recently.

5-39 A positive tuberculin test in an adult indicates either present or past infection. A positive test in early childhood is more likely to be caused by active tuberculosis. Patients with very advanced or terminal cases of tuberculosis may fail to show delayed-type hypersensitivity. A negative reaction in these patients is an example of *anergy*, or the inability to muster a hypersensitivity reaction. These patients have a very poor prognosis. A positive tuberculin reaction also may be suppressed by such drugs as cortisone and such infections as measles, pertussis, and infectious mononucleosis.

BCG Vaccine

X **5-40** BCG vaccine (bacille Calmette and Guérin) was prepared by Calmette and Guerin as a living attenuated vaccine. *Mycobacterium bovis*, which antigenically is indistinguishable from *M. tuberculosis*, was attenuated by growth on an unfavorable medium containing bile through several hundred serial transfers. BCG vaccine should not be given to tuberculin-positive patients because of the danger of causing a severe allergic reaction and the possible activation of a pulmonary lesion. Although BCG vaccine has been used in some countries, it has been used to a very limited extent in the United States. Immunized persons develop delayed-type hypersensitivity to *M. tuberculosis*; the tuberculin test becomes positive, so that the advantage of the tuberculin test for screening purposes is destroyed.

X **5-41** It has recently been observed that injection of BCG vaccine into experimental animals with tumors causes destruction or regression of the tumors. The underlying mechanism is believed to be that of delayed-type hypersensitivity. Lymphocytes occur at the site of injection and produce lymphokines. Some lymphokines act on macrophages, and angry macrophages destroy tumor cells nonspecifically. BCG vaccine is now being used experimentally for the treatment of patients with cancer. BCG vaccine acts as an adjuvant. The reticuloendothelial system of the host is stimulated so that there is a stronger host immune response to weak cancer antigens (see Chap. 10).

Freund's Adjuvant

5-42 Freund's adjuvant in its complete form contains killed *Mycobacterium* species in addition to an oil emulsion. It has the unique property that when it is mixed with a small amount of antigen, it induces a delayed-type hypersensitivity response to the antigen. The active component in *Mycobacterium* species appears to be a lipid, wax D. This fraction attracts cells concerned with production of delayed-type hypersensitivity. Because Freund's complete adjuvant contains *Mycobacterium* spp., it is used for research and not to prepare vaccines regularly used for immunization. The amount of antigen injected is critical for the induction of cell-mediated reactions. A large amount of antigen induces antibody formation. Freund's complete adjuvant induces an immune response to very weak antigens. Freund's incomplete adjuvant (without mycobacteria) is a water-in-oil emulsion and when mixed with antigen serves to retard local destruction and elimination of antigen, so that there is prolonged stimulation of the immune system. Without the addition of *Mycobacterium* spp. antibody production is the main response.

Questions for Secs. 5-33 to 5-42

27. (*a*) Are the basic underlying mechanisms of cell-mediated immunity and delayed-type hypersensitivity essentially the same? (*b*) What cells are effector cells for delayed-type hypersensitivity? (*c*) What is the Coombs and Gell classification for delayed-type hypersensitivity reactions? (*d*) What are lymphokines?

28. (*a*) What was the first demonstration of allergy of infection? (*b*) With what microorganism was this demonstration made? (*c*) What is the mechanism of the tuberculin skin test? (*d*) What causes induration, seen in a positive tuberculin skin test? (*e*) What substance is currently used in the tuberculin skin test? (*f*) What is the origin of this substance? (*g*) Who purified it? (*h*) Is the purified substance antigenic?

29. (*a*) If a large amount of PPD is injected intracutaneously into the forearm of a highly sensitized individual, what reaction(s) might be observed besides a positive delayed allergic skin reaction? (*b*) What strength tuberculin is chosen for routine use? (*c*) What method of skin testing is preferred for the tuberculin test?

30. What can cause the tuberculin reaction to be negative in a previously sensitized patient?

31. (*a*) What do the letters BCG of the BCG vaccine represent? (*b*) What microorganism does the BCG vaccine contain? (*c*) Is it attenuated? If your answer is yes, state how it was attenuated. (*d*) What are the main objections to using the BCG vaccine in the United States? (*e*) For what purpose has the vaccine been used experimentally?

32. (*a*) What is the composition of Freund's complete adjuvant? (*b*) Is it used in vaccines? (*c*) Is it used extensively for research? (*d*) What are the advantages of Freund's adjuvant?

Answers

27. (*a*) Yes, they appear to be. (*b*) T lymphocytes. (*c*) Type IV reactions. (*d*) Soluble protein substances which are released on encounter of sensitized T lymphocytes with antigen and which act as soluble mediators of delayed-type hypersensitivity. (Secs. 5-33 and 5-34.)

28. (*a*) Koch phenomenon. (*b*) Tubercle bacilli (*Mycobacterium tuberculosis*). (*c*) Delayed-type hypersensitivity. (*d*) Accumulation of mononuclear cells. (*e*) PPD. (*f*) From old tuberculin of Koch. (*g*) Seibert. (*h*) No. (Secs. 5-35 and 5-36.)

29. (*a*) Focal and systemic reactions. (*b*) Intermediate strength (5 TU). (*c*) Intradermal injection (Mantoux test). (Secs. 5-37 and 5-38.)

30. Patients with advanced tuberculosis may become anergic or desensitized by continual exposure of T lymphocytes to large numbers of tubercle bacilli. Negative tuberculin skin reactions are observed with cortisone therapy and infections such as measles, pertussis (whooping cough), and infectious mononucleosis. (Sec. 5-39.)

31. (*a*) Bacillus Calmette Guérin. (*b*) *Mycobacterium bovis*. (*c*) Yes, by growth through several hundred serial transfers on culture medium containing bile. (*d*) Its value as a vaccine is questionable; all immunized persons become tuberculin-positive; the value of the tuberculin test as a screen for persons with tuberculosis is destroyed. (*e*) To study its effect on regression of tumors. (Secs. 5-40 and 5-41.)

32. (*a*) *Mycobacterium* species and oil emulsion. (*b*) Not in vaccines prepared commercially for routine immunizations. Freund's adjuvant has been used in some vaccines for cancer but only on an experimental basis. (*c*) Yes. (*d*) It can induce delayed-type hypersensitivity as well as antibody formation; it induces an immune response even to very weakly antigenic substances. (Sec. 5-42.)

Assay for Specific Cell-mediated Reactivity

5-43 For a long time skin tests were the only method known to assay for cell-mediated reactions. Skin tests for infectious diseases (except those based on neutralization of exotoxin) show a delayed-type hypersensitivity reaction which develops slowly and is usually read at 48 h. A typical reaction shows erythema, induration, and sometimes necrosis. Skin tests are commonly used to test for present or past infection with microorganisms which cause diseases like

Tuberculosis

Coccidioidomycosis

Histoplasmosis

Echinococcosis

Brucellosis

Lymphogranuloma venereum (Frei test)

Chanchroid

A skin test like the tuberculin test has the advantage that the skin-test material, PPD in this case, is a hapten and does not induce an immune response and affect the results of subsequent tests. In contrast, skin-test material like that for brucellosis is antigenic and can affect the value of other diagnostic tests, e.g., agglutination, if the skin test is performed before they are.

5-44 Recently in vitro tests for cell-mediated reactions have been developed. The test for migration-inhibition factor (MIF), which has proved to be a very good test, was described in Sec. 2-28. When sensitized lymphocytes come in contact with specific antigen, MIF is produced. Assays for other lymphokines besides MIF have also been developed.

5-45 In the *lymphocyte-activation test*, another in vitro test for cell-mediated reactivity, a suspension of leukocytes from the patient is prepared and mixed with antigen. Upon exposure of sensitized lymphocytes to the specific antigen, the lymphocytes undergo a series of morphological and biochemical changes. An increase in deoxyribonucleic acid (DNA) synthesis can be measured by incorporation of tritiated thymidine into newly synthesized DNA. Several methods are available for preparation of lymphocyte suspensions for in vitro assays of cell-mediated reactivity. The Ficoll-Hypaque method is commonly used. For procedure see Boyum (1968) or Rose and Friedman (1976).

Assay for T-Lymphocyte Function

5-46 Many tests have been described to test for T-lymphocyte function; their purpose is not to test for specific sensitivity of a patient's lymphocytes to a particular antigen but to evaluate the general capacity of the patient to develop cell-mediated immunity or delayed-type hypersensitivity to many different antigens. Some of the tests most frequently used for T-cell function are summarized below.

In Vivo Tests for T-Cell Function

Skin tests for sensitivity to microorganisms to which a person may be exposed in the environment
Some antigens or haptens used are as follows:

Tuberculin (PPD)

Candida albicans, a common yeast

Trichophyton spp, cause of athletes foot

Mumps virus skin test material or inactivated mumps virus

Streptokinase and streptodornase, enzymes of beta-hemolytic streptococci

A suspension of an inactivated microorganism or a metabolic product may be used. These tests are based on preexposure of the patient and the ability to produce a delayed-type hypersensitivity reaction. Patients who show a positive reaction to some but not all of the antigens listed above appear to have been exposed to some but not all of the microorganisms represented and to have T-cell function. In contrast, patients who show no skin reaction to any of the antigens listed above appear to be anergic, or deficient in T-cell function. The remote possibility exists that they have not been previously exposed to any of the antigens. In this case, one of the antigens, say *C. albicans*, can be chosen and used to determine whether or not the patient can be sensitized to produce a delayed allergic skin reaction. PPD should not be used for trial sensitization because it is not antigenic.

Sensitization and skin testing with antigens not commonly found in the environment A patient can be tested for T-cell function by using for trial sensitization an antigen which is not prevalent in the environment. Such an antigen is *keyhole limpet hemocyanin* (KLH). After sensitization and subsequent skin testing with KLH, a positive delayed allergic reaction would show that the patient did have T-cell function. A hapten which has been used for sensitization and testing is 2,4-dinitrochlorobenze (DNCB). Sensitization and testing with DNCB can be carried out by application of filter paper saturated with an appropriate amount of DNCB in acetone. DNCB very easily sensitizes skin, but it is not without danger and should be used only in special cases. Use of DNCB requires approval of the Food and Drug Administration.

In Vitro Tests for T Cells and T-Cell Function

Rosette test on peripheral blood of patient to determine number of T cells T cells have receptors for sheep red blood cells and therefore form rosettes with them (see Sec. 2-11). This test only shows the presence of T cells; however, when T-cell function is deficient, there are usually very few T cells. The rosette test does not require either antibody or complement but only erythrocytes, so that is is often referred to as the *E-rosette test.*

Biopsy of lymph nodes of patients In a patient who has T-cell deficiency, stained sections of the nodes show very few lymphocytes in the thymus-dependent paracortical area of the lymph node. This is the area where mainly T lymphocytes are found (see Sec. 2-13). This test indicates either that T cells are present or that the node is deficient in T cells.

Response of lymphocytes to mitogens Response of lymphocytes to mitogens was discussed in Sec. 2-32. T cells characteristically undergo transformation, as shown by uptake of tritiated thymidine, when they are exposed to mitogens such as phytohemagglutinin (PHA) and concanavalin A (ConA). T lymphocytes which undergo transformation or become activated by mitogens are considered to have normal T-cell function.

Contact Dermatitis (Allergic Eczematous Contact Dermatitis)

5-47 Allergic contact dermatitis is a form of delayed-type hypersensitivity in which sensitization takes place as a result of exposure of the skin to simple chemical molecules of low molecular weight. Most of these chemicals are relatively hydrophobic and readily penetrate the intact skin and combine with epidermal proteins to form complete antigens. The complete antigen is formed by covalent bonding between chemical contactant and skin protein. The chemical substances bound to protein act as the determinant groups of the antigen and are responsible for specificity of skin sensitization, which develops in 7 to 14 days. When the chemical again comes in contact with the skin of a sensitized person, a delayed-type hypersensitivity reaction occurs in 48 h. It appears necessary for the chemical (hapten) to conjugate with protein not only to sensitize but also to elicit a reaction in already sensitized skin. The patch test usually is employed for diagnosis of allergic contact dermatitis.

In the patch test, the chemical is applied to a 1-cm-square piece of cloth or filter paper and taped to the arm for 48 h. In 48 h a delayed allergic reaction appears, and in contact dermatitis vesicles appear, which sometimes coalesce to form large blisters.

5-48 Some of the most common contact-sensitizing antigens met with in clinical practice are catechols, present in poison ivy, poison oak, and sumac; metal compounds, especially nickel; rubber compounds; and chemicals such as *p*-phenylenediamine and dichromates used in dyes. A patient may be sensitive to many different kinds of metals in jewelry, scissors, thimbles, etc., or to chemicals for dying clothing made of cloth, fur, or leather. Patients are also often sensitive to many different kinds of cosmetics. Analyses of the area of sensitization helps pinpoint the substance responsible for sensitization. The best way to cure contact dermatitis is to avoid the substance responsible for it. A form of contact dermatitis known as *photoallergic contact dermatitis* occurs on exposure of skin to sunlight or ultraviolet light if certain kinds of soaps or chemicals have been applied to the skin. Areas of the body which are covered by clothing usually are not affected. Chemicals shown to cause photoallergic dermatitis include halogenated salicylanilides, biothionol, chlorpromazine, and sulfonamides. The mechanism of photoallergic contact dermatitis is not clear.

5-49 It was shown in 1942 by Landsteiner and Chase that contact dermatitis is a form of delayed-type hypersensitivity. Allergic contact dermatitis can be transferred from sensitized guinea pigs to unsensitized pigs by the injection of peritoneal exudate cells but not by serum. The mechanism of contact dermatitis has been studied extensively in guinea pigs using dinitrochlorobenzene, which produces contact dermatitis in these animals.

Delayed-Type Hypersensitivity and Resistance to Infection

5-50 Resistance to infection may be antibody-mediated (humoral) or cell-mediated. Resistance to some infections, e.g., those caused by higher moldlike bacteria (tubercle and leprosy bacilli), fungi, parasites, and viruses, are mainly cell-mediated. There are exceptions; e.g., in poliomyelitis infection, virus released from infected cells in the intestinal tract is neutralized locally by specific antibodies if they are present in the intestinal tract. If poliomyelitis virus spreads beyond the intestinal tract, the virus can still be neutralized in the blood so that it does not reach the central nervous system to cause neurological symptoms of poliomyelitis. It is typical of poliomyelitis virus in patients and in cell culture that virus is released from infected cells and that infection of surrounding cells can be prevented by presence of specific antibodies. In contrast, herpes viruses spread directly from cell to cell, so that infection of surrounding cells is not prevented by specific antibodies. For many years it was not understood why fever blisters, cold sores, etc., caused by infection with herpes virus continued to recur even in the presence of a high titer of serum antibodies until it was shown that this virus can spread from cell to cell without coming in contact with tissue antibodies. Herpes virus persists as a latent infection at the site of invasion. After an infection is established, the mechanism of resistance to herpes and many other viruses is that of delayed-type hypersensitivity. Neutralizing antibodies do prevent the dissemination of herpes virus to different areas or organs.

5-51 Some viruses propagate by budding from the cell membrane of infected cells so that viral antigens are present at the cell surface. These viral antigens at the cell surface may be largely responsible for delayed-type hypersensitivity reactions seen in these viral infections.

5-52 The mechanism of resistance to leprosy and to fungi is cell-mediated and similar to that described for tuberculosis. Different degrees of resistance are apparent. For example, patients with tuberculoid leprosy show resistance and a positive skin reaction, while those with lepromatous leprosy have a disseminated infection and a negative skin-test reaction. The skin-test material prepared from homogenized leprous tissue is called *lepromin*. Likewise, in fungal infections such as coccidioidomycosis the skin reaction may be negative in advanced cases, indicating that the patient has become anergic and has little resistance. Chemotherapeutic agents are available for treating tuberculosis, leprosy, and most fungal infections. After treatment some persons who have had advanced cases and become anergic may regain the ability to muster a delayed-type hypersensitivity skin response. Although antibodies are produced during fungal infections and aid in diagnosis with serologic tests, antibodies do not appear to confer significant resistance here.

5-53 There is considerable evidence that resistance to, or recovery from, parasitic infections is often cell-mediated. However, antibodies are formed to antigens of the parasite during different stages of development, and in some cases these antibodies may be protective. Infestation with worms causes eosinophilia and production of IgE. The role of IgE in parasitic infections is not known, but there is some evidence that IgE is protective. Other classes of immunoglobulins may also be formed. An antibody known as *ablastin* appears to be IgG and its formation T-cell dependent. Ablastin was first described by Taliaferro (1924) as a substance which inhibited reproduction of *Trypanosoma lewisi.* This type of immune reaction is known also as *ablastic immunity*. In human malaria, infection with *Plasmodium* spp. induces formation of a complement-independent antibody which can inhibit entry of the merozoites into the host erythrocytes. This antibody is IgG; it crosses the placenta and in endemic areas serves to protect a child against malaria during the first few months of life. Although antibodies may contribute to protection against, or termination of, parasitic infections, it appears that resistance of the host to many parasitic infections is either cell-mediated or a combination of cell-mediated and antibody-mediated immunity. Resistance to *Toxoplasma* appears to be due to a combination of both.

Delayed-Type Hypersensitivity and Pathogenesis of Disease

5-54 Although, as discussed above, delayed-type hypersensitivity reactions may be associated with resistance, it is important to point out that delayed-type hypersensitivity also may be associated with pathogenesis of disease. For example, delayed-type hypersensitivity reactions can cause marked tissue damage, e.g., that seen in cases of advanced tuberculosis where there is cavitation of the lung. In typhoid fever perforation of the intestine is thought to be caused by delayed-type hypersensitivity. In schistosomiasis, eggs laid by the mature female parasites appear to be the main cause of pathogenesis of this disease; antigens secreted from the eggs cause delayed-type hypersensitivity reactions and the eventual formation of granulomas and fibrosis. The pathogenesis of a number of autoimmune diseases discussed in Chap. 6 appears to result from delayed-type hypersensitivity reactions.

Other Conditions Associated with Delayed-Type Hypersensitivity Reactions

5-55 Some of the other conditions and diseases in which delayed-type hypersensitivity appears to be an underlying mechanism are discussed as indicated below:

Some autoimmune diseases, Chap. 6

Graft-versus-host reaction, Chap. 9

Rejection of allografts, Chap. 9

Tumor immunity, Chap. 10

Immunopotentiation, Chap. 10

Summary of Main Features of Type I to IV Immune Reactions Responsible for Tissue Damage

5-56 See Table 5-1.

Questions for Secs. 5-43 to 5-56

33. (*a*) What is the general underlying mechanism of skin tests for infectious diseases (exception diphtheria)? (*b*) What is a disadvantage of using a skin test to help diagnose brucellosis?

34. (*a*) Name one in vivo method to test for a specific cell-mediated reaction. (*b*) Name two in vitro methods which could be used to test for specific cell-mediated reactions. (*c*) Give one method which is commonly used to measure activation or transformation of lymphocytes.

Table 5-1 Main Features of Type I to IV Immune Reactions Responsible for Tissue Damage.

Type (Coombs and Gell)	Description	Antibodies involved	Examples	Complement required?	Mechanism of damage: Cells involved	Mechanism of damage: Mediators released
I	IgE-dependent immediate-type hypersensitivity	IgE	Anaphylaxis, atopy	No	Mast cells, basophils	Histamine, serotonin, etc.
II	Cytotoxic or cell-stimulating	IgG, IgM	Blood-transfusion reactions; antibody-dependent cytotoxicity (ADC) by K cells*, long-acting thyroid stimulator (LATS)	For some reactions†	None for most transfusion reactions; phagocytes for opsonic adherence; K cells for ADC	None
III	Immune-complex formation	Mainly IgG	Arthus reaction, serum-sickness syndrome	Yes	Neutrophils	Lysosomal enzymes
IV	Delayed-type hypersensitivity	None	Tuberculin test, contact dermatitis	No	Sensitized T lymphocytes	Lymphokines

*K (killer) cells appear to be either monocytes or non-T lymphocytes with Fc receptors. Null cells are often called K cells.

†Complement is not required for opsonic adherence (binding to phagocyte through Fc receptors for IgG) or for antibody-dependent cytotoxicity (ADC) by K cells.

35. (*a*) Name five skin-test materials which often give a positive delayed-type hypersensitivity reaction in children and adults due to exposure in the environment and which therefore can be used to assay for T-cell function. (*b*) If five of the antigens cited in part (*a*) are used to skin-test a patient and a positive reaction is obtained only in two, what would your interpretation of these results be? (*c*) What could you do further to confirm that your patient has T-cell function? (*d*) What is the disadvantage of using the antigens mentioned in part (a)? (*e*) What other antigens could be used?

36. (*a*) Besides the skin-test method cited in Question 35 what other procedures can be used to test for potential T-cell function? (*b*) In normal peripheral blood are B lymphocytes or T lymphocytes more numerous? (*c*) What is the mechanism of the rosette test for T cells in peripheral blood? (*d*) Where are T cells mainly found in lymph nodes?

37. (*a*) Does contact dermatitis have the characteristics of immediate or delayed-type hypersensitivity? (*b*) What kind of substances are responsible for sensitization in contact dermatitis? (*c*) Are these substances complete antigens? If the answer is no, explain how they cause sensitization. (*d*) What method of skin testing is used to diagnose contact dermatitis? (*e*) What is the best way to cure contact dermatitis?

38. (*a*) What kinds of microorganisms generally cause diseases in which resistance is cell-mediated? (*b*) What is the significance of eosinophilia and elevated IgE in parasitic infections? (*c*) What is ablastin?

Answers

33. (*a*) Delayed hypersensitivity. (*b*) The skin-test material for brucellosis is antigenic and could effect the outcome of other diagnostic serologic tests for brucellosis. (Sec. 5-43)

34. (*a*) Skin tests. (*b*) Test for migration-inhibition factor (MIF) and lymphocyte activation. (*c*) Activated lymphocytes show an increase in DNA synthesis, which can be measured by the incorporation of tritiated thymidine into newly synthesized DNA. (Secs. 5-43 to 5-45.)

35. (*a*) Tuberculin, *Candida albicans*, *Trichophyton* spp., mumps virus, streptokinase-streptodornase. (*b*) The patient has T-cell function and has been sensitized to only two of the five skin-test antigens. (*c*) Carry out trial sensitization with one of the other antigens but not tuberculin which is not antigenic; repeat skin test with the antigen. (*d*) The skin-test antigen would no longer have any diagnostic value for this patient. (*e*) For trial sensitization, use antigens which are not common in the environment, e.g., keyhole limpet hemocyanin (KLH) and 2,4-dinitrochlorobenzene (DNCB). (Sec. 5-46.)

36. (*a*) Rosette test, biopsy of lymph nodes, response of lymphocytes to mitogens such as PHA or ConA. (*b*) T lymphocytes. (*c*) T cells have receptors for sheep red blood cells; B lymphocytes and null lymphocytes do not. (*d*) In the paracortical area. (Sec. 5-46.)

37. (*a*) Delayed type. (*b*) Low-molecular-weight chemicals of plants, metals, etc. (*c*) No; these chemicals are usually hydrophobic and readily penetrate the intact skin and combine with epidermal proteins to form complete antigens. (*d*) Patch test. (*e*) Avoid substance causing it. (Secs. 5-47 and 5-48.)

38. (*a*) Intracellular parasites such as viruses. Also higher moldlike bacteria, such as tubercle and leprosy bacilli; fungi; some protozoa and helminths. (*b*) Not known. There is some evidence that IgE may be protective. (*c*) Ablastin is an antibody which has been shown to interfere with reproduction of parasites such as trypanosomes. (Sec. 5-53.)

REFERENCES

Bigley, N. J. (1975): "Immunologic Fundamentals," Yearbook, Chicago.

Bloom, B. R., and P. R. Glade (eds.) (1971): "*In Vitro* Methods in Cell-mediated Immunity," Academic, New York.

Boyum, A. (1968): Isolation of Mononuclear Cells and Granulocytes from Human Blood, *Scand. J. Clin. Lab. Invest.*, **21** (suppl. 97):77-89.

Coombs, R. R. A., and P. G. H. Gell (1963): The Classification of Allergic Reactions Underlying Disease, pp. 317-337 in P. G. H. Gell and R. R. A. Coombs (eds.), "Clinical Aspects of Immunology," Davis, Philadelphia.

———and——— (1975): Classification of Allergic Reactions Responsible for Clinical Hypersensitivity and Diseases, pp. 761-781 in P. H. Gell, R. R. A. Coombs, and P. J. Lackmann (eds.), "Clinical Aspects of Immunology," 3d ed. Blackwell, Oxford.

D'Alesandro, P. A. (1975): Ablastin: The Phenomenon, *Exp. Parasitol.*, **38**:303-308.

Eisen, H. N. (1973): Antibody-mediated (Immediate-Type) Hypersensitivity, pp. 527-555, and Cell-mediated Hypersensitivity and Immunity, pp. 557-595 in B. D. Davis, R. Dulbecco, H. N. Eisen, H. S. Ginsberg, W. B. Wood, and M. McCarty (eds.), "Microbiology," 2d ed. Harper & Row, Hagerstown, Md.

Fudenberg, H. H., D. P. Stites, J. L. Caldwell, and J. V. Wells. (1976): "Basic and Clinical Immunology," Lange, Los Altos, Calif.

Gordon, B. L., II (1974): "Essentials of Immunology," 2d ed., Davis, Philadelphia.

Green, R. L., R. W. Scales, and S. J. Kraus (1976): Increased Serum Immunoglobulin E Concentrations in Veneral Diseases, *Br. J. Vener. Dis.*, **52**:257-260.

Ishizaka, I. 1977. Structure and Biologic Activity of Immunoglobulin E, *Hosp. Prac.*, **12**(1):57-67.

Johansson, S. G. O., H. H. Bennick, and T. Berg (1972): The Clinical Significance of IgE, *Prog. Clin. Immunol.*, **1**:157-181.

Landsteiner, K., and M. W. Chase (1942): Experiments on Transfer of Cutaneous Sensitivity to Simple Compounds, *Proc. Soc. Exp. Biol. Med.*, **49**: 688-690.

Miescher, P. A., andH. J. Muller-Eberhard (eds.) (1976): "A Textbook of Immunopathology," vol. 1, 2d ed., Grune and Stratton, New York.

Myrvik, Q. N., L. A. Kohlweiss, and D. Harpold (1975): Pathological Potential of Exaggerated Immunological Reactions, pp. 227-235 in D. Schlessinger (ed.), "Microbiology: 1975," American Society for Microbiology, Washington, D.C.

Nakamura, R. M. (1974): "Immunopathology, Clinical Laboratory Concepts and Methods," Little, Brown, Boston.

Nelson, D. S. (ed.) (1976): "Immunobiology of the Macrophage," Academic, New York.

Perlmann, P. (1976): Cellular Immunity: Antibody-dependent Cytotoxicity (K-Cell Activity), *Clin. Immunobiol.*, **3**:107-132.

Pinsky, C. M. (1976): Cell-mediated Immunity: *In Vivo* Testing, *Clin. Immunobiol.*, **3**:97-105.
Rajka, E., and S. Korossy (eds.) (1974*a*): "Immunological Aspects of Allergy and Allergic Diseases," vol. 1, "Basic Concepts in Experimental Immunology," Plenum, London.
———and ——— (eds.) (1974*b*): "Immunological Aspects of Allergy and Allergic Diseases," vol. 2, "Methods in Experimental Immunology," Plenum, London.
Rocklin, Ross E. (1976): Products of Activated Lymphocytes, *Clin. Immunobiol.*, **3**:195-220.
Rose, N. R., and H. Friedman (1976): "Manual of Clinical Immunology," American Society for Microbiology, Washington, D.C.
Rundles, S. C., J. A. Hansen, and B. Dupont (1976): Lymphocyte Transformation *in Vitro* in Response to Mitogens and Antigens, *Clin. Immunobiol.*, **3**:151-194.
Samter, M. (ed.) (1971): "Immunological Diseases," vols. I and II, 2d ed., Little, Brown, Boston.
Sell, S. (1975): "Immunology, Immunopathology, and Immunity," 2d ed., Harper & Row, Hagerstown, Md.
Tada, T. (1975): Regulation of Reaginic Antibody Formation in Animals, *Prog. Allergy*, **19**:122-194.
Taliaferro, W. H. (1924): A Reaction Product in Infection with *Trypanosoma Lewisi* Which Inhibits the Reproduction of the Trypanosomes, *J. Exp. Med.*, **39**:171-190.
Thaler, M. S., R. D. Klausner, and H. J. Cohen (1977): "Medical Immunology," Lippincott, Philadelphia.

6
Autosensitization as a Cause of Disease

AUTOIMMUNE RESPONSES AND AUTOIMMUNE DISEASES

Meaning and Use of the Term Autoimmunity

6-1 *Autoimmunity* (*auto-* means "self") refers to a condition believed to result from an immune response of a host against his own body constituents. The response may be humoral or cellular. Autoimmunity is not associated with resistance but is often associated with disease. It has been proposed that *autoallergy* should be used instead of autoimmunity and *autosensitization* instead of autoimmunization.

Distinction between Autoimmune Diseases and Autoimmune Responses

6-2 Autoimmune diseases These are diseases in which host reactions to self or autoantigens lead to a disease state. The autoimmune diseases may be mediated by antibodies or sensitized lymphocytes. Many autoimmune diseases have been recognized. In general, autoimmune diseases are of two kinds: (1) those which mainly involve a single organ and (2) those characterized by widespread pathologic changes in many different organs and tissues throughout the body. The division often is not sharp. Some examples are given in Table 6-1.

Autoimmune responses Autoimmune responses are the production of antibodies or sensitized T lymphocytes to self antigens. Some autoimmune responses may or may not be associated with disease.

Autoantibodies Not Associated with Autoimmune Disease

6-3 Syphilis reagin is an autoantibody, but syphilis is not an autoimmune disease. Syphilis reagins react with cardiolipin extracted from normal animal tissue, usually beef heart. During syphilitic infection with *T. pallidum* much destruction of tissue occurs, so that the immune system is exposed to antigens uncovered during tissue breakdown. One of the determinant groups exposed is cardiolipin.

Table 6-1 Examples of Autoimmune Diseases

Organ-specific	Not organ-specific*
Postinfection encephalitis (brain)	Systemic lupus erythematosus
Pemphigus (skin)	Rheumatoid arthritis
Addison's disease (adrenal)	Scleroderma (progressive systemic sclerosis)
Hashimoto's thyroiditis (thyroid)	
Goodpasture's syndrome (kidney and lung)	

*All are diffuse-connective-tissue or collagen diseases

The antibody (reagin) formed reacts with cardiolipin in vitro and serves as the basis for nonspecific serologic tests for syphilis such as VDRL, RPR, and other flocculation tests for syphilis using cardiolipin (Chap. 11). This antibody is not responsible for the disease process of syphilis but occurs as a result of it. This type of autoantibody occurs in some other diseases where there is similar tissue destruction (see Chap. 11). In mycoplasma pneumonia, which is not an autoimmune disease, autoantibodies known as *cold agglutinins* are formed to host red blood cells in about 50 percent of patients. Cold agglutinins cause agglutination of red blood cells at 5 to 10°C, but they appear to have no role in pathogenesis of mycoplasma pneumonia.

Autoantibodies Associated with Autoimmune Disease

6-4 Autoantibodies (*warm antibodies*) to red-blood-cell antigens such as Rh are responsible for anemia in the autoimmune disease known as *acquired hemolytic anemia*. Autoantibodies appear in many different autoimmune diseases, but it is often difficult to tell whether they cause the disease or are merely a result of it. Rheumatoid factor (RF) is an autoantibody to IgG and is found in patients with rheumatoid arthritis; formerly thought to be only IgM, RF may also be IgG. RF is useful for diagnosis; it can be detected by agglutination of latex particles coated with homologous or heterologous IgG. RF reacts with the Fc portion of IgG; it does not react with latex particles coated with IgM or IgA. Rheumatoid arthritis is thought to be caused by an Arthus type of reaction due to formation of complexes of RF with IgG in synovial fluid. It has been theorized that RF is formed to IgG in immune complexes such as virus-antibody complexes and that the structure of IgG is altered when it is aggregated with viruses or other antigens. That RF contributes to the pathogenesis of rheumatoid arthritis is questioned by some investigators. In synovial tissue of joints, RF may react with altered IgG or with IgG complexed with another antigen, bind complement, and subsequently lead to tissue injury. Complement levels of joint fluid are depressed in active cases of rheumatoid arthritis. RF may be found in other diseases such as systemic lupus erythematosus (SLE) but usually in lower titers than in rheumatoid arthritis. Many different kinds of antibodies are found in SLE. Patients with SLE often have a biologic false positive reaction for syphilis due to the formation of autoantibodies to cardiolipin. Antinuclear antibodies are especially characteristic of SLE: they are found in 95 to 100 percent of SLE cases. Immune complexes formed in SLE such as DNA-anti-DNA damage tissue wherever the immune complexes are deposited. Localization of immune complexes in glomeruli of the kidneys leads to glomerulonephritis, which usually is the cause of death in SLE. Glomerulonephritis in SLE is an example of an autoimmune disease in which the site of tissue damage is not directly related to the specificity of the autoantibody. In SLE, complexes also localize in blood vessels, causing vasculitis, and in serous membranes, causing arthritis and serositis.

Possible Mechanisms in Development of Autoimmunity

6-5 Loss of immunological tolerance In general, mechanisms involved in loss of immunological tolerance to self antigens are responsible for development of autoimmunity. It has been pointed out (Chap. 2) that the immune system recognizes host tissue as self and under ordinary circumstances cannot be induced to respond to it. In Chap. 3, when the characteristics of immunogens or antigens were discussed, one important characteristic was foreignness to host tissue. Immunological tolerance can be induced experimentally by injection of antigen in utero or by injection immediately after birth. It appears that tissue antigens present during in utero development of the host are not recognized as foreign after birth. In laboratory animals, the state during which tolerance can be induced persists for a short time after birth. The experimental induction of immunologic tolerance in rabbits is more easily achieved with soluble antigens like bovine serum albumin (BSA) than with antigens in a particulate structure like bacteria. Some diseases, e.g., rheumatoid arthritis, are seen more frequently in the older age group and may be due to a partial failure of the immune system with loss of tolerance to a particular antigen.

6-6 Exposure to sequestered or unmasked self antigens Antigens considered to be hidden or sequestered are those found in tissues inaccessible to blood and lymph circulation; therefore, they are not in contact with elements of the immune system such as B and T lymphocytes. Examples of sequestered antigens are sperm and lens protein. Sperm have an additional characteristic in that development is not complete at birth, so that antigens acquired after birth are recognized as foreign. These sperm antigens are called *maturation antigens.* In the host, maturation antigens act like altered or neoantigens because they have a different antigenic structure after birth. If physical injury or infection occurs, there is a breakdown between blood-tissue barriers in the damaged tissue and autosensitization occurs. Autosensitization to sperm may cause infertility. Leakage of lens protein into the eye during the course of cataract removal may cause autosensitization to lens protein and inflammatory changes in the other eye, so that a condition known as *uveitis* occurs. For many years thyroglobulin was thought to be a sequestered antigen, but this no longer appears to be true; however, autosensitization to thyroglobulin of the thyroid gland does occur and may result in thyroiditis.

6-7 Exposure to altered antigens Tissue antigens may be altered in a number of ways, e.g., by virus infection and reaction with toxins, drugs, and other chemicals. The body recognizes altered antigens as nonself. Drastic alteration in antigen structure is unlikely to cause autosensitization. Virus infection has been shown to be one of the main causes of tissue alteration leading to autoimmune disease. Postinfection encephalomyelitis sometimes may follow infection with viruses such as measles. Autoallergy to brain tisuse is cell-mediated. In viral hepatitis, autosensitization of the cell-mediated type is considered to be responsible for much of the liver damage. With regard to alteration by drugs, some forms of hemolytic anemia and thrombocytopenic purpura are brought on by binding of the drug to red blood cells and platelets, respectively. This alteration may be caused by such drugs as chlorpromazine, quinidine, quinine, and stibophen.

6-8 Exposure to exogenous antigens structurally similar to normal tissue components These antigens are considered to be shared or cross-reacting antigens. Group A beta-hemolytic streptococci have an antigen in common with human heart tissue. Antibodies to group A streptococci cross-react with human heart tissue. Many years before this sharing of antigens by streptococci and heart tissue was discovered, it was recognized that when rheumatic fever occurs, it characteristically follows about 2 weeks after group A streptococcal infection. Likewise, glomerulonephritis can be caused by certain strains of group A streptococci which share antigens with kidney tissue. It has been shown that a strain (O14) of *E. coli* shares a common antigen with tissue of human colon. Some strains of *E. coli* are part of the normal flora of the intestinal tract, but it is possible that cases of ulcerative colitis in which anticolon antibodies are found are due to a local immune response to this particular strain of *E. coli.* Antigens with similar structure may cause a break in immunologic tolerance by a mechanism first elucidated by Weigle (1961), who reported that after rabbits were made tolerant to bovine serum albumin (BSA), tolerance could be broken by immunization with a cross-reacting antigen, in this case human serum albumin (HSA). After the break in tolerance by injection of HSA, the rabbit made antibodies to BSA. Tolerance could also be broken by chemically modified BSA.

6-9 Alteration in cells of the immune system This mechanism would depend not on alteration of such tissue cells as heart, liver, etc., but on alteration in the cellular processes necessary for maintenance of normal tolerance. Here the effect of a drug or virus would have to be on lymphoid tissue containing B and T cells or their precursors. A number of changes in lymphoid tissue could possibly take place and lead to autoimmunity. Autoantibodies are found in infectious mononucleosis, which is believed to be caused by infection of B lymphocytes with Epstein-Barr (EB) virus. A very large number of mononuclear T lymphoblasts are formed by T cells, probably in response to new cell-surface antigens on virus-infected B cells.

Possible Mechanisms Affecting Cells of Lymphoid Tissue and Leading to Autoimmunity

6-10 Some of the mechanisms below are interrelated or related to mechanisms previously discussed.
Somatic mutation of lymphocytes into self-reacting cells Postulation of this change is based on the clonal-selection theory, which states that self-reacting lymphocytes are not present after birth unless a mutation occurs in an existing clone.
Stimulation of preexisting population of B lymphocytes capable of making autoantibodies Naturally occurring autoantibodies have been described by several investigators. According to them, small amounts of autoantibodies present in the blood of normal individuals facilitate the removal of debilitated cells by phagocytosis. The amount of antibody produced is in "physiologic" amounts and is controlled by suppressor T cells. It has also been postulated that tolerance to some antigens may depend on continuous low serum levels of autoantibody to these antigens and that when production of antibody ceases, autoimmunity ensues. The normal production of autoantibodies to clean up dying or damaged tissue cells or to maintain a state of tolerance is hard to explain on the basis of the clonal-selection theory, which states that forbidden clones capable of self-recognition are eliminated before birth.
Loss of suppressor-T-cell activity Suppressor T cells are lymphocytes which act as regulators of antibody production; these suppressor cells also appear to regulate cell-mediated immune reactions.
Nonspecific stimulation of helper-T-cell activity Tissue antigens require helper T cells for antibody production. Helper T cells are carrier-specific (review Sec. 2-19). Altered carrier protein on an antigen could stimulate T cells of different specificity to cooperate with B cells (hapten specificity same as tissue) to make autoantibodies. Infectious agents other than viruses also can act as carriers or adjuvants. When Freund's complete adjuvant is injected with homologous tissue into experimental animals, the adjuvant bypasses the need for helper T cells.

Association between Aging and Development of Autoimmune Diseases

6-11 Several events appear to be age-related and to occur more frequently as a person grows older, namely immunodeficiency states, the appearance of autoimmune diseases, and malignancy. When immunodeficiency occurs in young children, there is still the propensity to produce autoantibodies and malignancy. This association has been shown to occur not only in human beings but also in animals. Therefore, the production of autoimmunity cannot be considered only in terms of altered or shared antigens, etc. It appears that in at least some autoimmune diseases, there is perturbation of the immune system. Two theories which may explain a relationship between aging and autoimmunity are that aging results from a decline in an immune homeostatic mechanism or from somatic-cell variation of factors some of which determine self-recognition and eventually lead to the onset of autoimmunity.

Association between Histocompatibility Loci Antigens and Development of Autoimmunity

6-12 A number of autoimmune diseases, in addition to some other diseases, appear to be associated with genetic factors which determine tissue or transplantation antigens, known as HLA. This is a relatively new area of investigation; some of the diseases in which an association with HLA has been reported are listed in Table 6-2.

Autoimmune Diseases or Immune Disorders following Immunization

6-13 Autoimmune diseases or immune disorders sometimes follow immunization with licensed vaccines. In the cases discussed here, with the exception of rabies brain vaccine, it is not possible to predict an unfavorable outcome. In Sec. 1-30 it was pointed out that there is a greater chance of encephalomyelitis following immunization against rabies with Pasteur-type vaccine containing virus propagated in rabbit brain than when other rabies vaccines are used. The mechanism here is probably one of sharing of common antigens by rabbit and human brain tissue. Encephalomyelitis is not antibody-mediated but is caused by sensitized T lymphocytes. Experimental studies on encephalomyelitis have

Table 6-2 Diseases with a Reported Association with HLA

Disease	Antigen
Ankylosing spondylitis	HLA-B27
Reiter's syndrome	HLA-B27
Acute anterior uveitis	HLA-B27
Chronic hepatitis	HLA-B8
Dermatitis herpetiformis	HLA-B8
Graves' disease	HLA-B8
Addison's disease	HLA-B8
Multiple sclerosis	HLA-B7, HLA-A3

identified a myelin basic protein as being the major constituent which endows mammalian tissue of the central nervous system with encephlitogenic activity. Encephalomyelitis occurs more frequently in people who have been immunized previously against rabies. The other vaccines which are available for immunization against rabies were discussed in Sec. 1-30.

6-14 The *Guillain-Barrē syndrome*, which sometimes followed immunization during the 1976 national swine influenza immunization program, is possibly caused by autoallergy. This syndrome is called *idiopathic polyneuritis*. An autoimmune basis is supported by the observation that experimental allergic neuritis (EAN) produced in monkeys by injection of peripheral nerve tissue resembles idiopathic polyneuritis in human beings. Idiopathic polyneuritis and EAN are characterized by a latent period of about 6 to 14 days between exposure to the inciting agent and appearance of symptoms. Symptoms include a gradually ascending symmetrical polyneuropathy; pathologic lesions in the nerve roots and peripheral nerves; lymphocytic infiltration in the liver, heart, and other internal organs; and a tendency to spontaneous remission. Experimental transfer of EAN from an affected animal to a normal one can be accomplished by injection of a suspension of lymphoid cells, indicating that cell-mediated immunity (CMI) is responsible for pathogenesis. The inciting agent is frequently a virus. Certain viral infections are known to stimulate autoimmune phenomena directed against host-tissue antigens. In these viral infections, virus-specific antigens are at the host cell surface. Also, host-specific antigens are incorporated into the lipid envelopes of viruses such as influenza when they bud from the surface of the host cell. However, virus of the vaccine was inactivated and host tissue was that of chicken embryo and not human. The Gullain-Barrē syndrome appeared within 8 weeks after influenza vaccination in approximately 10 of every 1 million persons vaccinated; 5 to 10 percent of persons with the syndrome had residual weakness, and approximately 5 percent died.

6-15 Subacute sclerosing panencephalitis (SSPE) is a degenerative brain disease which is caused by infection of the central nervous system with measles virus or one very closely related to it. SSPE affects mainly young children, but it may not become apparent until several years after infection. In this respect, it has the characteristics of a slow virus disease. SSPE is eventually fatal. In patients with SSPE, very high titers of antibodies to measles virus are present in the serum and spinal fluid; viral inclusion bodies are in the brain. The establishment of measles virus in this way appears to be caused by a deficiency in cell-mediated immunity. SSPE also has occurred after immunization with the living attenuated measles vaccine, but the incidence is less than that after the disease. The pathogenesis of SSPE is not understood; although this disease appears to result from a lack of cell-mediated immunity, in vitro T-lymphocyte function to measles virus has been reported to be normal.

Questions for Secs. 6-1 to 6-15

1. (*a*) Are autoimmune responses considered to be favorable to the host? (*b*) What other term has been proposed for autoimmune? (*c*) For autoimmunization?

2. (*a*) What is an autoimmune disease? (*b*) Are autoimmune diseases antibody-mediated or cell-mediated? (*c*) Are autoantibodies found only in autoimmune diseases? Explain. (*d*) What are cold agglutinins? (*e*) Why are reagins of syphilis considered to be autoantibodies?

3. (*a*) What kinds of autoantibody is rheumatoid factor? (*b*) What autoantibody is characteristically found in SLE? (*c*) Is glomerulonephritis in SLE caused by autoantibodies, and if so are they kidney-specific? Explain your answer. (*d*) Do patients with SLE often show a biologic false positive (BFP) reaction for syphilis?

4. (*a*) What are sequestered, or hidden, antigens? (*b*) What causes hidden antigens to become unmasked? (*c*) What are maturation antigens? Give an example.

5. In rheumatic fever, what theory is used to explain an immune response to heart tissue and also to account for the fact that rheumatic fever characteristically follows infection with group A beta-hemolytic streptococci?

6. (*a*) According to the clonal-selection theory, what happens to self-reacting clones of lymphocytes before birth? (*b*) According to this theory, would you expect autoantibodies in physiologic amounts to be formed under normal conditions to aid in phagocytosis of old or damaged tissue cells?

7. (*a*) Name three abnormal conditions which are often associated with aging. (*b*) Name a well-known antigen which has certain specificities associated with autoimmune diseases.

8. (*a*) What is the Guillain-Barré syndrome? (*b*) Why is it thought to be an autoimmune disease? (*c*) Why are certain viruses especially likely to cause autoimmune diseases? (*d*) With what vaccine was the Guillain-Barré syndrome associated in 1976? (*e*) What does the abbreviation SSPE stand for? (*f*) What causes SSPE?

Answers

1. (*a*) No. (*b*) Autoallergic. (*c*) Autosensitization. (Sec. 6-1.)

2. (*a*) A disease caused by an immune response to self antigens. (*b*) Both. Some are antibody-mediated, but many are cell-mediated. (*c*) No. Some autoantibodies do not contribute to the pathogenesis of a disease but appear as a result of disease processes, e.g., tissue breakdown. (*d*) Cold agglutinins are autoantibodies which agglutinate human red blood cells at refrigerator temperature. (*e*) Reagins react with cardiolipin extracted from normal tissue; they also occur in other diseases where there is considerable destruction of tissue. (Sec. 6-3.)

3. (*a*) IgM or IgG to IgG. (*b*) Antinuclear. (*c*) Yes, glomerulonephritis in SLE is caused by autoantibodies such as anti-DNA, but they are not kidney-specific. Immune complexes such as DNA–anti-DNA fix complement and are deposited in capillaries of the renal glomeruli, where they cause tissue injury. (*d*) Yes. (Sec. 6-4.)

4. (*a*) Antigens which under normal circumstances are not accessible to blood and lymph circulation. (*b*) Infection or injury. (*c*) Antigens which are not fully developed until after birth, e.g., antigens of sperm. (Sec. 6-6.)

5. Human heart tissue and group A beta-hemolytic streptococci share a common antigen. (Sec. 6-8.)

6. (*a*) They are destroyed. (*b*) No. (Sec. 6-10.)

7. (*a*) Autoimmunity, immunodeficiency, and malignancy. (*b*) HLA. (Secs. 6-11 and 6-12.)

8. (*a*) Idiopathic polyneuritis. (*b*) Monkeys injected with peripheral nerve tissue develop the same symptoms. The Guillain-Barré syndrome follows some viral infections after a latent period. (*c*) Viruses such as influenza bud from the cell surface so that viral antigens at the cell surface make the cell appear altered to the host. Also viruses like influenza incorporate host-specific antigens into their lipid envelope as they are shed from the cell surface so that a suspension of influenza virus contains host-tissue antigens. (*d*) Influenza. (*e*) Subacute sclerosing panencephalitis. (*f*) Initially, SSPE is caused by infection of the central nervous system with measles virus or a virus very similar to it. The host appears to lack CMI to this infection. The pathogenesis of SSPE is not clear. (Secs. 6-14 and 6-15.)

Characteristics Associated with Autoimmune Diseases

6-16 The following characteristics are often cited as being associated with autoimmune diseases, but not all of the features listed would be expected for all autoimmune diseases:

Improvement of disease with immunosuppressive therapy

Inflammatory lesions with many lymphocytes and plasma cells

Autoantibodies in serum

Hypergammaglobulinemia

Coexistence with other conditions which appear to be autoimmune

Familial aggregation

Protracted course with exacerbations and remissions

Often no known precipitating cause

Serologic Tests for Diagnosis of Autoimmune Diseases

6-17 There are many kinds of serologic tests to aid in the diagnosis of autoimmune diseases. Some of the more frequently used tests are outlined below. The underlying mechanisms of most of these tests were discussed in Chap. 4..

Coombs test (direct) (Sec. 4-15). A sensitive method for the detection of antibodies on red blood cells.

Passive agglutination (Secs. 4-16 and 4-17). Latex particles or bentonite act as carriers for antigen to detect autoantibodies.

Passive hemagglutination (Secs. 4-16 and 4-17). Formalinized red blood cells act as carriers for antigen to detect autoantibodies.

Agar-gel diffusion (Ouchterlony) (Sec. 4-23). This is not a very sensitive method for detection of autoantibodies; it can also be used for the detection of immune complexes.

Counterelectrophoresis (Sec. 4-29). Used to detect autoantibodies.

Radioimmunoassay (Sec. 4-30). Used to detect autoantibodies and immune complexes. Talal and Pillarisetty (1976) used another technique besides those described in Chap. 4 for collection of radioactive complexes, i.e., cellulose ester (Millipore) filters.

Immunofluorescence (Sec. 4-41). Immunofluorescence can be used (1) to detect specific antibodies (or complement) deposited in tissue (antibodies to basement membrane of cells show a linear pattern of immunofluorescence like that seen in a renal biopsy from a patient with Goodpasture's syndrome); (2) to detect immune complexes (plus complement) deposited in tissue (the pattern of fluorescence is usually described as lumpy bumpy; this is the pattern seen in glomerulonephritis of SLE); (3) to detect antinuclear antibodies (ANA) and antibodies to other cell components in patients' sera. Indirect FA can detect at least four types of antinuclear antibodies. These four types and their characteristic pattern of nuclear fluorescence are anti-deoxyribonucleic acid (DNA), peripheral; antinucleoprotein (anti-DNA histone), homogeneous; anti-non-DNA, speckled; and anti-ribonucleic acid (RNA), nucleolar. The peripheral pattern is present only in SLE and is correlated with the severe form of SLE. Some of the other nuclear patterns of fluorescence are found in SLE and such diseases as rheumatoid arthritis, scleroderma, and Sjögren's syndrome.

Platelet aggregation, which has not been previously discussed, is based on the observation that when immune complexes are mixed with platelets, the surface of the platelets is altered, causing platelet aggregation. Aggregation is not due to cross linking of platelets by immune complexes but to changes in their adhesive properties.

Titration of complement (hemolytic assay) (Sec. 4-37). Complement is bound by immune complexes so that a low complement level in serum is an indication of immune-complex disease. The same general procedure is used to titrate complement in patient's serum as to titrate complement for the complement-fixation test. The patient's serum is diluted and mixed with sensitized sheep red blood cells (sheep rbc + specific hemolysin).

Complement-fixation test (Sec. 4-38). Used to detect autoantibodies. This technique, which is less frequently used than others, cannot be used with anticomplementary sera.

LE cell test This is an in vitro test which has been assocaited for many years with the diagnosis of SLE. The patient's blood is incubated at 37°C. Antibodies in SLE combine with the nuclear surface of damaged leukocytes and bind complement, with the release of chemotactic products which attract polymorphonuclear leukocytes. Cytoplasm of the damaged cell is lost, and the nuclear mass is phagocytized. LE cells appear as polymorphs which contain a large homogeneous nuclear mass intracellularly with the true nucleus of the cell pushed aside. Many of the tests described above are considered more satisfactory tests for SLE.

Experimental Studies with New Zealand Black Mice on Autoimmunity

6-18 In early experimental studies on laboratory animals such as rabbits, homologous tissue was injected with Freund's adjuvant in order to induce an autoimmune response. Through the years, various animal models have been obtained to study autoimmunity. One of the most interesting of these animal models is the New Zealand black (NZB) mouse strain; its outstanding characteristic is that after the age of 6 months mice spontaneously begin to develop typical autoimmune hemolytic anemia with a positive direct Coombs test. Many of the mice, particularly females, die with renal disease caused by deposition of immune complexes in the glomeruli. Older mice develop spleenic tumors, mostly of the reticulum type. The NZB strain is used to study autoimmune hemolytic anemia. A hybrid strain (NZB/NZW_{F_1}), frequently used to study SLE, was obtained by crossing NZB mice with NZW (W = white) mice. These mice develop autoantibodies and disease typical of SLE in human beings. Patients with SLE and NZB/NZW_{F_1} mice produce antibodies to double stranded DNA while in other human disease states and with other experimental animals, antibodies to only single-stranded DNA are produced.

Questions for Secs. 6-16 to 6-18

9. Name three general procedures which can be used to test for autoantibodies.

10. (*a*) If antibody is specific for glomerular basement membrane, what pattern of fluorescence is observed? Give an example (disease). (*b*) If soluble immune complexes which fix complement lodge in the glomeruli of the kidneys, what pattern of fluorescence is observed? Give an example (disease).

11. Why is the level of serum complement low in immune-complex diseases?

12. (*a*) What is an LE cell? (*b*) With what disease is it associated?

13. (*a*) What strain(s) of mice spontaneously develop a disease similar to autoimmune hemolytic anemia and SLE? (*b*) What kind of antibody is found in SLE and in NZB/NZW_{F_1} mice which is not found in other diseases or experimental animals?

Answers

9. Passive agglutination, radioimmunoassay, counterelectrophoresis, and immunofluorescence. (Sec. 6-17.)

10. (*a*) Linear pattern of fluorescence; Goodpasture's syndrome. (*b*) Lumpy-bumpy pattern of fluorescence; SLE. (Sec. 6-17.)

11. Complement is fixed to the immune complexes (provided they are of the Ag-Ab composition to fix complement). (Sec. 6-17.)

12. (*a*) A polymorphonuclear leukocyte with engulfed nuclear material of a damaged white cell which had reacted with antinuclear antibodies. (*b*) SLE. (Sec. 6-17.)

13. (*a*) New Zealand black (NZB) mice, autoimmune hemolytic anemia; a hybrid known as NZB/NZW_{F_1} mice, SLE. (*b*) Antibody to double-stranded DNA. (Sec. 6-18.)

REFERENCES

Agnello, V. (1976): Detection of Immune Complexes, pp. 669-675 in N. R. Rose and H. Friedman (eds.), "Manual of Clinical Immunology," American Society for Microbiology, Washington, D.C.

Barrett, J. T. (1976): "Basic Immunology and Its Medical Application," Mosby, Saint Louis.

Burnet, M. (1973): The New Zealand Mice, pp. 109-119 in M. Burnet, "Auto-immunity and Autoimmune Disease," Davis, Philadelphia.

Doniach, D. (1972): Autoimmunity in Liver Diseases, *Prog. Clin. Immunobiol.*, **1**:45-70.

Engelfriet, C. P. (1976): Autoantibodies in Hematological Disorders, *Clin. Immunobiol.* **3**:345-364.

Freedman, S. O., and P. Gold (ed.) (1976): "Clinical Immunology," 2d ed., Harper & Row, Hagerstown, Md.

Fudenberg, H. H., D. P. Stites, J. L. Caldwell, and J. V. Wells (eds.) (1976): "Basic and Clinical Immunology," Lange, Los Altos, Calif.

Jasin, H. E., and J. D. Smiley (1976): Rheumatoid Factors in Human Disease, *Clin. Immunobiol.*, **3**:365-373.

Lapointe, N., G. Geoffrey, B. McLaughlin, and J. G. Mongeau (1975): Subacute Sclerosing Panencephalitis (SSPE), *Birth Defects: Orig. Artic. Ser.* XI, pp. 239-243.

Miescher, P. A., and H. J. Müller-Eberhard (eds.) (1976): "Textbook of Immunopathology," vols. 1 and 2, Grune and Stratton, New York.

Nakamura, R. M. (ed.) (1974): "Immunopathology: Clinical Laboratory Concepts and Methods," Little, Brown, Boston.

Rajka, E., and S. Korossy (1975): "Immunological Aspects of Allergy and Allergic Diseases" vol. 3, "Clinical Aspects of Autoimmune Diseases," Plenum, London.

———and———(1975): "Immunological Aspects of Allergy and Allergic Diseases," vol. 4, "Clinical Aspects of Immune Pathology," Plenum, London.

Riott, I. (1977): "Essential Immunology," 3d ed., Blackwell, Oxford.

Rose, N. R., and H. Friedman (1976): "Manual of Clinical Immunology," American Society for Microbiology, Washington, D.C.

Talal, N. (1976): Antibodies to Nucleic Acids, *Clin. Immunobiol.*, **3**:375-385.

———and R. Pillarisetty (1976): Radioimmunoassay for Antibodies to Desoxyribonucleic Acid, pp. 652-655 in N. R. Rose and H. Friedman (eds.), "Manual of Clinical Immunology," American Society for Microbiology, Washington, D.C.

U.S. Department of Health, Education and Welfare/Public Health Service, Center for Disease Control (1977): Influenza Vaccine, *Morb. Mortal. Wkly. Rep.*, **26**(24):193-199.

Weigle, W. O. (1961): The Immune Response of Rabbits Tolerant to Bovine Serum Albumin to the Injection of Other Heterologous Serum Albumins, *J. Exp. Med.*, **114**:111-125.

———(1977): Immunologic Tolerance and Immunopathology, *Hosp. Pract.*, **12**(6):71-80.

Yunis, E. J., G. Fernandes, and L. J. Greenberg (1975): Immune Deficiency, Autoimmunity and Aging, *Birth Defects: Orig. Artic. Ser.* XI, pp. 185-192.

7
Failure of the Immune System, Hereditary and Acquired

DISORDERS OF THE IMMUNE SYSTEM

7-1 Disorders of the immune system appear to be responsible for many different kinds of immunological diseases, e.g., autoimmune diseases, discussed in Chap. 6. Others may be immunological deficiency diseases or immunoproliferative diseases like those characterized by hypergammaglobulinemia, in which malignant production of an immunoglobulin is associated with lack of immunity. In order to convey some idea of the general magnitude of diseases caused by, or associated with, disorders of the immune system, a list of many but not all of these disorders is given in Table 7-1. The diseases are listed according to the organs or tissues involved. Some diseases, e.g., systemic lupus erythematosus, involve more than one organ. In some of the diseases listed, an immunological basis of disease is suspected but not proved. The immunological disorders observed in connection with some of the diseases may be the result rather than the cause of the disease. Immunological disorders associated with many infectious diseases are not included in the table.

IMMUNOLOGIC DEFICIENCY DISEASES

Deficiences Attributed to Defects in Development of B and T or Stem Cells

7-2 Immunologic deficiency diseases are concerned with failures of specific resistance mechanisms, which may be antibody-mediated (humoral) or cell-mediated or both. Antibody-mediated and cell-mediated immunity are determined by B and T lymphocytes, respectively; however, T helper lymphocytes are necessary in addition to B cells for antibody production to certain antigens. A combined deficiency raises the question whether the defect in development occurred at the stem-cell level (see Fig. 1-2). For a review of the development of B and T cells and their interaction, see Chap. 2. Children born with B- or T-cell deficiencies usually die soon after birth unless measures are taken to reinforce their resistance or to reconstitute them immunologically. Recognition for the first time of an

Table 7-1 Diseases Caused by, or Associated with, Disorders of the Immune System

Region	Disease
Nervous system	Acute dissiminated encephalomyelitis (ADEM): Postvaccinal and postinfectious encephalitis Idiopathic polyneuritis (Guillain-Barré syndrome) Multiple sclerosis Myasthenia gravis Subacute sclerosing panencephalitis
Digestive system	
Salivary gland	Sjögren's syndrome
Gastrointestinal tract	Chronic atrophic gastritis and pernicious anemia Gluten-sensitive enteropathy Ulcerative colitis Granulomatous enterocolitis (Crohn's disease) Immune deficiency diseases and gastrointestinal disturbances
Liver	Chronic active hepatitis Primary biliary cirrhosis
Heart	Progressive systemic sclerosis (scleroderma) Acute rheumatic fever
Lung	Fibrosing alveolitis (diffuse interstitial pulmonary fibrosis) Goodpasture's syndrome (lung and kidney)
Endocrine system:	
Thyroid	Hashimoto's thyroiditis (chronic thyroiditis) Primary atrophic hypothyroidism Graves' disease (hyperthyroidism)
Adrenal	Addison's disease (primary adrenal atrophy)
Gonads	Premature ovarian failure Gonadal dysgenesis (Turner's syndrome) Infertility (sperm-agglutinating antibodies)
Pancreas	Diabetes mellitus
Eye	Endogenous uveitis Lens-induced uveitis Sympathetic ophthalmia
Kidney	Immune-complex glomerulonephritis, e.g., poststreptococcal glomerulonephritis, systemic lupus erythematosus, and cryoglobulinemia Antiglomerular basement-membrane disease, e.g., Goodpasture's syndrome Immunologic tubular and interstitial renal disease, e.g., drug-induced interstitial nephritis and hypergammaglobulinemia renal tubular acidosis Immunologic mesangial (intercapillary) renal disease, e.g., Bergen's nephropathy and anaphylactoid purpura
Skin	Hereditary angioedema Erythema nodosum Discoid lupus erythematosus Erythema multiforme

	Bullous diseases:
	Pemphigus vulgarius
	Bullous pemphigoid
	Dermatitis herpetiformis
	Vertiligo
	Papular mucinosis
Diffuse-connective-tissue or collagen diseases	Scleroderma (progressive systemic sclerosis)
	Systemic lupus erythematosus
	Sjögren's syndrome
	Polyarteritis nodosa
	Polymyositis and dermatomyositis
	Rheumatoid arthritis
	Juvenile rheumatoid arthritis
	Ankylosing spondylitis
	Reiter's syndrome
	Psoriatic arthritis
	Behcet's syndrome
	Relapsing polychondritis
Blood:	
Platelets	Autoimmune (idiopathic) thrombocytopenic purpura
	Drug-induced thrombocytopenic purpura
	Thrombocytopenia caused by antibodies to platelets and immune complexes
Red blood cells	Hemolytic diseases of the newborn:
	Rh or ABO incompatibility
	Autoimmune hemolytic anemias:
	Cold and warm antibody types
	Paroxysmal cold hemoglobinuria
	Drug-induced immune hemolytic anemias
	Paroxysmal nocturnal hemoglobinuria
	Pure-red-cell aplasia
	Pernicious anemia (autosensitization to parietal cells and intrinsic factor)
White blood cells	Leukemias
	Paraproteinemias (plasma-cell dyscrasias or monoclonal gammopathies)
	Biclonal gammopathy
	Malignant lymphomas:
	Hodgkin's disease
	Non-Hodgkin's lymphomas
	Chronic autoimmune neutropenia
	Drug-induced neutropenia
	Leukocytopenia

inherited antibody-deficient sex-linked trait by Bruton in 1952 coincided with the development of broad-spectrum antibiotics. It was found that these children could be maintained with antibiotic therapy and injections of normal adult human gamma globulin. The treatment of children with T-cell deficiencies is much more complex. Table 7-2 summarizes some of the deficiencies which may occur during development; some are genetically determined. They are called *primary immunodeficiency diseases.*

B-Lymphocyte Deficiency Diseases

7-3 Outstanding characteristics of some of the B-cell deficiency diseases are briefly described below.
Infantile sex-linked agammaglobulinemia (Bruton's type) This deficiency disease occurs only in

Table 7-2 Primary Immunodeficiency Diseases Attributed to Defects in Development of B, T, or Stem Cells and Their Relationship to Genetic Factors

Primary immunodeficiency disease*	Cells defective	Genetically determined	
		Sex-linked	Autosomal recessive
Infantile sex-linked agammaglobulinemia (Bruton type)	B	Yes	
Transient hypogammaglobulinemia	B		
Selective IgA deficiency	B (some)		
Thymic hypoplasia (pharyngeal pouch or DiGeorge syndrome)	T		
Immunodeficiency with ataxia telangiectasia	B and T		Yes
With thrombocytopenia and eczema (Wiskott-Aldrich syndrome)	B and T	Yes	
Severe combined immunodeficiency disease	Stem, B and T		Yes

*Not a complete list of all primary immunodeficiency diseases.

male children. They have normal T-cell function and resistance to viral infections but suffer from recurrent bacterial infections. Examination of their lymph nodes show that they lack germinal centers and plasma cells. Electrophoretic examination of their blood serum shows almost no gamma globulin. Examination of whole blood shows an absence of B lymphocytes. Immunization with vaccines fails to elicit antibody formation.

Transient hypogammaglobulinemia The newborn infant receives IgG antibodies transplacentally from the mother. The age at which different classes of immunoglobulins start to develop and finally reach normal levels was discussed in Sec. 3-26. Occasionally, gamma-globulin synthesis is delayed for the first 18 to 30 weeks of life, a condition called *transient hypogammaglobulinemia.*

Selective IgA deficiency The incidence of selective IgA deficiency is about 1 in 700 in the general population. The level of other immunoglobulins is normal. Clinical features are not characteristic for IgA deficiency. The deficiency is associated with recurrent sinopulmonary infections, allergy, gastrointestinal-tract disease, and autoimmunity. Patients with IgA deficiency develop antibodies to IgA and may go into anaphylactic shock if they receive a blood transfusion or are treated with gamma globulin following sensitization.

Dysgammaglobulinemia There is an imbalance of normal immunoglobulin concentrations. The immunoglobulins affected are usually IgG (or IgG subgroups), IgM, and IgA. This imbalance can occur in several different ways. Selective IgA deficiency is an example of dysgammaglobulinemia.

Treatment of B-Lymphocyte Deficiency Diseases

7-4 B-cell deficiency diseases are treated with antibiotic therapy and gamma globulin except for patients with selective IgA deficiency. Since they form antibodies to IgA and may already be sensitized to IgA through previous exposure, they should not be treated with gamma-globulin therapy. If a blood transfusion is needed, they can be given washed packed red blood cells, but even so, precautions should be taken in case some IgA remains after washing and anaphylaxis occurs. In some cases of IgA deficiency, there is also IgE deficiency, and in these cases anaphylaxis does not occur.

T-Lymphocyte Deficiency Disease

7-5 The first T-cell deficiency disease was described by DiGeorge. The characteristics of this disease are described below.

Thymic hypoplasia (pharyngeal pouch or DiGeorge syndrome) This deficiency is not genetically determined but results from the failure of the third and fourth pharyngeal pouches to develop. This failure may be caused by in utero infection. Its cause is not known. Neither the thymus nor parathyroid gland develops. B-cell function is normal, but T-cell function is lacking. These patients cannot be sensitized with 2,4-dinitrochlorobenzene (DNCB) (review Sec. 5-46). They are unable to reject allografts. They are very susceptible to viral and fungal infections. At autopsy, thymus-dependent areas of the lymph nodes and spleen are almost devoid of cells, a finding which shows failure of T-lymphocyte development.

Combined T- and B-Lymphocyte Deficiency Diseases

7-6 Outstanding characteristics of some of the combined B- and T-cell deficiency diseases are given below.

Immunodeficiency with ataxia telangiectasia This inherited autosomal recessive disease becomes manifest around the second year of life by an unsteady gait (ataxia). It is also characterized by oculocutaneous telangiectasia (dilatation of small blood vessels) and recurrent sinopulmonary infection. This disease develops slowly, accompanied by mental deterioration. T-cell function is absent or markedly decreased. With regard to B-cell function, there is often an IgA deficiency and also an IgE deficiency.

Immunodeficiency with thrombocytopenia and eczema (Wiskott-Aldrich syndrome) This syndrome is inherited as a sex-linked recessive disorder. The disease is characterized by bleeding due to thrombocytopenia, by eczema, and marked susceptibility to infection, especially with gram-negative organisms. The last symptom is associated with IgM deficiency because the body is unable to make IgM antibodies to polysaccharide antigens found in many gram-negative organisms. Also there are reduced titers of IgM isoagglutinins, anti-A and anti-B, to polysaccharide blood-group antigens A and B. T-lymphocyte and macrophage functions are decreased. These patients are prone to widespread lymphoreticular malignancies.

Severe combined immunodeficiency diseases (SCID) It appears now that this is a group of heterogeneous diseases which may be inherited either in a sex-linked or in an autosomal recessive fashion. Swiss-type agammaglobulinemia was first described by Swiss scientists as a severe combined immunodeficiency disease. Most investigators feel that stem cells are defective. Both B- and T-cell functions are markedly affected. When there is a B-cell deficiency, peripheral blood shows few, if any, lymphocytes with immunoglobulin receptors; when there is a T-cell deficiency, peripheral blood shows few, if any, lymphocytes which give an E-rosette test with sheep red blood cells. Deficiency of the enzyme adenosine deaminase (ADA) has been found in about 50 percent of patients with the autosomal recessive form of SCID. This deficiency was first found in red blood cells but also occurs in other tissues. Deficiency of ADA can be used as a genetic marker for early detection of certain forms of SCID.

Treatment of T-Lymphocyte Deficiences

7-7 Treatment of T-lymphocyte deficiencies can be accomplished by grafting thymus tissue and by adoptive immunization or transfer of T lymphocytes. Both these precedures are dangerous, often leading to a graft-versus-host reaction. Although transfer factor (an extract of immune leukocytes) was described in 1954 by Lawrence, transfer factor has been used only recently to any extent on an experimental basis to treat patients with T-cell deficiencies. Another preparation, called *thymosin,* an extract of the thymus gland, has also been used. Since transfer factor and thymosin do not contain intact cells, they do not cause the graft-versus-host reaction. The different kinds of tissues or extracts used to treat patients with T-cell deficiencies are listed below.

Fetal thymus transplantation Thymuses from aborted infants have been used successfully in a number of cases. Fetal thymus tissue is less likely to cause a graft-versus-host reaction than nonfetal thymus. Fetal thymuses taken during the first 16 weeks of gestation are preferable to older ones, although older ones have been used without notable graft-versus-host reaction.

Bone-marrow transplantation Bone-marrow cells of the donor must be histocompatible with HLA antigens of the recipient.

Dialyzable transfer factor (TFd) TFd is an extract of sensitized leukocytes. The person(s) from whom the leukocytes are obtained must have the desired cell-mediated immunity. This can be determined in a number of ways, e.g., by skin testing or by in vitro tests for activation of lymphocytes by antigen. The chemical nature and mode of action of TFd still are not clear. TFd does not cause a graft-versus-host reaction and it is not antigenic, so there is no problem with sensitization.

Thymosin, thymus factors, thymopoietins Multiple factors with thymic activity have been isolated and described. They can be extracted from calf or human thymuses; these factors have been reported to have a molecular weight between 1000 and 12,000. Thymosin promotes T-cell differentiation. Thymosin has the advantage of being easy to prepare on a large scale if clinical trials being carried out now continue to show that it has a beneficial effect.

Secondary T-Lymphocyte Deficiences

7-8 Other T-lymphocyte deficiencies have been described besides the primary immunologic deficiency disorders described above.

Disseminated mucocutaneous candidiasis *Candida albicans* is a pathogenic yeast which is widely distributed in the population, causes some unpleasant conditions, but usually is not too difficult to control. In certain children and adults with T-cell deficiency, *C. albicans* infection is difficult to control and may become widely disseminated throughout the body. Antibiotics like amphotericin B will decrease the infection temporarily but will not cure it. There are reports by Fudenberg and others that transfer factor has been effective in clearing up disseminated mucocutaneous candidiasis in T-cell immunodeficient patients.

Sarcoidosis Sarcoidosis is a chronic systemic granulomatous disease, the etiology of which is not known. It is fairly common in the eastern part of the United States. One of the most striking features of sarcoidosis is the depression of cell-mediated immunity; however, resistance to infection is not greatly impaired. Noncaseating granulomatous lesions are characteristic of sarcoidosis. The Kveim reaction, used to aid in diagnosis, is carried out with a suspension of lymph-node tissue from a patient with sarcoidosis. A papulonodular lesion which contains epitheloid-cell follicles and reaches its maximum development (3 to 8 mm in diameter) in 4 to 6 weeks constitutes a positive test. This test is positive in about 80 percent of patients with sarcoidosis.

Complement Deficiences

7-9 Complement is very important to host resistance. Complement deficiencies were discussed in Sec. 3-38.

Disorders of Phagocytosis

7-10 The importance of phagocytosis to host resistance was discussed in Secs. 1-7 to 1-12. There are a number of disorders which affect phagocytes, e.g., those concerned with chemotaxis, migration, opsonization, and intracellular killing of microorganisms. Most of these disorders are only indirectly related to immunologic deficiency disorders and will not be discussed here.

Questions for Secs. 7-1 to 7-10

1. For each condition listed indicate whether it is associated mainly with function of B or T lymphocytes, both, or neither: (*a*) infantile sex-linked agammaglobulinemia (Bruton's type), (*b*) resistance to viral infections, (*c*) resistance to bacterial infections, (*d*) lymph nodes with well-developed germinal centers, (*e*) presence of plasma cells in lymph nodes, (*f*) production of antibodies in response to vaccines, (*g*) selective IgA deficiency, (*h*) dysgammaglobulinemia, (*i*) allograft rejection, (*j*) skin sensitization to DNCB, (*k*) DiGeorge syndrome, (*l*) immunodeficiency with ataxia telangiectasia, (*m*) Wiskott-Aldrich syndrome, (*n*) severe combined immunodeficiency (SCID).

2. (*a*) What disease is associated with IgM deficiency and the inability to produce antibodies to polysaccharide antigens? (*b*) To what group of bacteria are these patients very susceptible?

3. In general, what two different kinds of preparations are used to treat B-lymphocyte deficiences?

4. (*a*) What four methods have been used to treat T-cell deficiencies? (*b*) Which method is most likely to cause a graft-versus-host reaction? (*c*) What kind of cells are used for the preparation of transfer factor? (*d*) Is transfer factor antigenic?

Answers

1. (*a*) Lack of B. (*b*) T. (*c*) B but also T. (*d*) B. (*e*) B. (*f*) B (T helper cells may be needed). (*g*) lack of B. (*h*) lack of B. (Sec. 7-3.)
(*i*) T. (*j*) T. (*k*) lack of T. (Sec. 7-5.)
(*l*) Lack of B and T. (*m*) lack of B and T. (*n*) lack of B and T (possibly at stem-cell level). (Sec. 7-6.)

2. (*a*) Wiskott-Aldrich syndrome. (*b*) Gram-negative bacteria. (Sec. 7-6.)

3. Antibiotics and adult human gamma globulin. (Sec. 7-4.)

4. (*a*) Transplantation of fetal thymuses; bone-marrow transplantation; injection of transfer factor; injection of thymosin. (*b*) Injection of bone marrow unless HLA antigens of donor and recipient are very carefully matched. (*c*) Immune or sensitized leukocytes taken from a person or persons with the desired cell-mediated immunity. (*d*) No. (Sec. 7-7.)

HYPERIMMUNOGLOBULINEMIA

7-11 Hyperimmunoglobulinemia refers to an abnormal increase in production of immunoglobulins. The term hypergammaglobulinemia also has been used to refer to this condition. Although antibodies which contribute to resistance of the host are present in the gamma-globulin fraction of serum, hypergammaglobulinemia is often associated with a decrease in resistance. When abnormally large amounts of pathological immunoglobulins are produced, the normal production of all antibodies is depressed but especially that of IgG.

Polyclonal Gammopathies

7-12 Some cases of hyperimmunoglobulinemia are classified as polyclonal gammopathies. The increased amount of immunoglobulin comes from several clones of antibody-producing cells. The increase in gamma globulin is believed to be due to antigenic stimulation. Some of the antibodies may be autoantibodies, etc., and not associated with resistance, but others may be antibacterial, antiviral, etc., and associated with resistance. Hypergammaglobulinemia of the polyclonal type may be found in such disease states as the collagen-vascular diseases, infectious diseases, liver diseases, gastrointestinal disease, renal disease, and miscellaneous diseases such as sarcoidosis. Figure 7-1 shows the electrophoresis patterns obtained for patients' sera with polyclonal and monoclonal gammopathies compared with that of normal human serum (review Sec. 3-12).

Monoclonal Gammopathies

7-13 Hyperimmunoglobulinemia may be caused by the abnormal production of immunoglobulins by a single plasma-cell clone which is malignant. These cases of hyperimmunoglobulinemia are called *monoclonal gammopathies.* The homologous immunoglobulins produced have also been called paraproteins, and their production is associated with depression of the normal immune response of the host. Monoclonal gammopathies, also known as *plasma-cell dyscrasias,* include such diseases as multiple myeloma, macroglobulinemia, and heavy-chain disease. These plasma-cell dyscrasias were discussed in Sec. 3-27. Monoclonal proteins in serum can be detected by electrophoresis or im-

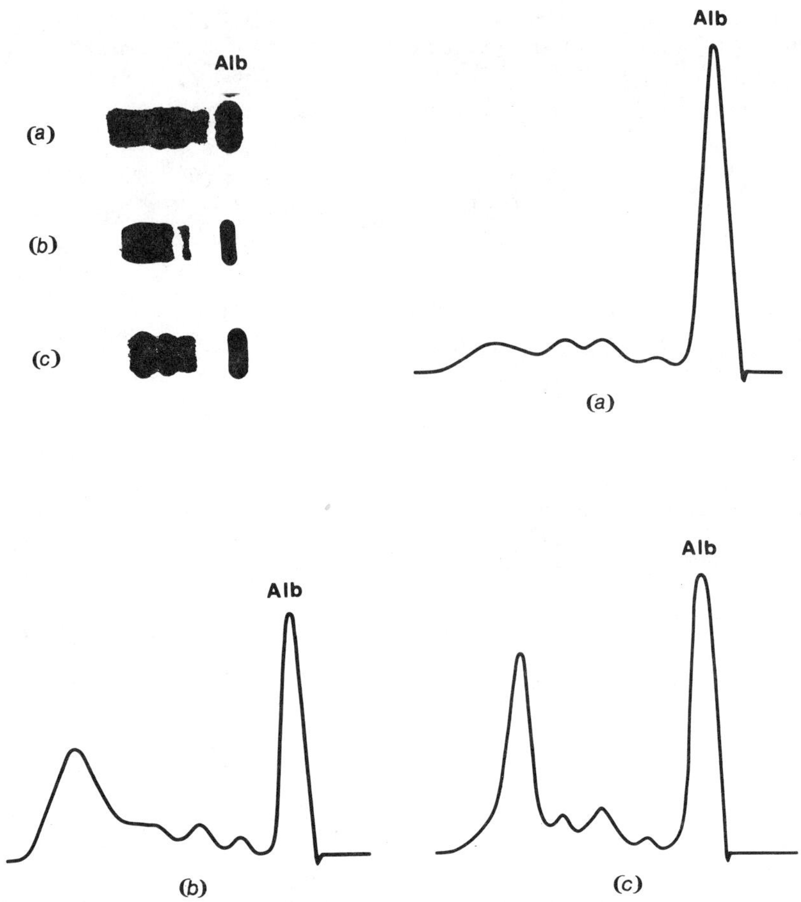

Figure 7-1 Electrophoresis patterns obtained for patients' sera with polyclonal and monoclonal gammopathies compared with that of normal human serum: (*a*) normal, (*b*) polyclonal, and (*c*) monoclonal. (*Courtesy of B. P. Barton, Department of Pathology, Medical College of Georgia.*)

munoelectrophoresis (review Sec. 4-28). Clones producing IgG are the most common; IgA is more common than IgM, while IgD or IgE are the least common. Figure 7-2 shows immunoelectrophoresis studies on the monoclonal protein detected by electrophoresis as shown in Fig. 7-1. Monoclonal gammopathies may lead to conditions known as hyperviscosity and cryoglobulinemia. *Hyperviscosity* refers to the property of the blood to resist flow. In *cryoglobulinemia* proteins in serum are precipitated when the temperature of the patient is reduced and may lead to thrombus formation. In the laboratory, cryoglobulins can be detected by placing the patient's serum in the refrigerator at 4°C for 48 h and examining for gel formation. Cryoglobulinemia is often observed with Waldenström's macroglobulinemia and may be helped by plasmapheresis. Cryoglobulinemia may also be polyclonal and associated with autoimmune diseases and immune-complex formation. Another condition, known as *amyloidosis,* is associated with monoclonal gammopathies but also occurs in other diseases. Amyloid is deposited in tissue and has a fibrillar structure in electron micrographs. The kind of amyloid deposited varies with the disease. With multiple myeloma, amyloid appears to be composed of light chains, or variable regions, of the pathological immunoglobulin.

Questions for Secs. 7-11 to 7-13

5. In the following diseases, state whether hyperimmunoglobulinemia is usually monoclonal or polyclonal: (*a*) systemic lupus erythematosus, (*b*) rheumatoid arthritis, (*c*) multiple myeloma, (*d*) macroglobulinemia.

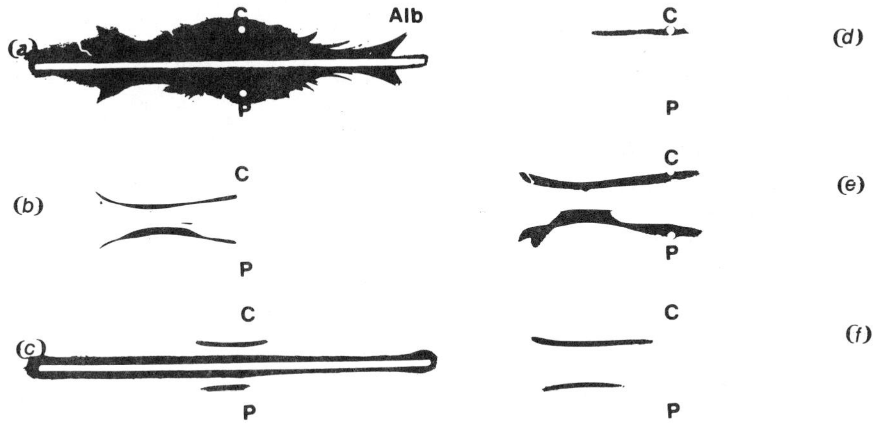

Figure 7-2 Immunoelectrophoresis studies on the serum of a patient with multiple myeloma. The patient has an IgG kappa-light-chain monoclonal gammopathy. After electrophoresis, control (C) and patient (P) sera were tested against (*a*) anti-normal human serum, (*b*) anti-IgG heavy chain, (*c*) anti-IgA heavy chain, (*d*) anti-IgM heavy chain,(*e*) anti-kappa light chains, and (*f*) anti-lambda light chains. Note the increased thickness and bowing of precipitin arcs with patient serum in (*b*) and (*e*). (*Courtesy of B. P. Barton, Department of Pathology, Medical College of Georgia.*)

6. What immunoglobulin is most frequently observed with monoclonal gammopathies?
7. What is a plasma-cell dyscrasia?

Answers

5. (*a*) and (*b*) polyclonal. (*c*) and (*d*) monoclonal. (Secs. 7-12 and 7-13.)
6. IgG. (Sec. 7-13.)
7. An excessive or disproportionate synthesis of immunoglobulin by a plasma-cell clone. (Sec. 7-13.)

REFERENCES

Barber, H. R. K. (1977): "Immunobiology for the Clinician," Wiley, New York.
Barrett, J. T. (1974): "Textbook of Immunology," 2d ed., Mosby, St. Louis.
Biggar, W. D., B. H. Park, O. Stutman, K. Gajl-Peczalska, and R. A. Good (1975): Fetal Thymus Transplantation: Experimental and Clinical Observations, *Birth Defects*: *Orig. Artic. Ser.* XI, pp. 361-366.
Franklin, E. C. (1976): Electrophoresis and Immunoelectrophoresis in the Evaluation of Homogeneous Immunoglobulin Components, *Clin. Immunobiol.*, 3:21-36.
Freedman, S. O., and P. Gold (eds.) (1976): "Clinical Immunology," 2d ed., Harper & Row, Hagerstown, Md.
Fudenberg, H. H., D. P. Stites, J. L. Caldwell, and J. V. Wells (eds.) (1976): "Basic and Clinical Immunology," Lange, Los Altos, Calif.
Goldstein, A. L., G. B. Thurman, G. H. Cohen, and J. A. Hooper (1975): The Role of Thymosin and the Endocrine Thymus on the Ontogenesis and Function of T Cells, *Miami Winter Symp.*, 9:243-265.
Good, R. A. (1975): Bone Marrow Transplantation: Cellular Engineering to Correct Primary Immunodeficiency, Aregenerative Anemia and Pancytopenia, *Birth Defects*: *Orig. Artic. Ser.* XI, pp. 377-379.
Kirkpatrick, C. H. (1975): Restoration of Cell-mediated Immune Responses with Transfer Factor, *Birth Defects*: *Orig. Arti. Ser.* XI, pp. 441-444.
Levin, A. S., L. E. Spitler, and H. H. Fudenberg (1975): Transfer Factor, I: Methods of Therapy, *Birth Defects*: *Orig. Artic. Ser.* XI, pp. 445-448.
Meuwissen, H. J. and B. Pollara (1974): Adenosine Deaminase Deficiency: The First Inborn Error of Metabolism Noted in Immunodeficiency Disease, *J. Pediatr.*, **84**:315-316.

Miescher, P. A., and H. J. Müller-Eberhard, (eds.) (1976): "Textbook of Immunopathology," 2 vols., Grune and Stratton, New York.
Nakamura, R. M. (ed.) (1974): "Immunopathology: Clinical Laboratory Concepts and Methods," Little, Brown, Boston.
Rose, N. R., and H. Friedman (1976): "Manual of Clinical Immunology," American Society for Microbiology, Washington, D.C.
Spitler, L. E., A. S. Levin, and H. H. Fudenberg (1975): Transfer Factor, II: Results of Therapy, *Birth Defects*: *Orig. Artic. Ser.* XI, pp. 449–456.
Waldmann, T. A., and W. Strober (1976): Metabolism of Immunoglobulins, *Clin. Immunobiol.*, 3:71-95.

8

General Immunosuppression and Specific Immunosuppression

IMMUNOSUPPRESSION

Distinction between Specific and Nonspecific Immunosuppression

8-1 Immunosuppression refers to a decrease in the immune response(s) of the host. In specific immunosuppression response to a particular antigen is abolished, but all other host immune responses are unaffected. Specific suppression or specific immunological unresponsiveness was cited in Sec. 2-1 as one of the four possible immune responses of the host. Other terms such as immunological tolerance and immunological paralysis refer to this same state of unresponsiveness to a single antigen. For transplantation of allografts to the human host, the ideal situation would be to suppress the host's immune response only to the transplanted tissue in order to prevent rejection without affecting the host immune responses to bacterial, viral, or fungal infection or to transformed cancer cells, etc. This type of specific suppression in the human host to allografts has not yet been accomplished. Nonspecific immunosuppression refers to a general suppression of immune responses. When nonspecific suppression is carried out for transplantation, suppression of host immune response to the graft to prevent its rejection is accompanied by a decrease in host resistance to bacteria, viruses, fungi, etc.

NONSPECIFIC SUPPRESSION OF IMMUNE RESPONSES

8-2 Since the immune response is dependent on B and T lymphocytes, it seems evident that the way to bring about a general suppression of immune responses would be to try to remove or destroy as many B and T lymphocytes as possible and still maintain the host. B and T lymphocytes are somewhat more susceptible to irradiation and certain cytotoxic drugs than other tissue cells. Nonspecific suppression of immune responses is carried out as outlined below.

1. Suppression by removal of lymphocytes
   a. Thoracic-duct drainage
   b. Surgical removal of lymphoid tissue such as spleen
2. Suppression by destruction of lymphocytes
   a. Irradiation
   b. Drugs
   c. Antilymphocyte globulin: (ALG): antibodies are specific for T lymphocytes; cell-mediated immunity (CMI) is mainly affected, but suppression of CMI is nonspecific, i.e., not for a particular antigen

Thoracic-Duct Drainage

8-3 One method which has been used to decrease the number of lymphocytes is thoracic-duct drainage. Lymphocytes are separated, so that lymph can be reinfused. This procedure leads to a marked decrease in the number of T lymphocytes in peripheral blood, a depletion of thymus-dependent areas in lymph nodes and spleen, and a depression of cellular immunity. Humoral immunity appears not to be affected significantly. The procedure of thoracic-duct drainage has been used before organ transplantation.

Surgical Removal of Lymphoid Tissue

8-4 The spleen has been removed in some severe cases of autoimmune disease. This procedure is not highly effective and is not without danger. Many of these patients die with postsplenectomy sepsis.

X-Irradiation

8-5 Many immunosuppressive agents act by impairing reproductive integrity of immunocompetent cells. Radiation damage to cells may not become apparent until weeks or months later, when the cells fail to replicate. X-irradiation was one of the first methods used for immunosuppression. Irradiation has been reported to have more effect on antibody formation than on cell-mediated responses. Immunosuppression by irradiation is more effective if irradiation takes place before sensitization; the secondary immune response is relatively resistant to irradiation. Irradiation causes scission of the DNA chain so that synthesis of DNA does not occur. Irradiation exerts its effect not only on lymphocytes but also on stem cells, which are necessary for repopulation of lymphoid tissue. Irradiation therapy has been carried out by whole-body irradiation, but this is too dangerous. Local irradiation of an allograft immediately after transplantation helps to prolong its survival. Extracorporeal irradiation of blood has been reported to result in T lymphocytopenia.

Drugs Used for Immunosuppression

X **8-6** Cortisone, a corticosteroid drug, was reported in 1951 to delay rejection of allografts in experimental animals. Since then other corticosteroids such as prednisone have been used to prevent rejection of transplants. In contrast to irradiation corticosteroids are able to suppress a preexisting state of sensitivity. Corticosteroids have anti-inflammatory and antiphagocytic properties; they also suppress antibody formation. Corticosteroids cause lymphocytopenia, which in human beings results from redistribution of lymphocytes from the peripheral blood to some other area. Macrophage circulation patterns and access to sites of potential immunologic reactions are suppressed. In the presence of steroids, antigens can activate T lymphocytes to produce lymphokines such as MIF, but the macrophages are not able to respond to these lymphokines. Corticosteroids have been used not only to prevent graft rejection but also to treat a number of autoimmune diseases. Cortisone has dangerous side effects, one of which is increased susceptibility to infection.
8-7 *Cytotoxic drugs* are used for immunosuppression and are classified as antimetabolites and as

alkylating agents. Antimetabolites are substances that resemble natural enzyme substrates but are not identical to them, so that they can compete with them for the substrate-binding sites on enzyme molecules. Azathioprine and 6-mercaptopurine are purine antagonists; methotrexate is a folic acid antagonist. Biological alkylating agents are chemicals which can substitute alkyl radicals in other molecules under biological conditions of temperature, pH, etc. Alkylating agents which have at least two alkyl radicals interact with nucleophilic centers of molecules and link them together. Alkylating agents cross-link native DNA, DNA with proteins, DNA with RNA, RNA with RNA, or RNA with proteins to interfere with nucleic acid synthesis and cell function. Cyclophosphamide is a biological alkalating agent. Since most cytotoxic drugs used for immunosuppression also cause tumor inhibition, many of these drugs were first used to treat malignancies. The drugs are more effective on cells undergoing proliferation.

Antilymphocyte Globulin (ALG)

8-8 Antilymphocyte serum (ALS) is prepared by injecting T lymphocytes into animals, usually horses. This antiserum is absorbed to remove possible antibodies to other blood-cell components besides lymphocytes. The globulin fraction is separated to obtain antibodies to T lymphocytes and to remove as much foreign serum or protein as possible. It has been difficult to standardize the activity of antilymphocyte serum, but recently the amount of antibody to T lymphocytes has been determined by inhibition of the E-rosette test (for the principle of the E-rosette test, review Sec. 2-11). Also, antilymphocyte globulin has been standardized recently by prevention of graft rejection in higher primates. The advantage of antilymphocyte globulin is that it suppresses cell-mediated immunity more than humoral immunity. Graft rejection is usually caused by cell-mediated hypersensitivity reactions, so that antilymphocyte globulin helps to prevent graft rejection while having little effect on humoral immunity. However, host resistance to viruses, fungi, and cancer cells is affected. Antilymphocyte globulin causes lysis of lymphocytes in the presence of complement. Lympholysis causes lymphopenia and a transient depletion of the thymus-dependent areas in lymph nodes. Antilymphocyte globulin is more selective in its action than any of the other immunosuppressive agents discussed above. With regard to the lymphocyte, the action of antilymphocyte globulin is specific, but with regard to the host, the action of antilymphocyte globulin is nonspecific in that it suppresses not only the host immune response to an antigen such as HLA in an organ but also indiscriminately suppresses host-specific immune responses to viruses, fungi, cancer cells, etc.

Possible Complications of Nonspecific Immunosuppression

8-9 The complications listed below have been observed with nonspecific immunosuppression.

Increased susceptibility to infection Patients who are treated with immunosuppressive drugs are very susceptible to infection. This is especially true of viral and fungal infections when cell-mediated immunity is suppressed. Some viral infections, e.g., those caused by herpes simplex and cytomegalovirus, may appear as a result of reactivation of a latent infection. Infection occurs not only with pathogenic organisms but also with opportunists because they can invade only when resistance of the host is depressed. One common opportunist is *Pneumocystis carinii.*

Increased susceptibility to cancer From data available, it appears that patients treated with nonspecific immunosuppressive drugs show a higher incidence of cancer. From what is known about resistance to transformed cancer cells, host resistance depends on cell-mediated reactions or rejection of the transformed cells.

Malformations of fetus All drugs affecting nucleic acid and protein metabolism exhibit teratogenecity in animals. Although the number of malformed children born to women taking cytotoxic immunosuppressive drugs during pregnancy has not been high, there appears to be a potential danger to the child. It has been reported that teratogenecity may also be caused by the father's taking cytotoxic immunosuppressive drugs at the time of conception.

Hypersensitivity reactions Antilymphocyte globulin is a foreign protein and can cause immediate-type hypersensitivity reactions.

SPECIFIC SUPPRESSION OF IMMUNE RESPONSE TO A SINGLE ANTIGEN

8-10 Specific suppression of an immune response to a particular antigen has been accomplished in two ways: (1) passive transfer of specific antibodies and (2) exposure to the specific antigen.

Specific Suppression by Passive Transfer of Specific Antibodies

8-11 The use of a commercial preparation called RhoGAM to prevent sensitization to Rh was described in Sec. 3-7. RhoGAM consists of specific antibodies (gamma globulin) to Rh_0 (or D) antigen. When an Rh-negative mother gives birth to an Rh-positive child, sensitization usually occurs at parturition. Sensitization can be prevented if specific antibodies are given within 72 h after delivery. These antibodies appear to react with Rh-positive red blood cells so that they are removed by phagocytosis and sensitization does not occur. The same procedure can be used if an Rh-negative patient is inadvertently transfused with Rh-positive blood.

8-12 In feedback inhibition a high level of antibodies exerts a homeostatic effect and keeps additional antibodies from being formed. It was pointed out in Sec. 1-25 that passive immunization might interfere with active immunization. This type of specific suppression or feedback inhibition could have a harmful effect, especially on active immunization against rabies when combined immunization is required.

8-13 The effect which antibodies to HLA or transplantation antigens might have on survival or rejection of organ transplants such as kidney is not clear at present. Studies on tumors have shown that antibodies to certain tumor antigens may cause a state of immunosuppression in experimental animals (see Chap. 10). Several mechanisms appear to be responsible; e.g., antibodies to the tumor may cover the tumor antigens in such a way as to block either induction of cell-mediated immunity or expression of cell-mediated immunity (destruction by sensitized lymphocytes). This phenomenon from the standpoint of tumor growth has been called *immunologic enhancement.* In contrast to tumor growth and survival, if a similar type of reaction could be obtained with specific antibodies to transplantation antigens, this would be a favorable reaction and could facilitate survival of tissue grafts or organ transplants. There are a few studies to show that graft enhancement takes place sometimes; if antibodies bound to surface histocompatibility antigens are not cytotoxic, they may be able to protect cells of the graft from destruction by sensitized lymphocytes. As previously stated, the effect of specific tissue antibodies on graft survival is not yet clear.

Specific Suppression by Exposure to the Specific Antigen: Immunological Tolerance

8-14 Burnet (1959) and Medawar (1958) independently concluded that if fetal exposure to an antigen occurs before birth, exposure to the antigen after birth does not stimulate the production of antibodies or sensitized T lymphocytes. This type of specific unresponsiveness is called *immunological tolerance.* This state of tolerance was the basis of Burnet's clonal-selection theory, which states that clones of cells capable of responding to self antigens are destroyed during fetal life. Owen reported (1945) that when cattle have genetically different twin calves, the calves sometimes prove to be chimeras because they share the same placenta and there are anastomoses of placental blood vessels. The blood of each calf contains some blood cells of its twin. Normally, genetically different blood cells would be destroyed. When blood cells from other calves were injected, they were destroyed. It was later shown that these chimeras accept skin grafts from each other because of specific tolerance induced before birth.

8-15 Felton (1949) reported that the injection of a large amount (1000 μg) of pneumococcal polysaccharide into mice caused a state of immunological unresponsiveness which was called *immunologic paralysis.* The injection of a small amount (0.01 to 1.0 μg) of pneumococcal polysaccharide induced antibody formation. At one time, immunologic paralysis was viewed as being distinct from immunological tolerance, but now they are viewed as part of the same mechanism.

Induction of Immunological Tolerance in Experimental Animals

8-16 It was previously pointed out that immunological tolerance can be induced by injection of an antigen in utero. Tolerance also can be easily induced by injection of an animal soon after birth. An animal has functional B and T cells at this time, but the immune system is not fully developed. Adult animals can also be rendered tolerant, especially if nonspecific immunosuppressive drugs are given before injecting antigen. By nonspecific immunosuppression, the adult lymphoid system is made to resemble the immature lymphoid system of the newborn animal. Several factors affect the establishment of tolerance.

Physical state of antigen It is easier to induce tolerance with soluble antigens such as bovine serum albumin (BSA) than with particulate antigens such as bacteria, viruses, etc., or even with aggregated proteins such as aggregated BSA. The latter have many repeating copies of a given determinant per particle and are more immunogenic.

Route of injection The intravenous route is the most effective for establishing tolerance.

Amount of antigen Tolerance is usually achieved with a large amount of antigen, and this is called high-dose (or high-zone) tolerance. Tolerance can also be induced with a very small, subimmunogenic amount of antigen; this is called low-dose (or low-zone) tolerance. The term *tolerogen* is sometimes used to refer to the antigen which induces tolerance.

Maintenance of tolerant state The persistence of antigen in tissues is necessary to maintain tolerance induced by injection after birth. Less antigen is required to maintain tolerance than to induce it.

The Role of B and T Lymphocytes in Immunological Tolerance

8-17 In studies on experimental animals made tolerant to an antigen and examined at intervals thereafter, several conclusions were reached:

Tolerance is more easily established with T cells.

Only T cells are made unresponsive by low-dose tolerance.

Both B and T cells are made unresponsive by high-dose tolerance.

T cells remain tolerant about 3 times longer than B cells.

In Sec. 5-52 several examples of anergy which may occur during infection were cited, including anergy during advanced tuberculosis and coccidioidomycosis and in patients with lepromatous leprosy. Anergic patients lose their ability to develop a positive delayed allergic skin reaction to the infecting microorganisms. In these diseases, T cells become tolerant or unresponsive to the antigens of these microorganisms. With regard to B-cell tolerance, it appears that if a fairly large amount of antigen with many combining sites, e.g., pneumococcal polysaccharide, is present, there is excessive or complete cross linking of immunoglobulin B-cell receptors so that a cap is not formed (see Sec. 2-16) with subsequent endocytosis and antibody induction. If antigen molecules with few combining sites are present along with specific antibody so that Ag-Ab complexes are formed in antigen excess, the complexes can act as described above to give excessive cross linking of Ig receptors on B cells and induce tolerance. This may be a mechanism of immunologic enhancement of tumor growth (Chap. 10) observed with cancer-antigen complexes; however, mainly T cells appear to be affected, and little is known about receptors on T cells.

Questions for Secs. 8-1 to 8-17

1. What is meant by nonspecific suppression of immune responses?
2. What is meant by specific immunosuppression?
3. At what tissue is immunosuppression directed?
4. State whether the following procedures are specific or nonspecific with regard to suppression of host immune responses: (*a*) thoracic-duct drainage, (*b*) use of corticosteroid

drugs, (*c*) present procedures used for kidney transplantation, (*d*) use of antilymphocyte globulin, (*e*) prevention of sensitization with anti-Rh antibodies, (*f*) induction of immunological tolerance in experimental animals.

5. Does antilymphocyte globulin (ALG) have more effect on antibody production or cell-mediated immunity?

6. List four complications of nonspecific suppression.

7. What is the difference between immunological tolerance and immunological paralysis?

8. Is tolerance easier to induce with soluble or particulate antigens?

9. Can low-dose tolerance be induced with both B and T lymphocytes?

10. Can high-dose tolerance be induced with both B and T lymphocytes?

11. After induction of tolerance in experimental animals, do B or T cells remain unresponsive for a longer period of time?

Answers

1. There is a general suppression of host immune responses. (Sec. 8-1.)

2. There is suppression of immune responses of the host to one particular antigen; other immune responses are not affected. (Sec. 8-1)

3. Lymphoid tissue containing B and T cells or their precursors. (Sec. 8-2.)

4. (*a*) Nonspecific. (Sec. 8-3.) (*b*) Nonspecific. (Sec. 8-6.)
(*c*) Nonspecific. (Secs. 8-6 and 8-7.) (*d*) Nonspecific. (Sec. 8-8.)
(*e*) Specific. (Sec. 8-11.) (*f*) Specific. (Sec. 8-16.)

5. Cell-mediated immunity. (Sec. 8-8.)

6. Increased susceptibility to infection; increased susceptibility to cancer; malformations of fetus; hypersensitivity with ALG, if used. (Sec. 8-9.)

7. The mechanisms are believed to be essentially the same. (Sec. 8-15.)

8. Soluble. (Sec. 8-16.)

9. No, only with T cells. (Sec. 8-17.)

10. Yes. (Sec. 8-17.)

11. T cells remain unresponsive longer. (Sec. 8-17.)

REFERENCES

Allen, J. C. (ed.) (1976): "Infection and the Compromised Host," Williams & Wilkins, Baltimore.

Bach, J. F. (1975): "The Mode of Action of Immunosuppressive Agents," North-Holland, Amsterdam.

Burnet, F. M. (1959): "The Clonal Selection Theory of Acquired Immunity," Cambridge University Press, London.

Felton, L. D. (1949): The Significance of Antigen in Animal Tissue, *J. Immunol.*, **61**:107-117.

Freedman, S. O., and P. Gold (eds.) (1976): "Clinical Immunology," Harper & Row, Hagerstown, Md.

Medawar, P. B. (1958): The Immunology of Transplantation, *Harvey Lect.*, **52**:144-176.

———(1969): Antilymphocytic Serum: Its Properties and Potential, *Hosp. Pract.*, **4**(5):26-33.

Miescher, P. A., A. Gerebtzoff, and P. H. Lambert (1976): Immunosuppressive Therapy, pp. 343-365 in P. A. Miescher and H. J. Müller-Eberhard (eds.), "Textbook of Immunopathology," vol. 1, 2d ed., Grune and Stratton, New York.

Munster, A. M. (ed.) (1976). "Surgical Immunology," Grune and Stratton, New York.

Owen, R. D. (1945): Immunogenetic Consequences of Vascular Anastomoses between Bovine Twins, *Science*, **102**:400-401.

Sarles, H. E., A. R. Remmers, Jr., J. C. Fish, C. D. Canales, F. D. Thomas, K. R. T. Tyson, G. A. Beathard, and S. E. Ritzman (1970): Depletion of Lymphocytes for the Protection of Renal Allografts, *Arch. Intern. Med.*, **125**:443-450.

Schreiber, A. D. (1977): Clinical Immunology of the Corticosteroids, *Prog. Clin. Immunol.*, **3**:103-114.

Schwartz, R. S. (1969): Immunosuppression: The Challenge of Selectivity, *Hosp. Pract.*, **4**(2): 42-49.

Waldemann, T. A., and S. Broder (1977): Suppressor Cells in the Regulation of the Immune Response, *Prog. Clin. Immunol.*, **3**:155-199.
Wolf, J. S. (1973): Extracorporeal Irradiation of Blood as an Immunosuppressive Agent, *Transplant. Proc.*, **4**:469-474.

9 Immune Reactions Affecting Tissue Transplants

TRANSPLANTATION IMMUNOLOGY

Different Kinds of Grafts

9-1 The transfer of tissue from one individual to another is referred to as *grafting* of tissue or *transplantation.* The transferred tissue is called a *graft* or a *transplant.* In an *autograft* a graft is transferred from one site of the body to another, and no tissue of another individual is involved. Provided an autograft is carried out properly, it should not be rejected because the donor and recipient cells are genetically and antigenically the same. Grafts which are genetically different will be rejected. If there are only minor antigenic differences, immunosuppressive measures (Chap. 8) may allow grafts to be accepted rather than rejected. The different kinds of grafts with a brief description of each are listed in Table 9-1. The name allograft is preferred to homograft because allograft (*allo*-means "other") calls attention to individual differences whereas homograft calls attention to the same or homologous species. The name homograft (*homo*- means "same") is misleading since this type of graft will be rejected. In contrast, a syngraft is not rejected. The name is preferred to isograft because isoantigens are different antigens within the same species. Blood-group antigens such as A, B, and Rh are isoantigens, but there is an increased tendency to refer to them as *alloantigens.* Syngeneic cells are cells with the identical genetic constitution; hence, the name syngraft is preferred to isograft since isoantigens have been associated with antigenic differences within the same species. The term syngraft has not been universally accepted, and isograft continues to be used by many investigators and surgeons. In previous chapters when antigenicity, anaphylactic shock, etc., were discussed, emphasis usually was on species differences. In transplantation, individual antigenic differences in the same species cause graft rejection.

Table 9-1 Different Kinds of Grafts

New term	Old term	Description	Genetic and antigenic state	Subject to rejection
Allograft	Homograft	Graft from same species but with individual specificity	Different from recipient	Yes*
Syngraft	Isograft	Graft from identical, i.e., monozygotic, twin; inbred animal strains for experimental purposes (considered syngeneic)	Same	No
Autograft (unchanged)	Autograft	Graft from one site to another on same individual	Same	No
Xenograft†	Heterograft	Graft from different species	Very different	Yes‡

*Histocompatibility testing and immunosuppression are used to prevent rejection.

†*Xeno-* means "foreign"

‡Tissue match not possible.

Antigens Responsible for Graft Rejection

9-2 Graft rejection is caused by certain antigenic differences between donor and recipient cells. General terms for antigens responsible for graft rejection are *histocompatibility* or *transplantation antigens.* Although blood-group antigens must be matched for transplantation, blood-group antigens are not usually considered transplantation antigens. Transplantation or histocompatibility antigens in human beings have been designated HLA antigens and are found at four different loci, A, B, C, and D, on the sixth chromosome; the HLA antigens at the different loci are known as HLA-A, HLA-B, HLA-C, and HLA-D. A number of alleles have been recognized at each of these loci and will be discussed later in this chapter. Although HLA is the designation for histocompatibility loci antigens, the letters H and L as originally derived stand for "human leukocyte" because transplantation antigens are on white blood cells; lymphocytes are the cells used for histocompatibility testing. As originally used, the A of HLA represented the first defined genetic locus for human leukocyte antigens, and the name was written as HL-A; now, however, it is usually written HLA, in accordance with terminology recommended by WHO.

9-3 HLA antigens are not found to any extent on red blood cells, but they are present on leukocytes and other nucleated cells and also on platelets. The HLA antigens present on leukocytes are also present on cells of solid tissue or organs. HLA antigens have been reported to be globular glycoproteins with a molecular weight of about 45,000 to 50,000 daltons. HLA molecules can be dissociated into two fragments (MW $\approx$ 33,000 and 11,000 daltons), linked by noncovalent bonds. The heavier fragment is a glycopeptide and is responsible for allotypic specificity of HLA; the lighter fragment is β_2-microglobulin, which has the same structure of the C_3H domain of IgG and therefore has been considered as a possible antigen receptor on T lymphocytes, as discussed in Sec. 2-30. However, B lymphocytes also have HLA antigens with β_2-microglobulin. The nature of the T-cell receptor for antigen has not been resolved.

Rejection of Solid Tissue or Organs

9-4 Rejection of grafts is considered to be mainly cell-mediated; however, antibodies also appear to take part in some rejection processes. Rejection of grafts known as white grafts is mainly antibody-mediated. Some of the outstanding features of different kinds of graft rejection are described below.

First-set rejection (primary rejection) In this reaction, the grafted tissue at first appears to be accepted. Blood supply to the tissue is reestablished (tissue revascularized), and the tissue appears healthy. When the tissue begins to be rejected depends partly on the kind of tissue and the host. In many animals rejection takes place in about 10 days. The tissue becomes infiltrated with mononuclear cells, including lymphocytes, macrophages, and some plasma cells. Polymorphonuclear leukocytes are also observed. Lymphocytes are the predominant infiltrating cell. Sensitized T lymphocytes are mainly responsible for primary rejection. Rejection is initiated when HLA antigens from the graft reach lymph nodes, where these antigens come in contact with T and B lymphocytes and cause their activation (review Chap. 2). The activated lymphocytes undergo clonal expansion. B cells differentiate into plasma cells, which produce antibodies. Activated (or sensitized) T lymphocytes enter the blood and infiltrate the graft, as just described, and cause its rejection. When sensitized T lymphocytes meet up with antigen, lymphokines are released. They exert many different effects which lead to tissue damage such as attracting and holding macrophages in the area. Antibodies also reach the graft; however, it appears that first-set rejection reactions are mainly cell-mediated. One of the ways HLA antigens may leave the graft is by way of lymphocytes of the donor present in the graft at time of transplantation. These lymphocytes are known as *passenger lymphocytes.* It has been shown experimentally that destruction of passenger lymphocytes before transplantation increases graft survival time.

Second-set rejection (accelerated rejection) If tissue from the same donor is again grafted, the series of events associated with rejection described for first-set rejection takes place at an accelerated rate. This reaction is an example of an anamnestic or memory response. Second-set rejection is caused not only by sensitized T lymphocytes but also by cytotoxic antibodies. Second-set rejection is donor-specific and systemic. Any kind of tissue from the donor will be rejected regardless of the kind of tissue (skin, kidney, etc.) which caused the first-set rejection.

White graft (hyperacute rejection) A white graft is one which is rejected so quickly that it never becomes vascularized and therefore appears white. This type of rejection occurs when there are preexisting cytotoxic antibodies which bring about rapid injury to cells in the presence of complement. Cells which infiltrate the tissue are mainly polymorphonuclear leukocytes. This type of rejection is sometimes seen when donor and recipient are mismatched with regard to the major blood-group antigens.

Chronic or slow rejection Experimentally, chronic rejection occurs when tissue is matched with regard to major histocompatibility determinants but not with minor ones. With regard to human transplantation, chronic rejection of a kidney may take place months or years after what appeared to be a successful transplant. Chronic rejection is not fully understood but is probably influenced in the case of an allograft by the fact that it is impossible to achieve complete immunosuppression and still maintain the patient.

Other cases of rejection Sometimes, regardless of how good a tissue match appears to be, rejection occurs for no apparent reason. It is quite probable that not all the tissue antigens associated with rejection have been recognized. Immunosuppression of the host often leads to some bizarre types of infection, e.g., with *Pneumocystis carinii.* Infections in the transplant patient are usually different from those in patients who are not receiving immunosuppressive therapy. Bacterial infections usually can be controlled with antibiotics, but if latent viruses, e.g., cytomegaloviruses, are activated, these infections are difficult to control. Also, in the case of organ transplantation such as kidney, rejection of the transplanted organ may occur later due to the disease process which originally caused the patient's own organ to become nonfunctional.

Specific Immunological Tolerance

9-5 It has been shown experimentally that if animals such as mice are exposed in utero or even immediately after birth to foreign tissue antigens, these animals can be grafted with tissue containing the same foreign antigens without rejection. Failure of the host to recognize tissue with different histocompatibility antigens as foreign and to muster an immunological response against it is known as *immunological tolerance* or *immunological unresponsiveness.* This kind of tolerance is antigen-specific. Tolerance can also be induced in adult animals under appropriate experimental conditions (review Secs. 8-14 to 8-16). With regard to the human host, it has not yet been possible to adapt the reactions leading to tolerance in the animal model so that they can be used in the human host. Experiments along these lines are going on, but meanwhile nonspecific immunosuppression (Sec. 8-2) must be used in order to prevent rejection of allografts.

Immunological Enhancement of Allografts by Noncytotoxic Antibodies

9-6 Immunological enhancement by antitumor antibodies is a well-known phenomenon in tumor immunology (Chap. 10). At first it was proposed that antibodies to tumor antigens react with and cover tumor-cell antigens in such a way that sensitized T lymphocytes cannot react with tumor cells and destroy them. More recent evidence indicates that antitumor antibodies may react with soluble tumor antigens to form complexes and that reaction of T lymphocytes with antigens in the complexes causes inactivation of lymphocytes. Whatever the mechanism may be, this reaction is very undesirable to the host with regard to tumor cells but would be very desirable if enhancement could be induced for grafted tissue or organs. In a few cases, immunological enhancement of tissue grafts by antibodies has been induced experimentally. It has also been shown that when $F(ab')_2$ (divalent fragments of pepsin-digested antibodies) specific for transplantation antigens are separated and allowed to react with grafted tissue, the tissue is not destroyed by sensitized T lymphocytes. Enhancing antibodies act differently from cytotoxic antibodies. Cytotoxic antibodies are known to destroy tumor cells in the presence of complement. Enhancing antibodies have been reported to be IgG and to have little complement-fixing ability. $F(ab')_2$ fragments can react with antigen but not fix complement. Complement-fixing ability is associated with the Fc fragment (review Chap. 3). It has been postulated that enhancing antibodies may act (1) in the afferent limb of the immune response by "covering" histocompatibility antigens and preventing sensitization of T lymphocytes or (2) in the efferent limb of the immune response by "covering" histocompatibility antigens and thus preventing cells containing these antigens from reacting with, and being destroyed by, sensitized T lymphocytes. It has recently been reported that patients who have received previous blood transfusions are more likely to accept than to reject grafted tissue. These reports are contrary to previously held views on transfusion before transplantation. In addition to HLA matching before transplantation, the serum of the patient to receive the transplant should be tested to make sure that cytotoxic antibodies are not already present. Much remains to be learned about possible immunological enhancement of tissue and organ transplants.

Graft-versus-Host Reaction

9-7 The graft-versus-host reaction, discussed in several other chapters, occurs when an animal is injected with allogeneic cells against which it is incapable of mounting an immune response. Since the host cannot destroy the mismatched donor cells, the donor T lymphocytes are free to act against the host. For example, if adoptive immunization with the transfer of immunocompetent T lymphocytes into immunodeficient children is carried out with imperfectly matched cells, the donor T lymphocytes may become activated by HLA antigens of the host and develop a cell-mediated immune response against host cells. This is known as the graft-versus-host reaction (GVH). Tissues of the host mainly affected are skin, gastrointestinal tract, liver, and lymphoid tissue. In young animals, this reaction causes a condition known as *runt disease*. The GVH reaction is often fatal. It may occur when any type of graft containing immunologically competent T lymphocytes is transferred into a patient who lacks a normal immune system. In some extremely immunodeficient patients, even a blood transfusion has caused a GVH reaction. In some such cases, whole blood has been irradiated before use in an attempt to destroy lymphocytes responsible for GVH reactions without altering red blood cells.

Clinical Use of Transplantation

9-8 Many different kinds of transplantations are used in the practice of medicine, ranging from blood transfusions (cell suspensions) to organ grafts (solid tissue). Various aspects of some of these grafts are briefly discussed below.

Blood transfusion Red blood cells do not have HLA antigens, but white blood cells do. It was pointed out above that in some cases of extreme immunodeficiency, e.g., congenital immunodeficiency (review Chap. 7), even blood transfusions containing immunocompetent T lymphocytes can cause a GVH reaction. In most patients who receive whole blood, T lymphocytes are treated as an allograft and rejected. In some patients in whom granulocytes are abnormal, and consequently phagocytosis as well, it would be helpful to be able to concentrate and transfuse granulocytes from a normal individual. However, granulocytes also contain HLA antigens, and antibodies to granulocytes can cause severe reactions. The same is true of platelets, which carry the largest proportion of HLA antigens in whole blood; antibodies to HLA antigens cause platelet destruction.

Bone-marrow transplantation Because of the severe GVH reaction which frequently follows bone-marrow transplantation, this procedure must be considered an experimental and potentially dangerous one. Bone marrow sometimes is used to supply stem cells not only for lymphoid cell lines in cases of immunodeficiency but also for hemopoietic cell lines in cases of aplastic anemia (review Fig. 1-2). Bone-marrow transplantation should not be attempted without histocompatibility testing and reasonable assurance that a match for HLA antigens has been obtained between donor and recipient, especially their HLA-D antigens.

Cornea transplants Corneal transplantation is an accepted clinical procedure. Neither HLA typing nor immunosuppression is required although corneas do contain tissue and serum protein antigens. The cornea exists in a *privileged site* because under normal conditions (absence of injury or infection) it is avascular and not subject to rejection. Corneas may be taken several hours after death and stored in a tissue bank.

Cartilage transplants Transplantation of cartilage is used in plastic surgery. Neither histocompatibility testing nor immunosuppression is required. Chondrocytes (cartilage cells) are considered privileged cells because they can be transplanted without matching into nonprivileged sites and still survive. Lack of rejection is not fully understood but is attributed to the structure of cartilage.

Skin transplants Allografts of skin are readily rejected. Autografts of skin are not rejected. Allogeneic skin is used in burn cases in an attempt to cover the skin long enough for it to heal although it is known that an allograft will be rejected.

Organ transplants Attempts have been made to graft many different kinds of organs, including kidney, heart, lung, liver, pancreas, and intestine. The greatest success in terms of organ survival and function in the new host has been with kidney, for a number of reasons. Surgically, the transplantation of kidneys is a simple technique. During a period of rejection or renal failure, a patient can be maintained on a dialysis machine. If a kidney is rejected, the patient can be maintained until another donor is found. There is no such safety factor built into other kinds of organ transplantation. Since the body has two kidneys, a kidney donation may be obtained from a sibling or in a few cases even from an identical twin. The latter is a syngraft and has the best chance of not being rejected. Cadaver kidneys may also be used. A cadaver kidney is one which is removed immediately after death of a donor and maintained in a viable condition until used. Donors are often young healthy adults who die following an automobile accident. Many people carry a card indicating that they wish to be organ donors in case of accidental death.

Immunosuppression for Allograft Transplantation

9-9 Drugs which may be used for nonspecific suppression of immune responses were discussed in Secs. 8-6 and 8-7. Antilymphocyte or antithymocyte globulin may also be used for immunosuppression (review Sec. 8-8). In some cases, grafts may be pretreated or perfused with drugs to destroy passenger lymphocytes before transplantation since these donor lymphocytes in the graft carry donor HLA antigens and appear to be one of the main causes of sensitization after transplantation.

Questions for Secs. 9-1 to 9-9

1. Why is the term allograft preferred to homograft?

2. (*a*) Do the following components of blood contain HLA antigens: red blood cells, B lymphocytes, T lymphocytes, neutrophils, and platelets? (*b*) Which of the above cells are used for histocompatability testing?

3. (*a*) What is the difference between transplantation antigens, histocompatibility antigens, and HLA antigens? (*b*) What is the origin of the letters HLA? (*c*) What is the relationship of β_2-microglobulin to HLA antigen? (*d*) Is β_2-microglobulin responsible for allotypic specificity?

4. (*a*) What are passenger lymphocytes in a graft, and why is an attempt made to destroy them before transplantation? (*b*) Is the main mechanism which causes primary rejection of most grafts considered to be cell-mediated or antibody-mediated? (*c*) Are second-set rejections donor-specific? (*d*) What is a white graft?

5. With regard to graft survival, how does the action of enhancing antibodies differ from that of cytotoxic antibodies?

6. (*a*) In what type of individuals does the GVH reaction occur? (*b*) What is the GVH reaction? (*c*) In the GVH reaction, would cells of the graft be termed allogeneic, syngeneic, or neither? (*d*) What other term besides GVH has been used to describe this condition in animals?

Answers

1. The derivation of term allograft calls attention to antigenic differences between individuals of the same species. The individual specific HLA antigens determine whether or not a graft will be accepted. The term homograft is misleading because grafts of the same species can be very different antigenically and are not accepted unless carefully matched with recipient tissue by histocompatibility testing. (Sec. 9-1.)

2. (*a*) All except red blood cells. (*b*) Lymphocytes. (Sec. 9-2.)

3. (*a*) In general, these terms are usually employed to refer to the same antigens. (*b*) Human leukocyte locus A. (*c*) HLA antigens can be dissociated into two components with molecular weights of about 33,000 and 11,000 daltons. β_2-microglobulin is the lighter fragment. (*d*) No, the heavier fragment is responsible for allotypic specificity. (Secs. 9-2 and 9-3.)

4. (*a*) Passenger lymphocytes are donor lymphocytes which are in the graft at the time of transfer. Since they have HLA antigens of the donor and can easily leave the graft after transplantation to reach lymphoid tissue, they cause the patient to become sensitized to graft HLA antigens. HLA antigens of the graft may eventually reach lymphoid tissue of the host but not as quickly as when passenger lymphocytes are present. (*b*) Cell-mediated. (*c*) Yes. (*d*) One which is rejected so quickly that it never becomes vascularized; rejection is caused by cytotoxic antibodies which were already present before transplantation. (Sec. 9-4.)

5. Enhancing antibodies seem to protect the graft, while cytotoxic antibodies destroy it. Enhancing antibodies appear to react with antigen on cells of the graft without fixation of complement and to cover antigen sites so that sensitized T lymphocytes cannot react with the cells and destroy them. (Sec. 9-6.)

6. (*a*) Immunodeficient. (*b*) A reaction in which donor T lymphocytes are activated by antigens on cells of the host and react against the host cells; since the host is immunodeficient, the host cannot destroy these incompatible lymphocytes. (*c*) Allogeneic. (*d*) Runt disease. (Sec. 9-7.)

IMMUNOGENETICS OF TRANSPLANTATION

HLA Antigens and the Major Histocompatibility Complex of Human Beings

9-10 So far as is known, HLA antigens of human beings are responsible for rejection of allografts. HLA antigens present on surface membranes are the ones most responsible for causing rejection. The natural function(s) of HLA antigens in the body have not been well studied, but they are believed to be associated with such vital functions as maintenance of cellular integrity, recognition of specificity, etc. A great deal has been learned from studying mouse transplantation antigens called H-2 antigens. The major histocompatibility complex (MHC) of mice has contributed much to our understanding of the MHC of human beings but will not be discussed in this chapter. HLA was derived from human leukocyte locus A and was originally written HL-A. Since then human transplantation antigens have become known as HLA antigens. Now that four different loci, A, B, C, and D are recognized, these antigens are written HLA-A, HLA-B, HLA-C, and HLA-D. These loci are very close together; crossing-over rarely occurs. Table 9-2 lists some of the alleles recognized at these loci, which determine different antigen specificities of HLA. The A locus was formerly designated LA (locus A) or SD-1 (SD means "serologically defined"). The B locus was formerly called "four" or SD-2. The old terminology for locus C was SD-3 or AJ. The D locus formerly was known as LD-1 (LD means "lymphocyte-defined") or MLC-S. Specificity at the D locus is determined by the mixed-lymphocyte-culture (MLC) or mixed-lymphocyte-reaction (MLR) test. Recent studies indicate that matching for HLA-D antigen compatibility is the most important in preventing allograft rejection.

9-11 Genes determining HLA antigens in human beings appear to be very closely associated with genes which determine the immune response to certain antigens. Present evidence indicates that the HLA-D locus is closer to the immune-response gene than the other HLA loci are. With regard to the position of the other loci on the chromosome, HLA-B is the closest to HLA-D and HLA-A is the farthest away. Genes for complement components C2, C4, and C8 and factor B (Chap. 3) are also located within the major histocompatibility complex. There appears to be a relationship between HLA antigens and genes which determine susceptibility to certain diseases. It was pointed out in Sec. 6-12 that certain autoimmune diseases are associated with certain HLA antigens, and some of these associations were cited, notably ankylosing spondylitis and HLA-B27.

Inheritance of HLA Haplotypes

9-12 An HLA haplotype represents HLA specificity on one chromosome. The HLA tissue specificity of an individual is determined by one haplotype received from the mother and one from the father. The letters a and b are often employed to represent the paternal haplotypes and c and d the

Table 9-2 Four HLA loci showing alleles or specificities recognized at each locus

HLA-A	HLA-B	HLA-C	HLA-D
HLA-A1	HLA-B5	HLA-Cw1*	HLA-Dw1*
HLA-A2	HLA-B7	HLA-Cw2	HLA-Dw2
HLA-A3	HLA-B8	HLA-Cw3	HLA-Dw3
HLA-A9	HLA-B12	HLA-Cw4	HLA-Dw4
HLA-A10	HLA-B14	HLA-Cw5	HLA-Dw5
HLA-A11	HLA-B18		HLA-Dw6
HLA-A28	HLA-B27‡		
HLA-A29†			

*The letter w stands for "workshop" and indicates designation given at the workshop on histocompatibility testing; the w is removed when the terminology is officially accepted by WHO.

†Plus 10 workshop-designated alleles

‡Plus 11 workshop-designated alleles

Table 9-3 Inheritance of HLA Haplotypes

Family member	Paternal haplotypes a* and b* and maternal haplotypes c* and d*	HLA haplotypes at A, B, C† and D† loci
Father	ab	A1, B8, C3, D5; A3, B7, C2, D6
Mother	cd	A2, B12, C1, D6; A9, B5, C4, D6
Child 1	ac	A1, B8, C3, D5; A2, B12, C1, D6
2	ad	A1, B8, C3, D5; A9, B5, C4, D6
3	bc	A3, B7, C2, D6; A2, B12, C1, D6
4	bd	A3, B7, C2, D6; A9, B5, C4, D6
5	ac	A1, B8, C3, D5; A2, B12, C1, D6

*Letters usually employed to designate haplotypes of mother and father and the possible combinations of their haplotypes in siblings. a = A1, B8, C3, D5; b = A3, B7, C2, D6; c = A2, B12, C1, D6; d = A9, B5, C4, C6.

†For convenience of expressing haplotypes for this example, w for workshop numbers has been omitted (see Table 9-2).

maternal haplotypes. Table 9-3 shows the inheritance of HLA antigens in a family with five siblings. For HLA genes, each parental haplotype is completely expressed. With reference to Table 9-3, if child 1 required a transplant, child 5 would be the best match for HLA antigens. Child 4 would be completely unsuitable, having no haplotypes in common with child 1. In a family like that here, if the HLA types of two siblings are determined, there is 1 chance in 4 that they will have the same haplotypes; 1 in 4 that they will have completely different haplotypes, and 2 in 4 that they will share one of two haplotypes. Although crossing-over rarely occurs at the HLA loci, it is possible to observe combinations besides ac, ad, bc, and bd in a family like this.

Source of Antisera for Histocompatibility Testing

9-13 One of the best sources of antisera for HLA typing has been the sera of multiparous women, i.e., those who have given birth to several children. These women develop antibodies to HLA antigens determined by the haplotype of the father. During gestation, the mother is exposed to the HLA antigens of the child and develops antibodies to HLA antigens not of her own haplotype. Usually these antibodies have no effect on the development of the child. The fetus can be considered an allograft which is not rejected for reasons still unknown. Since there are so many different alleles which may exist at the four loci, the chance of the mother's and father's having the same haplotypes is very small. In some cases, however, the father and mother share all but one or two HLA antigenic determinants, so that the mother's antiserum shows a fairly high degree of specificity for these HLA antigens. Antisera for HLA typing have also been obtained from people who have received several blood transfusions, but their sera usually contain antibodies to many different HLA antigens. In some cases, antisera can be made more specific by absorption with the appropriate lymphocytes. Purified preparations of transplantation antigens for immunization of experimental animals are not available at present. In addition, to the above antisera for typing, antisera have been produced by immunization of human volunteers with blood leukocytes or by skin grafts. This type of sensitization is potentially dangerous and carries with it the risk of transferring hepatitis virus.

Histocompatibility Testing for Transplantation

9-14 Recent studies indicate that differences in HLA-D antigens of the donor and recipient are more likely to cause allograft rejection than differences in HLA antigens A, B, and C. Differences in HLA-D antigens can be detected by mixed-lymphocyte-culture (MLC) test but not by cytotoxic tests. Cytotoxic tests detect differences in HLA antigens A, B, and C. Until recently, most histocompatibility testing has been for HLA antigens A and B. For renal allografts obtained from siblings, there has been a good success rate with matching only for HLA antigens A and B; however, whenever A and

B were matched in siblings, D probably was also (see Table 9-3 and discussion in Sec. 9-12). The same is not true for cadaver kidneys, which have been used less successfully, especially in the United States, where there is a more heterogenous population than in western European countries. Although matching for HLA-D antigens appears at present to be the most important, matching for HLA antigens A, B, and C is believed to contribute to graft survival. The serum of a recipient should be tested for cytotoxic antibodies to the HLA antigens of the prospective donor. If cytotoxic antibodies for the prospective donor cells are already present, transplantation should not be carried out.

9-15 Lymphocytes obtained from peripheral blood of the donor and recipient are used for HLA typing; about 75 percent in peripheral blood are T lymphocytes. Lymphocytes are separated by the Ficoll-Hypaque gradient method. It has been stated many times that lymphocytes contain HLA antigens on their surface membranes. In addition to having the appropriate antisera for typing (see Sec. 9-13), it is also necessary to have lymphocytes of known HLA specificity (frozen by liquid nitrogen). Tests currently used for typing are described below.

Lymphocyte cytotoxicity test The cytotoxicity test for tissue typing was developed by Terasaki. The test is usually carried out with micro amounts and will identify HLA-A, HLA-B, and HLA-C antigens. In the presence of specific antibodies and rabbit complement, injury to the cell membrane occurs. Cell injury can be detected by the dye-exclusion test in which dye (trypan blue or eosin Y) is excluded from normal cells but taken up by injured cells. In addition to identifying HLA antigens of donor and recipient, the cytotoxicity test can be used to determine whether or not cytotoxic antibodies for donor cells are already present in the recipient's serum.

Antibody-dependent cell-mediated cytotoxicity test The class of antibody responsible for this reaction appears to be IgG. Complement is not required. It is not clear what cells act as effector cells to bring about destruction of target cells. The effector cells are usually described as being small mononuclear cells with Fc receptors. These cells are referred to as K (killer) cells. They do not have receptors for antigens of the target cells and are not T lymphocytes. They are found mainly in the peripheral blood and the spleen. The Fc receptors allow immunoglobulins (antibodies) to be bound at their Fc region to the cell surface. Antibody-dependent cell-mediated cytotoxicity also has been called *lymphocyte-dependent antibody-mediated lysis* (LDA). When this reaction is used in an assay, the test procedure is designed to expose target cells to antibodies in the absence of complement and then to determine the extent of target-cell injury which occurs after addition of effector cells (mononuclear leukocytes). In histocompatibility testing, target cells are the graft or donor cells. Radioactive markers are often used to measure target-cell lysis. One frequently used is chromium 51. Target cells are labeled with ^{51}Cr. The amount of cell injury is measured by the amount of isotope released. Hyperacute rejection (Sec. 9-4) sometimes occurs even when the conventional cross-match lymphocyte cytotoxicity test described above was negative. It appears that cytotoxic antibodies in the serum of the recipient may not always cause injury to donor cells in the presence of complement but may act on donor cells and render them susceptible to the action of K cells, which have an Fc receptor for immunoglobulins and can cause cell injury in the absence of complement.

Mixed-lymphocyte-culture (MLC) test This test is also referred to as the mixed lymphocyte reaction (MLR). It is used to test for differences between HLA-D antigens of the prospective donor and the recipient. Donor and recipient lymphocytes are mixed together in tissue-culture medium. Aseptic technique is required throughout the procedure since bacterial contamination can cause false results. If HLA-D antigens of donor and recipient lymphocytes are different, lymphocytes of both may be stimulated by antigen of each other to form blast cells and to undergo proliferation and clonal expansion. In order to make this a one-way reaction, donor lymphocytes are usually treated with mitomycin C. These treated lymphocytes can no longer become activated, but they can stimulate the recipient cells. The degree of activation and proliferation of recipient (responding) cells is measured by their rate of DNA synthesis as reflected by the incorporation of tritiated thymidine (^{3}H-thymidine) into DNA. Results are read on a scintillation counter. Since the standard MLC test requires 4 to 7 days to complete, it cannot be used for typing when a cadaver kidney becomes available because the kidney must be transplanted within a few days. Modifications of the MLC test are being devised to allow testing for HLA-D antigen in less time.

Cell-mediated-lymphocytolysis (CML) test Differences in HLA-D antigens of the donor and recipient are believed to be responsible for the outcome of this test, but other HLA antigens also may be involved. The procedure described below tests for the formation of killer lymphocytes, which are capable of destroying a graft or causing the GVH reaction. Lymphocytes of the prospective donor and the recipient are mixed in tissue culture. The donor lymphocytes are pretreated with mitomycin C; after treatment, they act as stimulating cells but cannot be transformed into lymphoblasts. At the same time the mixed culture is prepared, donor lymphocytes are cultured separately and labeled with ^{51}Cr to be used later as target cells. If HLA differences existed between the prospective donor lymphocytes (stimulating cells) and recipient lymphocytes (responding cells) in mixed culture, the recipient lymphocytes should have been stimulated to form lymphoblasts or sensitized lymphocytes capable of reacting against the donor target cells. The amount of ^{51}Cr released from the donor target cells is a measure of the amount of injury caused by the recipient killer lymphocytes.

Lymphocytotoxicity test for Ia antigens and possibly HLA-D Ia (I-region-associated) antigen determinants closely linked with the HLA-D locus appear to be responsible for the development of helper T lymphocytes and also cytotoxic T lymphocytes. There appears to be a very close relationship between Ia antigens and MLC-stimulating determinants. The MLC and CML tests for HLA-D differences described above are difficult to perform compared with cytotoxicity tests for HLA-A, HLA-B, and HLA-C. Since HLA-D antigens and Ia antigens are coded for by intimately related gene regions within the major histocompatibility complex, a cytotoxicity test for Ia antigens to test for HLA differences at the D locus has been used. B lymphocytes have a lot of Ia antigen, but T lymphocytes have very little. Since platelets have no Ia antigens but are rich in HLA antigens, they can be used to absorb anti-Ia sera to remove anti-HLA antibodies from sera to be used for cytotoxicity tests for Ia antigens. Whether or not a cytotoxicity test for Ia antigens (with B lymphocytes) based on the close association between Ia antigens and MLC-stimulating determinants will prove to be a reliable indication of HLA differences at the D locus remains to be shown. Such a test is much simpler to perform than the MLC and CML tests.

Questions for Secs. 9-10 to 9-15

7. (*a*) How many loci have been recognized in the major histocompatibility complex (MHC) of human beings? (*b*) How are these loci designated? (*c*) Does crossing-over occur within the major histocompatibility complex? If the answer is yes, state whether it occurs often or rarely. (*d*) Which loci were originally designated as serologically defined or SD-1, SD-2, and SD-3? (*e*) Which locus was known as lymphocyte defined or LD-1? (*f*) Have several alleles been recognized at each locus?

8. (*a*) Which HLA locus is closest to the gene known as the immune-response gene? (*b*) What might be an explanation of the association between certain HLA antigens and susceptibility to certain diseases?

9. (*a*) What is an HLA haplotype? (*b*) Are all HLA genes expressed equally? (*c*) What are the chances that two siblings will have identical haplotypes? (*d*) What are the chances that two siblings will have completely different haplotypes? (*e*) What are the chances that two siblings will have one identical and one different haplotype?

10. What has proved to be one of the best sources of antisera for HLA typing?

11. (*a*) What cells from donor and recipient are used for histocompatibility testing? (*b*) At present what HLA antigen is thought to be the most important to match in order to prevent graft rejection? (*c*) What test can be used to determine whether or not differences exist between donor and recipient with regard to this antigen? (*d*) What test is used to detect HLA antigens A, B, and C?

12. What two tests are used to try to be sure that the recipient's serum does not contain cytotoxic antibodies for the prospective donor's cells?

Answers

7. (*a*) Four. (*b*) HLA-A, HLA-B, HLA-C, and HLA-D. (*c*) Yes, rarely. (*d*) HLA-A, HLA-B, and HLA-C. (*e*) HLA-D. (*f*) Yes. (Sec. 9-10.)

8. (*a*) HLA-D. (*b*) The genes which determine HLA antigens are very close to a gene which governs an individual's immune response to certain antigens. This immune-response gene could influence susceptibility to disease and being very close to the HLA loci could cause a relationship between HLA antigens and susceptibility to disease. (Sec. 9-11.)

9. (*a*) Half of a type which is found on a single chromosome. One haplotype is inherited from the mother and one from the father. (*b*) Yes. (*c*) 1 in 4. (*d*) 1 in 4. (*e*) 2 in 4. (Sec. 9-12.)

10. Sera from multiparous women. (Sec. 9-13.)

11. (*a*) Lymphocytes from peripheral blood. (*b*) HLA-D. (*c*) Mixed lymphocyte culture (MLC) test. (*d*) Lymphocyte cytotoxicity test. (Secs. 9-14 and 9-15.)

12. Lymphocyte cytotoxicity test and antibody-dependent cell-mediated cytotoxicity (ADCC) test. (Sec. 9-15.)

REFERENCES

Abelson, L., P. Henkart, and D. Mann (1976): Typing for Specific B Lymphocyte Antigens, pp. 811-813 in N. R. Rose and H. Friedman (eds.), "Manual of Clinical Immunology," American Society for Microbiology, Washington, D.C.

Amos, D. B. (1976): An Interpretation of the Major Histocompatibility Complex, pp. 884-889 in N. R. Rose and H. Friedman (eds.), "Manual of Clinical Immunology," American Society for Microbiology, Washington, D.C.

———and P. Pool (1976) HLA typing, pp. 797-804 in N. R. Rose and H. Friedman (eds.), "Manual of Clinical Immunology," American Society for Microbiology, Washington, D.C.

Bach, F. H., and J. J. van Rood (1976): The Major Histocompatibility Complex, *N. Engl. J. Med.*, **295**:806-813, 872-878, and 927-936.

Barnstable, C. J., E. A. Jones, W. F. Bodmer, J. G. Bodmer, B. Arce-Gomez, D. Snary, and M. J. Crumpton (1976): Genetics and Serology of HL-A–linked Human Ia Antigens, *Cold Spring Harbor Sympo. Quant. Biol.*, **41**(2):443-455.

Benacerraf, B. (ed.) (1975): "Immunogenetics and Immunodeficiency," Medical and Technical, Lancaster, England.

Bigley, N. J. (1975): "Immunologic Fundamentals," Year Book, Chicago.

Billingham, R., and W. Silvers (1971): "The Immunobiology of Transplantation," Prentice-Hall, Englewood Cliffs, N.J.

Bodmer, W. F. (1975): Histocompatibility Testing International, *Nature*, **256**:696-697.

Dobias, G. (1974): Human Transplantation Antigens: System and Heredity, pp. 681-706 in E. Rajka and S. Korossy (eds.), "Immunological Aspects of Allergy and Allergic Diseases," vol. 2, "Methods in Experimental Immunology," Plenum, London.

Ferreira, E. (1976): Reactions Involving Cytolytic Antibody and Normal Lymphocytes, pp. 858-867 in N. R. Rose and H. Friedman (eds.), "Manual of Clinical Immunology," American Society for Microbiology, Washington, D.C.

Freedman, S. O., and P. Gold (eds.) (1976): "Clinical Immunology," 2d ed., Harper & Row, Hagerstown, Md.

Fudenberg, H. H., D. P. Stites, J. L. Caldwell, and J. V. Wells (eds.) (1976): "Basic and Clinical Immunology," Lange, Los Altos, Calif.

Gomori, P., and I. Varga (1975): Clinical Aspects of Organ Transplantation, pp. 75-95 in E. Rajka and S. Korossy (eds.), "Immunological Aspects of Allergy and Allergic Diseases," vol. 4, "Clinical Aspects of Immune Pathology," Plenum, London.

Lichtiger, B. (1977): Blood Component Therapy for Cancer, *Cancer J. Clin.*, **27**:194-204.

Lightboy, J. (1976): Use of the Cell-mediated Lympholysis Test in Transplantation Immunity, pp. 851-857 in N. R. Rose and H. Friedman (eds.), "Manual of Clinical Immunology," American Society for Microbiology, Washington, D.C.

Lovchik, J. C., and R. Hong (1977): Antibody-dependent Cell-mediated Cytolysis (ADCC): Analyses and Projections, *Prog. Allergy*, **22**:1-44.

O'Leary, J., N. Reinsmoen, and E. J. Yunis (1976): Mixed Lymphocyte Reaction, pp. 820-832 in

N. R. Rose and H. Friedman (eds.), "Manual of Clinical Immunology," American Society for Microbiology, Washington, D.C.
Opelz, G., D. P. Sengar, M. R. Mickey, et al. (1973): Effect of Blood Transfusion on Subsequent Kidney Transplants, *Transplant. Proc.*, **5**:253-259.
———, M. R. Mickey, and P. I. Terasaki (1972): Identification of Unresponsive Kidney-Transplant Recipients, *Lancet*, **1972**(1):868-871.
Park, B. H., and R. A. Good (1974): "Principles of Modern Immunobiology: Basic and Clinical," Lea & Febiger, Philadelphia.
Ritzmann, S. E., T. M. Vyvial, J. C. Daniel, C. M. Townsend, Jr., and G. A. Beathard (1974): Transplantation Immunology, pp. 461-507 in R. M. Nakamura (ed.), "Immunopathology: Clinical Laboratory Concepts and Methods," Little, Brown, Boston.
———,———, H. Sakai, and J. C. Daniels (1974): Tissue Typing Techniques in the Clinical Laboratory, pp. 508-526 in R. M. Nakamura (ed.), "Immunopathology: Clinical Laboratory Concepts and Methods," Little, Brown, Boston.
Rood, J. J. van, A. van Leeuwen, J. J. Keuning, A. Blusse van Oud Ablas (1975): The Serological Recognition of the Human MLC Determinants Using a Modified Cytotoxicity Technique, *Tissue Antigens*, **5**:73-79.
Woods, J. E. (1976): Clinical Organ Transplantation, pp. 93-144 in A. M. Munster (ed.), "Surgical Immunology," Grune and Stratton, New York.

10

Immune Reactions Concerned with Tumor Growth and Destruction

CANCER IMMUNOLOGY

Cancer or Tumor Antigens

10-1 It has been shown experimentally that when normal animal cells are transformed into cancer or tumor cells, they assume the characteristic of abnormal growth. The agents responsible for transforming cells to produce tumors are called *tumorgenic* or *oncogenic* (*onkos* means "mass") agents. Some agents tumorgenic in animals have been viruses or chemicals such as methylcholanthrene. It has also been shown experimentally that the transformed cells acquire surface antigens not possessed by the normal adult tissue cells. Tumor antigens have been called *tumor-specific antigens* (TSA) or *tumor-specific transplantation antigens* (TSTA) because it appears that they are recognized as foreign by the host and rejected in a manner similar to that of graft rejection (see Chap. 9). Recognition of the new tumor antigens as foreign and immediate rejection of cells carrying these antigens has been proposed as the basis of *immune surveillance*, a term used to describe the general process by which the host keeps its body free of cancer cells whenever normal cells are transformed by certain stimuli in the environment. The concept of immune surveillance has been challenged by several investigators.

10-2 The general feeling among scientists has been that if tumor antigens arise in transformed cells of experimental animals, tumor antigens should also be present in transformed human cells and in human tumor masses. This appears to be true. Although only a few human cancer antigens have been recognized at present, finding them has encouraged a search for others. The fact that tumor antigens have been found in blood serum makes serologic testing for cancer possible. These tests are discussed in Sec. 10-6. Although these tests are not highly reliable, it is expected that future research will yield tests that are.

Human Cancer Antigens Characterized by Antigenic Reversion to Fetal Antigens

10-3 In 1965 Gold and Freedman extracted an antigen from human cancer of the colon which was present in malignant colon tissue but not in nonmalignant colon tissue of the same person. Further study of this antigen revealed that it is present in normal fetal gut, liver, and pancreas between 2 and 6 months' gestation but disappears during the last trimester of pregnancy. This antigen was called *carcinoembryonic antigen* (CEA) and was considered to have arisen by reversion or dedifferentiation. This antigen is also referred to as *tumor-associated antigen* (TAA). An antigen which is found in both malignant and fetal tissue is sometimes called *oncofetal antigen* or *marker*. CEA is a glycoprotein complex with a molecular weight of about 200,000 daltons; it is soluble in perchloric acid, which is used for extraction of CEA from tumors. CEA is located, in part at least, at the cell surface on the plasma membrane. Antibodies to CEA can be removed by absorption with blood-group A substance. It appears that blood-group A substance and specific CEA determinants may be present on the same molecule.

10-4 Another human cancer antigen, α-fetoprotein (AFP), was recognized as a fetal antigen several years before it was recognized as a cancer antigen. Abelev (1969) and associates reported that AFP is present in the serum of adult mice with chemically induced hepatomas (cancer of the liver). Later, it was shown that AFP is present in the serum of patients with cancer. Under normal conditions, AFP is an embryonic alpha globulin found in human fetal serum during gestation. During the neonatal period, AFP completely disappears. The reappearance of AFP in human serum is frequently associated with primary cancer of the liver and embryonal carcinomas. AFP is secreted by the cell but is not found on the cell surface, as CEA is. AFP is another case of antigen reversion or dedifferentiation in association with cancer.

10-5 The reappearance of fetal antigens in malignant disease is not understood. It has been postulated that the loss of repressor mechanisms, as described by Jacob and Monod (1961), could account for the transformation of a previously normal cell into a malignant cell. The reappearance of fetal antigens may be caused by derepression of inherent genetic information. Besides CEA and AFP, there are other less well studied examples of oncofetal antigens or antigenic reversions in patients with cancer. Fetal sulfoglycoprotein (FSA) has been reported to be in the gastric juice of 90 percent of patients with carcinoma of the stomach, but it is also found in about 10 percent of patients with other gastric disorders. Other tumor markers detectable by immunological methods but not actually cancer antigens are fetal isozymes and hormones produced ectopically (out of normal place) by malignant tissue. The placental isozyme of alkaline phosphatase (also called Regan isoenzyme) is in the maternal but not fetal serum during the third trimester of pregnancy. It has been reported that about 15 percent of patients with malignant disease have this placental enzyme in their serum, but this enzyme is also present in patients with other conditions, e.g., cirrhosis, hepatitis, and ulcerative colitis. The enzyme may be present in cancer tissue without being present in the serum of the patient. Another marker, the beta subunit of human chorionic gonadotropin (HCG), is produced by a variety of neoplasms and has been used to help diagnose testicular tumors and other malignancies.

Cancer Antigens in Laboratory Diagnosis of Malignant Disease

10-6 Radioimmunoassay is the procedure currently used for the detection of most cancer markers. Carcinoembryonic antigen (CEA), discussed in Sec. 10-3, has been extensively used in tests with sera from cancer patients. Results of these tests indicate that future use of CEA to screen for malignant disease has limited value. It was originally thought that CEA could be used to detect cancer of the colon. CEA values are found in a high percentage of patients with colorectal carcinoma but not all, and also in many patients with cancer of the pancreas, lung, and stomach. CEA is also found in other types of cancer but in a smaller percentage of patients. Low values of CEA have been found in the sera of heavy smokers and in patients with various inflammatory disorders such as ulcerative colitis. High levels of CEA indicate dissemination or metastasis of cancer cells to other organs. In general, the lower the level of CEA in serum of a patient with malignant disease before surgery or chemotherapy, the greater the chance that the CEA level in serum will return to normal. CEA tests have been used to monitor patients who have undergone surgery. A rise in CEA values indicates recurrence of the tumor. With regard to the use of AFP as a cancer antigen, AFP has found greatest use in the diagnosis of primary cancer of the liver, but it is also produced when metastasis to the liver occurs. In addition to use of AFP in serologic tests for cancer, a high concentration of AFP in maternal serum during pregnancy is an indication of fetal distress or even fetal death. High concentrations in amniotic fluid often indicate fetal abnormalities. Detection of human chorionic gonadotropin (HCG) in urine by radioimmunoassay allows the early diagnosis of choriocarcinomas. In general, the use of cancer antigens recognized to date has had limited diagnostic value; however, there is reason to believe that continued research in this area will yield cancer antigens of greater diagnostic value.

Possible Causes of Human Cancer

10-7 Although most of the evidence relating viruses to the cause of human cancer is indirect, viruses are viewed as being one of the likely causes. Experimentally, it can be shown that certain viruses are tumorgenic, but after they transform the cell, the virus can no longer be isolated from the cell. Tumor antigens present on the surface of a cell transformed by a virus are present on all cells transformed by the same virus, but the tumor antigens are different from the viral antigens. Only recently has it been reported that it is also possible to demonstrate a viral antigen in virus-transformed cells. When normal cells are transformed into tumor cells, they not only acquire new antigens but also may suffer deletion of some normal surface antigens such as blood-group antigens and transplantation antigens. It has been proposed that the loss of normal tissue-specific antigens may interfere with homeostatic control mechanisms. One human tumor for which there is convincing evidence that it is caused by a virus is Burkitt's lymphoma, believed to be caused by Epstein-Barr virus (EBV), apparently a herpes virus. It has been shown that adeno viruses, which cause human respiratory illnesses, induce tumors in newborn hamsters. Whether or not certain human viruses such as adeno viruses may also transform human cells of the very young is not known. It is known that many viruses are capable of passing the placenta and reaching the fetus in utero. Also it has been shown that an animal tumor virus (mouse mammary-tumor virus) can be transmitted to the newborn in mother's milk. Many studies have shown that newborn animals are susceptible to animal tumor viruses in that these animals subsequently show tumor formation. In contrast, adult animals do not form tumors when injected with tumor viruses but usually do produce tumors when injected with tumor cells.

10-8 Certain chemicals have been shown to induce malignant tumors in experimental animals. From these experiments it has been concluded that many chemicals in our environment, e.g., insecticides and various pollutants, are oncogenic. In early studies on tumors induced by chemicals it was reported that a single chemical carcinogen induced many different types of surface tumor antigens. Now it appears that tumor antigens induced by chemicals are less diverse than originally supposed. It is possible that chemicals induce mutations in different clones of cells which give rise to different tumor antigens. It is also possible that chemicals activate latent oncogenic viruses in tissue which transform the cells to produce tumor antigens characteristic for that virus. Other possible causes of cancer are physical agents (such as ionizing radiation) and genetic factors. Susceptibility to certain kinds of cancer, e.g., medullary thyroid carcinoma, seem to be genetically transmitted.

10-9 Associated with the above factors in the development of cancer is impairment of the immune system. The incidence of cancer is high in persons with spontaneous immunodeficiency disorders and also in those who receive immunosuppressive drugs for organ transplantation. The significance of the observation that tumors developing in patients receiving immunosuppressive therapy very often involve the lymphoreticular system more than other organs is not known. Age also seems to be a factor associated with development of malignancy. It was pointed out in Sec. 6-11 that the development of malignancy, immunodeficiency states, and autoimmune diseases appears to be age-related and to occur more frequently in old age. It was stated that in some autoimmune diseases there appears to be a perturbation of the immune system. This also appears to be the case in malignancy. In advanced cancer a patient often becomes anergic, as demonstrated by failure to develop delayed-type hypersensitivity skin reactions, failure to reject skin allografts, etc. Also in vitro tests for lymphocyte function such as response to mitogens may be negative. In contrast to the above situation, some forms of cancer are observed mainly in young children, e.g., Wilms' tumor of the kidney. It has even been proposed that cancer may occur in the very young as the result of an overactive immune system. It should be apparent from what has been stated above that even though much has been learned about cancer, its exact cause or causes are not known. Possibilities now being investigated are viruses, chemicals in the environment, physical agents, inheritance of genetic factors, breakdown of homeostatic control, and impairment or alteration of immune responses.

Mechanisms of Host Resistance to Cancer

10-10 For many years the main mechanism of host resistance to cancer has been considered to be cell-mediated. Cell-mediated immunity, in which thymus-derived T lymphocytes react to tumor antigens and reject or destroy transformed cells whenever they arise, is considered to be the underlying mechanism of immune surveillance. The opinion has been expressed that the almost unanimous acceptance of the concept of immune surveillance hindered investigation of other mechanisms of host resistance or immunity to cancer. Although tumor immunity is still considered to be mainly cell-mediated, it is possible that mechanisms involving antibodies may also contribute to the destruction of tumor cells. Table 10-1 summarizes some of the mechanisms of destruction of tumor cells demonstrated in vitro which are believed to be responsible for host resistance. The mechanisms of resistance are divided into three categories: those cell-mediated by T lymphocytes or lymphokines produced by T cells (Sec. 2-27); those based on the combined action of antibodies and non-T lymphocytes or antibodies and macrophages; and those antibody-mediated by cytotoxic antibodies capable of destroying tumor cells in conjunction with fixation of complement. The action of these antibodies is different from that of antibodies which enhance tumor growth. (Sec. 10-13).

10-11 T cells can act directly with tumor cells to bring about cytolysis of the tumor cells. These T cells are sometimes called killer cells and after reacting with a tumor cell to destroy it can subsequently react with other tumor cells. T-lymphocyte killer cells should not be confused with K cells (killer cells), which are antibody-dependent for cytolysis and not considered to be T lymphocytes (Sec. 10-12). It has been observed that patients whose tumors are infiltrated with lymphocytes have a better prognosis than those whose tumors are free of lymphocytes. Lymphocyte-mediated cytolysis can be measured by the release of ^{51}Cr from radiolabeled tumor cells after the latter are allowed to react with T lymphocytes. This type of measurement is similar to that described in Sec. 9-15 for the cell-mediated-lymphocytolysis (CML) test for histocompatibility. Another test for lymphocyte destruction of tumor cells is a tissue-culture method based on colony inhibition. Lymphocytes are mixed with tumor cells, and then the number of colonies of tumor cells which grow is compared with the controls. T lymphocytes are stimulated to become cytotoxic after contact with tumor antigens. When T lymphocytes are stimulated by tumor antigens, they form lymphoblasts, which proliferate and differentiate into killer cells and memory cells, as described in Fig. 2-8. In vitro, it can be shown that direct destruction of tumor cells by T lymphocytes is rapid, with cytolysis occurring within 1 h after contact. In contrast, destruction of tumor cells by lymphokines, e.g., lymphotoxin, requires several hours. Recent studies indicate that even nonsensitized and therefore nonselective lymphocytes may be cytotoxic for tumor cells. With regard to destruction of tumor cells by direct contact with T lymphocytes, Allison and Ferluga (1976) have reported that plasma membranes isolated from T lymphocytes can have a cytotoxic effect on tumor cells. They attributed at least part of this effect to a membrane-associated proteinase. Direct killing of tumor cells by T lymphocytes has been observed to take place in several stages:

1. Movement of T cells so that the plasma membrane of the lymphocyte establishes intimate contact with the tumor cell; agents which depress cell motility decrease destruction of tumor cells.
2. Establishment of firm adhesion between the lymphocyte plasma membrane and tumor cell membrane; shaking with ethylenediaminotetraacetic acid (EDTA) disrupts this union.
3. Intimate contact for several minutes between the lymphocyte and tumor cell in the presence of calcium ions.

Table 10-1 Host Mechanisms of Cytotoxicity for tumor cells

Cytotoxicity	*Reactions*
Cell-mediated reactions	
T lymphocyte	T lymphocytes (activated by tumor antigens) + tumor cells $\xrightarrow[\text{to target cell}]{\text{direct adherence}}$ cytolysis of tumor cells*
Lymphokine	T lymphocytes (activated) + tumor cells or tumor antigens $\xrightarrow[\text{from T cells}]{\text{lymphokine release}}$ lymphotoxin (also MIF, etc.) + tumor cells → killing of tumor cells
SMAF†-armed macrophage	Macrophage armed with SMAF + tumor cells → destruction of tumor cells
Combined cell- and antibody-mediated reactions	
Non-T-lymphocyte (K-cell) antibody-dependent (ADC)	Effector cells‡ with Fc receptors for IgG + tumor cells with bound antibody (IgG) $\xrightarrow[\text{target cell}]{\text{adherence to}}$ cytolysis of tumor cells
Antibody-armed macrophage	Macrophages with Fc receptors + antitumor antibodies (aggregated) → "armed" macrophages + tumor cells → destruction of tumor cells
Antibody-mediated reactions	
Antitumor antibodies (plus complement) §	Antitumor cytotoxic antibodies + complement + tumor cells → tumor cells with bound antibody and complement → tumor-cell injury

*T cells can dissociate from dying tumor cell and proceed to other tumor cells.

†SMAF is specific macrophage arming factor, released during interaction of T cells with tumor cells; SMAF originates from T cells and may be T-cell receptors.

‡Some effector cells may also have receptors for IgM bound to tumor cells; not all cells with Fc receptors are effector cells; they appear to be a heterogeneous population of small mononuclear cells mainly found in peripheral blood and in the spleen.

§The role of antitumor antibodies and complement acting against tumor cells is not clear.

4. Lysis of the tumor cell, which can occur in the absence of the lymphocyte and does not require Ca or Mg ions; as stated above, it appears that after a lymphocyte has interacted with a tumor cell to destroy it, the lymphocyte can dissociate itself and react with still other tumor cells.

Direct killing of tumor cells is also brought about by macrophages armed with specific macrophage arming factor (SMAF), released when T cells and tumor cells interact. SMAF originates from the T cells and may actually be T-cell receptors.

10-12 In vitro, it can be shown that cells other than T lymphocytes can bring about destruction of tumor cells which have reacted with antitumor antibodies. The exact identity of these cells, often called K cells, is not known; they may be white blood cells, e.g., monocytes, neutrophils, B cells, or null cells. Null cells are lymphocytes which lack identifying surface markers for either T or B cells but do have Fc receptors. The cell responsible for antibody-dependent cytolysis (ADC) has Fc receptors for antibodies (immunoglobulins). Since T cells mostly lack Fc receptors, the responsible cell is not a T lymphocyte. The responsible cell has been described by some scientists as being a B cell, but this view has not been widely accepted. Whatever kind of cells act as the effector cells here, their Fc surface receptors bind antibodies on the surface of the tumor cells so that the effector cells and tumor cells are held together in a way that facilitates their interaction and destruction of the tumor cells. It is not necessary for the effector cells to be immune cells or sensitized lymphocytes. Another reaction in which both cells and antibodies are involved is one in which aggregated antitumor antibodies react with Fc receptors on the surface of macrophages so that the macrophages are spoken of as being *armed*. The macrophages are thus prepared, or armed, to interact with tumor cells and destroy them. Killing is extracellular rather than intracellular following phagocytosis. With regard to destruction of tumor cells by antibodies without the help of cells, experiments carried out in vitro indicate that antibodies called *cytotoxic antibodies* can bring about destruction of tumor cells with the help of complement.

Mechanisms by Which Tumor Cells Evade Host Defenses

10-13 It was demonstrated several years ago in experimental animals that a high concentration of circulating antibodies to tumor surface antigens protects the tumor against destruction by T lymphocytes. This phenomenon was called *immunological enhancement*, and the antibodies were called *enhancing* or *blocking antibodies.* It was proposed that antibodies protect the tumor by reacting with surface tumor antigens in such a way that T lymphocytes cannot react with the tumor cell and destroy it. It is now considered more likely that tumor-enhancing antibodies react with soluble tumor antigens to form soluble complexes (in the region of antigen excess) and that the antigen of these complexes reacts with T-lymphocyte receptors and thus deactivates the lymphocytes. The presence of these complexes has been demonstrated.

10-14 Another possible mechanism proposed to account for evasion of host defenses by the tumor is the lack of the appropriate host immune-response gene for responding to certain tumor antigens. Still another mechanism for which there is some support is antigenic modulation, in which there is a decrease in expression of tumor antigens. If such a change should take place in vivo, tumors with weak surface antigens would be more likely to persist than tumors with strong surface antigens. The latter would induce an immune response and be destroyed. It is also possible that soluble cancer antigens can induce immunological tolerance in the host, so that there would be no host immune response to these cancer antigens. Immunological tolerance (specific suppression of the immune response) might occur because many tumor antigens are of fetal origin or because the tumor-antigen load in advanced cases is great.

Host-Tumor Interactions and Spontaneous Regression

10-15 It should be clear from what was said in Secs. 10-10 to 10-12 that the host has fairly effective defense mechanisms against tumor cells so long as they can be destroyed as they arise. But sometimes the tumor cells are not destroyed. As the tumor increases in size, the chance of destruction by immune mechanisms of the host becomes less. Chemotherapy for cancer seems to be more effective if the tumor can be surgically removed because excision usually allows immune function to be restored at least partially. In very rare instances, some malignant tumors which were not surgically removed have undergone spontaneous regression. In the documented cases reported in the literature, the cause for regression was not known. Regression may have had an immunological basis or have been caused by other factors. Some cases were stated to have followed bacterial or viral infections. The observation in 1891 that a lymphosarcoma of the neck regressed in a patient who had erysipelas (an infection caused by *Streptococcus pyogenes*) prompted Coley to prepare bacterial filtrates of streptococci and also other bacteria such as *Serratia marcescens* (formerly *Bacillus prodigiosus*). These preparations were known as Coley toxins and were often used mixed. At first, Coley toxins received much attention. Not all preparations were equally effective, and interest declined. There was a reinvestigation of Coley toxins during the 1940s. Coley toxins were given by several injections directly into the tumor; some preparations were described as having a Shwartzman effect. The Shwartzman reaction (Sec. 5-31) is usually associated with endotoxins of gram-negative bacteria. Coley toxins are not used now. Bacterial preparations which exert a nonspecific effect on cell-mediated immunity are being used and are described below. The fact that malignant tumors, sometimes considered inoperable, have been known to regress gives hope that a way can be found to cause tumors to regress under controlled conditions. To eliminate the need for cancer surgery was recently stated as the long-range objective of the group of immunologists appointed by the National Institutes of Health to a task force in immunology and disease.

10-16 The action of cytotoxic antibodies which with complement destroy tumor cells was described in Sec. 10-12. The action of blocking antibodies which enhance tumor growth was described in Sec. 10-13. A substance called *unblocking factor* has been reported to be in the sera of some animals "cured" of cancer or patients in remission. Unblocking factor may be the same as what others have termed deblocking antibody. Very little is known about unblocking factor or deblocking antibodies at present. The specificity of the deblocking antibodies has been suggested to be directed to the variable region (antigen combining site), or idiotype, of the blocking antibodies (review Chap. 3 on antibody structure). Deblocking antibodies presumably react with blocking antibodies so that the latter can no longer interfere with destruction of tumor cells by cell-mediated reactions. There is much that remains to be learned about the interaction of antitumor antibodies, cells (lymphocytes, etc.), and tumor antigens, both those on tumor cells and those shed into the circulation. It appears that tumor antigens shed into the circulation also have a blocking effect on host resistance. In Sec. 10-6 it was pointed out that tumor antigens like CEA are present in large amounts in the patient's serum in the late stages of cancer or when matastasis occurs. It appears that the initial host response to transformed cancer cells with nonself antigens is cell-mediated and these cancer cells are rejected just as a foreign graft would be rejected. If tumor cells escape this mechanism of immune surveillance and continue to grow, so that tumor antigens are shed into the circulation and blocking antibodies are formed, mechanisms of host resistance and interaction with tumor cells becomes quite complicated. Experimentally, it has been shown that immune complexes of soluble cancer antigens formed with antibody excess instead of antigen excess do not block immune destruction of tumor cells.

Questions for Secs. 10-1 to 10-16

1. (*a*) When a tissue cell is transformed by an oncogenic agent, does it become malignant? (*b*) What is another name for an oncogenic agent? (*c*) What are cancer antigens called which are responsible for rejection of cancer cells? (*d*) What is the general term for the body's mechanism to keep itself free from cancer?

2. (*a*) What kind of antigen reversion has been observed with cancer antigens of human beings and animals? (*b*) What is an oncofetal antigen? (*c*) Which human cancer antigen is associated with cancer of the colon but is also found in other kinds of cancer? (*d*) Is this cancer antigen found on the cell membrane of tumor cells and in sera of patients with certain types of cancer including cancer of the colon and pancreas?

3. (*a*) Which human cancer antigen is associated with primary cancer of the liver but is

also found with other kinds of cancer, especially embryonal cancer? (*b*) Is this cancer antigen found on the surface of tumor cells and in the sera of patients?

4. (*a*) Why have cancer antigens found on human cancer cells been disappointing as diagnostic aids? (*b*) What is the present use of CEA?

5. (*a*) Is there a change in normal surface components when tissue cells are transformed? Explain. (*b*) List some of the possible causes of human cancer for which there is support. (*c*) Is the incidence of cancer related to age?

6. (*a*) What cell is considered to be the most important cell in host resistance to cancer? (*b*) Explain the mechanism(s) of killing of cancer cells by the cell specified in part (a). (*c*) Is the in vitro destruction of cancer cells rapid? Explain your answer.

7. (*a*) With what kind of cells have antitumor antibodies been shown to react with in vitro to bring about destruction of tumor cells? Explain the mechanisms involved. (*b*) Can antitumor antibodies kill tumor cells in vitro without the help of the above-mentioned effector cells? Explain the mechanism involved.

8. What is meant by the term immunological enhancement of tumors? Explain the mechanism(s) involved.

9. (*a*) Explain how antigen modulation in vivo could affect host resistance to tumor cells. (*b*) What mechanisms could account for specific suppression of the immune response or immunological tolerance in patients with cancer?

10. (*a*) What is meant by spontaneous regression, and what causes this type of regression to occur? (*b*) Does spontaneous regression occur frequently?

Answers

1. (*a*) Yes. (*b*) Tumorigenic. (*c*) Tumor-specific antigens (TSA) and tumor-specific transplantation antigens (TSTA). (*d*) Immune surveillance. (Sec. 10-1.)

2. (*a*) Reversion to fetal antigens. (*b*) An antigen found in both cancer and fetal tissue. (*c*) Carcinoembryonic antigen (CEA). (*d*) Yes, on the cell membrane and in sera. (Sec. 10-3.)

3. (*a*) α-Fetoprotein (AFP). (*b*) It is not a surface antigen but is excreted by cells and found in sera of some patients. (Sec. 10-4.)

4. (*a*) Cancer antigens are found in the sera not only of patients with cancer but also in small amounts in the sera of some patients without cancer. Not all patients with cancer have cancer antigens in their sera during the early stages. Cancer antigens are present in patients' sera in large amounts during advanced stages and during metastasis. (*b*) CEA is not present in all patients with cancer during the early stages. After surgery and after chemotherapy, the serum level of CEA often returns to normal but rises again during metastasis. The test for CEA in serum appears to be more reliable for prognosis of a case than for diagnosis. (Sec. 10-6.)

5. (*a*) Yes, when tissue cells become malignant, they acquire tumor antigens but they also lose some normal cell antigens, e.g., some transplantation antigens and some blood-group antigens. The loss of these normal surface antigens may affect homeostatic control adversely. (*b*) Some viruses, some chemicals, some physical factors such as ionizing radiations, genetic factors, and impairment of immune function. (*c*) Cancer occurs in all age groups. Some forms occur in the very young. In general, the incidence of cancer increases as a person ages. (Secs. 10-7 to 10-9.)

6. (*a*) T lymphocyte. (*b*) Activated T lymphocytes are able to react directly with tumor cells to cause cytolysis; lymphokines such as lymphotoxin released by activated T lymphocytes can bring about the destruction of tumor cells. (*c*) Both the reactions cited in part (b) have been demonstrated in vitro; the former occurs rapidly within 1 h, but the latter requires several hours for destruction. (Sec. 10-11.)

7. (*a*) In vitro, it has been shown that antitumor antibodies combine with the Fc receptors for antibodies on macrophages, so that the macrophages are capable of reacting directly

with tumor cells to destroy them. These macrophages are called armed. It has been shown also that other types of cells not yet identified but with Fc receptors react with antibodies on tumor cells to cause cytolysis. This reaction is called antibody-dependent cytolysis. The cells involved here may be monocytes, B lymphocytes, or null cells, all of which have Fc receptors. (*b*) Yes; cytotoxic antibodies react with tumor cells with the fixation of complement and cause damage to the tumor cell membrane. (Sec. 10-12.)

8. Tumor growth is enhanced as the result of an immune response if antibody production occurs and cancer antigens are shed into the circulation. Earlier it was postulated that these antibodies act as blocking antibodies by covering the antigen sites on the tumor so that T lymphocytes cannot act directly with the tumor cells. Now it appears that the blocking antibodies react with soluble tumor antigens in antigen excess so that T lymphocytes react with antigens of the immune complexes and are inactivated before they can react with tumor cells. (Sec. 10-13.)

9. (*a*) If tumor antigens are weakened, they do not exert as strong an immune response and may escape being destroyed by the host immune system. (*b*) Since some cancer antigens contain fetal antigens present in the host in utero, the host may not recognize them as foreign, so that these cancer antigens may not be able to induce an immune response. Also the amount of cancer antigen present in the circulation during the latter stages of cancer may be great enough to induce a state of specific immunological unresponsiveness. (Sec. 10-14.)

10. (*a*) Spontaneous regression refers to the disappearance of a tumor (often nonoperable) without treatment. The mechanism or mechanisms of regression are not known. (*b*) No, very infrequently. There have been about 175 documented cases of spontaneous regression reported in the literature. (Sec. 10-15.)

IMMUNOPOTENTIATION AND IMMUNOTHERAPY OF CANCER

Nonspecific Immunopotentiation and Host Resistance to Cancer

10-17 BCG vaccine for tuberculosis contains an attenuated strain of *Mycobacterium bovis*, formerly called *M. tuberculosis* var. *bovis* because it causes tuberculosis not only in cattle but also in human beings. Antigenically *M. bovis* and *M. tuberculosis* (human strain) cannot be differentiated. BCG vaccine is not used now in the United States for immunization against tuberculosis, but it is being used in the treatment of cancer. It was one of the first preparations used for nonspecific stimulation of cell-mediated immunity of cancer patients. *Mycobacteria* spp. have been used in Freund's adjuvant, a powerful adjuvant, for many years (Sec. 5-42). Freund's complete adjuvant has the property of inducing an immune response even to very weak antigens. The use of BCG vaccine for treatment of cancer patients is also known as *adjuvant immunotherapy*. The exact role of adjuvants in cancer therapy is not understood. Adjuvants are known to cause a stimulation of the reticuloendothelial system. Other preparations which have an adjuvant effect and are being used in cancer therapy include a methanol-extractable residue of BCG known as MER and formalin-killed *Corynebacterium parvum.** One of the disadvantages of BCG is that it is a living attenuated strain and can actually cause an infection in immunodeficient patients. *C. parvum* is a gram-positive anaerobic bacillus which has a powerful adjuvant effect even when formalin-inactivated.

10-18 Several factors appear to affect the success of BCG vaccine in cancer therapy. BCG seems to be more effective when it is injected directly into the tumor, so that there is direct contact between BCG and tumor cells; however, BCG is also administered by scarification and intradermal injection. Tumor size is also a critical factor in limiting the effectiveness of BCG immunotherapy; it is more effective when the tumor burden can be lowered by excision. It appears necessary for the patient to be capable of developing an immune response to BCG and also to tumor antigen(s). BCG vaccine is often

*In the 8th edition of "Burgey's Manual" (1974) this organism is classified as *Propionibacterium acnes.*

used after surgery or chemotherapy in an attempt to destroy any tumor cells still remaining. When injected into tumors, BCG may induce a local delayed-type hypersensitivity reaction with tumor cells being killed as innocent bystanders due to the release of lymphokines and the action of macrophages. In other cases, BCG may induce a host immune response to tumor antigen(s), so that the mechanisms outlined in Table 10-1 take part in tumor destruction. BCG appears to have been especially effective in the treatment of malignant melanoma. It has been somewhat effective in treating leukemia and some solid tumors.

10-19 The action of *C. parvum* is similar to that of BCG. It has an advantage over BCG in that it can be used as a formalin-killed vaccine. Both BCG and *C. parvum* have been reported to convert the skin reactions of anergic patients from negative to positive in cases where the patients had been sensitized before they became anergic. *C. parvum* appears to have been used with success in combination with chemotherapy. Another substance recently used for cancer immunotherapy is Levamisole, an effective antihelmintic with few toxic effects. It has been reported that Levamisole can restore delayed-type hypersensitivity reactions in anergic patients within a very short time. This drug has not been used long enough for us to know just what impact it will have on cancer therapy. Still other substances which have been used are bacterial endotoxins and Lentinan,* a polysaccharide extracted from the mushroom *Lentinus edodes.*

10-20 In the section on delayed-type hypersensitivity skin reactions, it was pointed out that 2,4-dinitrochlorobenzene (DNCB) can be used to sensitize the skin by application (Sec. 5-46). This reaction has been used in local nonspecific immunotherapy for skin cancer. In patients with basal- and squamous-cell carcinoma of the skin, it has been demonstrated that the application of DNCB to the tumor tissue induces a delayed-type hypersensitivity reaction to DNCB which results in destruction of the cancer cells.

Active Immunotherapy for Cancer

10-21 The action of adjuvants described above may be considered a combination of nonspecific immunopotentiation and active immunization to cancer antigens. It was pointed out previously (Sec. 10-14) that cancer antigens probably undergo modulation in vivo, so that cancer antigens of tumor cells are weakened and the tumor cells thereby escape destruction by the host. BCG and *C. parvum* have a strong adjuvant effect and when used for therapy should allow even these weak cancer antigens to induce an immune response. Many types of cancer vaccines have been prepared, but in general they have had little value. It is almost impossible to prepare an effective vaccine when so little is known about human cancer antigens and the cause of human cancers. Some of the general approaches to active immunotherapy and the composition of the vaccines are outlined below.

Whole-tumor-cell vaccines (unmodified) Autologous tumor tissue has been mixed with Freund's adjuvant and injected back into the host with some favorable responses. Allogeneic tumor cells also have been used; however, for immunization of human beings, these tumor cells have been inactivated in various ways, e.g., irradiation.

Whole tumor cells (modified) In these vaccines, the tumor cells have been treated in various ways in attempts to increase their antigenicity. The modifications include addition of a carrier protein such as rabbit gamma globulin, chemical modification, treatment with neuraminidase, and treatment with concanavalin A.

Subcellular components of tumor cells These include crude cell extracts, isolated cell membranes, and solubilized-cell surface tumor antigens. As stated above, the use of cancer vaccines has been disappointing. If viruses cause cancer, viral vaccines should be effective in preventing cancer if the viruses could be neutralized before they had a chance to transform the cells. In animals studies even when it is known that transformation is caused by a virus, the virus cannot be isolated. Recently it has been reported that a virus antigen as well as the cancer antigen can be recognized in tumor cells. It has been suggested that it may be possible to isolate viral antigens from tumor cells and to use the viral antigens for immunization even though it is not possible to isolate the virus.

Passive Immunotherapy for Cancer

10-22 Antitumor serum has been used in attempts to give passive immunity against cancer. In general, it has not been effective. In a few cases reported, the sera of patients who had experienced regression of their tumors caused regression of tumors of the recipients. The role of antibodies in resistance to cancer is not clear. Cytotoxic antibodies and deblocking antibodies are associated with host resistance, and blocking antibodies are associated with tumor enhancement. Recent experimental evidence indicates that if the antibody titer is high enough for immune complexes of soluble cancer antigens to be formed in antibody excess instead of antigen excess, cell-mediated immune responses are not impaired. Cell-mediated reactions appear to be most responsible for destruction of tumor cells. The kinds of cells or cell extracts used for passive immunotherapy are outlined below.

Activated and nonactivated lymphocytes The transfer of lymphocytes is known as *adoptive immunization.* The problem with lymphocytotherapy is that unless the lymphocytes are HLA-matched, serious reactions like the GVH reaction can occur. Patients' lymphocytes have been grown in tissue culture and then reinfused. Experimental studies indicate that many lymphocytes are necessary to kill a tumor cell. Lymphocytes have been activated in vitro before transfusion, nonspecifically by mitogens or by tumor antigens. Recent studies indicate that normal nonactivated lymphocytes from healthy immunocompetent individuals should contribute to resistance of the cancer patient provided the HLA types of both donor and recipient are compatible. It seems reasonable that these lymphocytes could become activated in vivo, especially with the use of BCG or *C. parvum.* In general, lymphocytotherapy has not been very effective with either sensitized or nonsensitized lymphocytes.

Extracts from sensitized lymphoid cells; transfer factor and immune RNA Transfer factor is one substance which has been extracted from sensitized lymphocytes and used to treat cancer patients. If lymphocytes are taken by leukophoresis from cancer patients who have recovered from cancer, care must be taken not to upset the patient's state of resistance. The nature, preparation, and use of transfer factor in patients lacking cell-mediated immunity have previously been discussed. With transfer factor, there is no danger of the GVH reaction's occurring. The use of transfer factor for treating cancer patients and patients with other diseases is now being actively investigated. Thymosin, which is extracted from the thymus gland of animals, is also being evaluated for its effectiveness in cancer therapy. It contains a hormone which appears to stimulate cellular immunity. Immune RNA, still another substance which has been extracted from lymphoid tissues, has been obtained following immunization of animals with tumor cells; it was found to induce immunity in syngeneic recipients of tumor transplants. Being investigated at the present time is the possibility of isolating immune RNA from lymphoid tissue of "cured" cancer patients and using it for immunotherapy of cancer.

Subpopulations of Lymphocytes Affecting Host Resistance to Cancer

10-23 T lymphocytes and non-T lymphocytes responsible for destruction of tumor cells were discussed in Secs. 10-10 to 10-12. It has been shown that in some cases of human cancer besides the cytotoxic lymphocytes there are lymphocytes which act as inhibitors of cytotoxic lymphocytes. A patient's peripheral blood which is noncytotoxic in vitro and which appears to contain no cells capable of tumor-specific lysis may contain both inhibitor lymphocytes and cytotoxic lymphocytes. The two populations of lymphocytes can be separated on discontinuous gradients of bovine serum albumin. Most patients in whom inhibitor lymphocytes were found had already shown metastasis. Lymphocytes which enhance tumor growth or which suppress tumor-specific cytotoxic lymphocytes also have been identified in animal models.

Questions for Secs. 10-17 to 10-23

11. (*a*) What two microorganisms are used more frequently now than others for nonspecific immunopotentiation of host resistance to cancer? (*b*) Are these organisms used in the living or killed state? (*c*) Why is the use of these organisms referred to as adjuvant immunotherapy? (*d*) What adjuvant often used in research contains *Mycobacteria* spp.?

12. List several factors which appear to affect the successful use of BCG.

13. How has DNCB been used in the treatment of skin cancer?

14. (*a*) What kinds of vaccines have been prepared in an attempt to actively immunize against cancer? (*b*) In general, have these vaccines been effective?

15. (*a*) List the different kinds of passive immunotherapy which have been used for cancer and briefly state their effectiveness. (*b*) What advantage does transfer factor as a therapeutic agent have over the injection of lymphocytes?

Answers

11. (*a*) *Mycobacterium bovis* in BCG vaccine and *Corynebacterium parvum*. (*b*) *M. bovis* is used as a living attenuated microorganism and *C. parvum* is formalin-killed. (*c*) Both nonspecifically stimulate the reticuloendothelial system as Freund's adjuvant does. It is also believed that they allow weak cancer antigens to become immunogenic and induce an immune response. (*d*) Freund's. (Secs. 10-17 and 10-18.)

12. Intralesion injection; contact with tumor cells; reduction of tumor burden by surgery or chemotherapy; ability of host to develop an immune response to BCG and to tumor antigens. (Sec. 10-18.)

13. DNCB painted on skin cancer causes a delayed-type hypersensitivity reaction which destroys tumor cells. (Sec. 10-20.)

14. (*a*) Vaccines containing whole cells, autologous or syngeneic, have been prepared; vaccines containing tumor cells treated in various ways in order to make them more immunogenic, and vaccines containing subcellular components of tumor cells. (*b*) In general they have not been effective. (Sec. 10-21.)

15. (*a*) Antitumor sera; lymphocytotherapy with sensitized and nonsensitized lymphocytes; extracts of sensitized lymphoid cells such as transfer factor and immune RNA. In general, passive immunotherapy has not been very effective; however, transfer factor for cancer and immune RNA are just beginning to be used and evaluated. (*b*) Transfer factor cannot cause the GVH reaction. (Sec. 10-22.)

REFERENCES

Abelev, G. I. (1974): Alpha-fetoprotein as a Marker of Embryo-specific Differentiation in Normal and Tumor Tissues, *Transplant. Rev.*, **20**:3–37.

Allison, A. C., and J. Ferluga (1976): How Lymphocytes Kill Tumor Cells, *N. Engl. J. Med.*, **295**:165–167.

Bast, R. C., B. Zbar, T. Borsos, and H. J. Rapp (1974): BCG and Cancer, *N. Engl. J. Med.*, **290**:1413–1420 and 1458–1469.

Burnet, F. M. (1970): The Concept of Immunological Surveillance, *Prog. Exp. Tumor Res.*, **13**:1–27.

Cerottini, J. C. (1977): Lymphoid Cells as Effectors of Immunologic Cytolysis. *Hosp. Pract.*, **12**(11):57–68.

Ferluga, J., and A. C. Allison (1975): Cytotoxicity of Isolated Plasma Membranes from Lymph Node Cells, *Nature*, **255**:708–710.

Freedman, S. O., and P. Gold (1976): "Clinical Immunology," 2d ed., Harper & Row, Hagerstown, Md.

Fudenberg, H. H. (1976): Dialyzable Transfer Factor in the Treatment of Human Osteosarcoma: An Analytical Review, *Ann. N.Y. Acad. Sci.*, **277**:545–558.

———and C. L. Smith (1977): Human Lymphocyte Subpopulations and Metastatic Neoplasia, *N. Engl. J. Med.*, **297**:162–163.

———, D. P. Stites, J. L. Caldwell, and J. V. Wells (eds.) (1976): "Basic and Clinical Immunology," Lange, Los Altos, Calif.

Fujimoto, S., M. I. Greene, and A. H. Sehon (1976): Regulation of the Immune Response to Tumor antigens, I: Immunosuppressor Cells in Tumor-bearing Hosts; II: The Nature of Immunosuppressor Cells in Tumor-bearing Hosts, *J. Immunol.*, **116**:791–806.

Gold, P., and S. O. Freedman (1965): Demonstration of Tumor-specific Antigens in Human Colonic Carcinomata by Immunologic Tolerance and Absorption Techniques, *J. Exp. Med.*, **121**:439–462.

Hellstrom, K. E., and I. Hellstrom (1974): Lymphocyte-mediated Cytotoxicity and Blocking Serum Activity to Tumor Antigens, *Adv. Immunol.*, **18**:209-277.
———and——— (1977): Cellular Immunity to Tumor-associated Antigens in Man, *N. Engl. J. Med.*, **296**:874-875.
Henle, W., and G. Henle (1974): Epstein-Barr Virus and Human Malignancies, *Cancer,* **34**:1368-1374.
Horwitz, D. A., and M. A. Garrett (1977): Distinctive Functional Properties of Human Blood L Lymphocytes: A Comparison with T Lymphocytes, B Lymphocytes and Monocytes, *J. Immunol.*, **118**:1712-1721.
Immunopotentiation, *Ciba Found. Sym.* 18, *1973*, Associated Scientific Publishers, Amsterdam.
Jacob, F., and J. Monod (1961): Genetic Regulatory Mechanisms in the Synthesis of Proteins, *J. Molec. Biol.*, **3**:318-356.
Klein, E., (1969): Hypersensitivity Reactions at Tumor Sites, *Cancer Res.*, **29**:2351-2362.
Kopersztych, S., and M. T. Rezkallah, S. S. Miki, C. K. Naspitz, and N. F. Mendes (1976): Cell-mediated Immunity in Patients with Carcinoma: Correlation between Clinical Stage and Immunocompetence, *Cancer,* **38**:1149-1154.
Morton, D. L. (1973): Immunotherapy of Cancer: Present Status and Future Potential, *Cancer,* **30**:1647-1655.
Nauts, H. C., G. A. Fowler, and F. H. Bogatko (1953): A Review of the Influence of Bacterial Infection and of Bacterial Products (Coley's Toxins) on Malignant Tumors in Man: A Critical Analysis of 30 Inoperable Cases Treated by Coley's Mixed Toxins, in Which Diagnosis Was Confirmed by Microscopic Examination: Selected for Special Study, *Acta. Med. Scand.*, **145** (suppl. 276):5-103.
———, W. E. Swift, and B. L. Coley (1946): The Treatment of Malignant Tumors by Bacterial Toxins as Developed by the Late William B. Coley, M.D., Review in the Light of Modern Research, *Cancer Res.*, **6**:205-216.
Nelson, D. S. (ed.) (1976): "Immunobiology of the Macrophage," Academic, New York.
Prehn, R. T. (1976): Do Tumors Grow Because of the Immune Response of the Host?, *Transplant. Rev.*, **28**:34-42.
Putnam, R. S. (1976): Cancer Antigens in Laboratory Diagnosis of Malignant Disease, pp. 1-14 in G. T. Race (ed.), "Laboratory Medicine," vol. 2, chap. 30, Harper & Row, Hagerstown, Md.
Rocklin, R. E., R. Gagel, Z. Feldman, and A. H. Tashjian (1977): Cellular Immune Responses in Familial Medullary Thyroid Carcinoma, *N. Engl. J. Med.*, **296**:835-838.
Roitt, I. (1977): "Essential Immunology," 3d ed., Blackwell, Oxford.
Rosenberg, S. A. (1976): Cancer Immunology, pp. 231-281 in A. M. Munster (ed.), "Surgical Immunology," Grune and Stratton, New York.
Schwartz, M. K. (1976): Detection of Tumor-associated Antigens in Plasma or Serum, *Clin. Immunobiol.*, **3**:405-426.
Schwartz, R. S. 1975. Current Concepts: Another Look at Immunologic Surveillance, *N. Engl. J. Med.*, **293**:181-184.
Sellers, A. H. (1971): The Clinical Classification of Malignant Tumors: The TNM System, *Can. Med. Ass. J.*, **105**:836-843.
Sjögren, H. O., I. Hellstrom, S. C. Bansal, and K. F. Hellstrom (1971): Suggestive Evidence That the "Blocking Antibodies" of Tumor-bearing Individuals May Be Antigen-Antibody Complexes, *Proc. Natl. Acad. Sci. USA*, **68**:1372-1375.
Takasugi, M., A. Ramseger, and J. Takasugi (1977): Decline of Natural Nonselective Cell-mediated Cytotoxicity in Patients with Tumor Progression, *Cancer Res.*, **37**:413-418.
———, M. R. Michey, and P. I. Terasaki (1974): Studies on Specificity of Cell-mediated Immunity to Human Tumors, *J. Natl. Cancer Inst.*, **53**:1527-1538.
Tse, H., and R. W. Dutton (1976): Separation of Helper and Suppressor T Lymphocytes on a Ficoll Velocity Sedimentation Gradient, *J. Exp. Med.*, **143**:1199-1210.
U.S. Department of Health, Education and Welfare, Public Health Service, National Institute of Allergy and Infectious Diseases (1976): Immunology: Its Role in Health and Disease: Summary Report of the Task Force on Immunology and Disease. *DHEW Pub.* (NIH)77-940.
Yonemoto, R. H., and P. I. Terasaki (1972): Cancer Immunotherapy with HLA-compatible Duct Lymphocyte Transplantation: A Preliminary Report, *Cancer,* **30**:1438-1443.
Yu, A., H. Watts, N. Jaffe, and R. Parkman (1977): Concomitant Presence of Tumor-specific Cytotoxic and Inhibitor Lymphocytes in Patients with Osteogenic Sarcoma., *N. Engl. J. Med.*, **297**:121-127.

11

Appendix: Syphilis Serology and Its Value in Diagnosis

APPENDIX: SEROLOGIC TESTS USED IN THE DIAGNOSIS OF SYPHILIS

Etiologic Agent of Syphilis and Factors Influencing Serologic Diagnosis

11-1 It is probably more important for the physician to understand the principles underlying laboratory tests used to help diagnose syphilis than for any other disease. Since 1949 great advances have been made in the development of specific serologic tests for syphilis, but there is still no completely satisfactory test. *Treponema pallidum*, the etiologic agent of syphilis, is a spirochete. Many conventional laboratory procedures used for diagnosis of infectious diseases cannot be applied to the diagnosis of syphilis. *T. pallidum* is stainable and fairly long, but its width is only 0.2 μm, just at the limit of the resolving power of the light microscope. *T. pallidum* is a spiral microorganism which can flex and bend; it is motile by rotation along the long axis, by bending and twisting, or by undulation from side to side. *T. pallidum* has not been grown on bacteriologic media, in tissue culture, or in the embryonated egg, but it does multiply in vivo in rabbit testicular tissue. There are recent reports of its growth in vitro, but the success of a method for cultivation of *T. pallidum* for antigen remains to be confirmed. *T. pallidum* is serologically related, if not serologically identical, to *T. pertenue* and *T. carateum,* which cause yaws and pinta, respectively. Since yaws and pinta occur mainly in the tropics and not in the United States, serologic cross reactions between pathogenic species of *Treponema* are not a major problem of laboratory diagnosis in this country.

Stages of Syphilitic Infection and Relationship to Serologic Diagnosis

11-2 Infection with *T. pallidum* induces two kinds of antibodies important for diagnosis: (1) nontreponemal antibodies, which react with cardiolipin, a nonspecific lipid hapten extracted from beef heart, and (2) species-specific antibodies, which react with *T. pallidum.* Group specific antibodies for the genus *Treponema* are also produced. Since tests used in diagnosis of syphilis often depend on the stage of the disease, the stages of syphilitic infection are reviewed below.

Primary syphilis The incubation period of syphilis is 2 to 8 weeks. Spirochetes multiply locally at the site of entry; some spread to lymph nodes and then to blood. The characteristic lesion of syphilis, known as a *chancre*, contains numerous spirochetes, persists for 10 to 14 days, and then heals spontaneously without leaving a scar. Blood serology is negative (nonreactive) during the first part of primary syphilis but becomes positive (reactive) before the chancre disappears.

Secondary syphilis Following healing of the primary lesion, the patient is asymptomatic for varying lengths of time (2 to 12 weeks) before the appearance of multiple secondary lesions in skin and mucous membranes. Secondary lesions also contain numerous spirochetes. Serologic tests for syphilis on infected individuals are reactive at this stage. The secondary lesions subside spontaneously.

Latent syphilis In latent syphilis there are no clinical symptoms of the disease. Serologic tests on blood serum are reactive, but those on spinal fluid are nonreactive. Latent syphilis may or may not be followed by tertiary syphilis.

Tertiary syphilis Not all untreated cases of syphilis progress to this stage. Tertiary syphilis may appear years later and is characterized by the development of granulomatous lesions (called *gummas*) in the skin, bones, and organs such as liver. These lesions probably are caused by cell-mediated hypersensitivity reactions to infection. Paresis and tabes dorsalis are caused by degenerative changes of the central nervous system. Clinical manifestations of tertiary syphilis are highly diverse. Spirochetes are present in the tertiary lesions but only in small munbers. At this stage, serologic tests for syphilis usually are positive if tests with specific antigen are employed. Serologic tests on blood serum with the nonspecific cardiolipin hapten are not reliable for diagnosis of tertiary syphilis.

Congenital syphilis A child may be infected in utero if the mother has syphilis. Adequate treatment of an infected woman before the fifth month of pregnancy prevents congenital syphilis. Syphilitic infection of the fetus may result in miscarriage, stillbirth, an infant with lesions at birth, or an infant who may not develop signs of congenital syphilis until childhood. Early diagnosis of congenital syphilis is very important.

Identification of *T. pallidum* in Lesions of Primary and Secondary Syphilis

11-3 Two procedures used at present for identification of *T. pallidum* in lesions are (1) dark-field examination and (2) direct fluorescent-antibody (FA) technique. The primary lesion of syphilis is a chancre, which appears where the spirochete enters the body and multiplies. Spirochetes usually are numerous enough in chancre fluid to be detectable by microscopic examination. When the primary lesion of syphilis first becomes manifest, serologic tests for syphilis on the blood serum may still be negative; therefore, detection in chancre fluid of spirochetes with characteristics of *T. pallidum* may allow the earliest possible diagnosis of syphilis. Material for examination of chancre fluid should be collected before antibiotics are given because the treponemes usually disappear from the lesion within a few hours after administering antibiotics. Material should be collected from the base of the chancre. When collecting chancre fluid, physicians should wear rubber gloves to protect against accidental infection. The lesion should be cleansed with a gauze sponge wet with physiological saline or water but not with antiseptics or soap. The lesion is dried and abraded with a dry gauze sponge to cause exudation of tissue fluid. The clear serous exudate collected with capillary tubing from the base of the lesion is the material that should be examined because this fluid is more likely to contain motile treponemes.

11-4 Dark-field examination of chancre-fluid wet mount This is not a serologic test but is discussed here in order to compare the technique with direct FA for detection of *T. pallidum* in lesions of syphilis. Material collected as described in Sec. 11-3 is placed on a clear glass slide, and a cover glass is applied.

This preparation is called a *wet mount.* At least two slides should be prepared and examined immediately. An ordinary light microscope with a dark-field condenser is required; the treponemes appear bright against a dark background. Although it is difficult to observe *T. pallidum* in stained smears with the light microscope, this organism shows up fairly well by dark-field examination of wet mounts. *T. pallidum* can be seen as a very thin, delicate corkscrew-shaped organism with an average of 8 to 14 regular, rigid, tightly coiled, deep spirals. *T. pallidum* is usually 6 to 14 μm long with an average of 10 μm; its width is approximately 0.2 μm. Motility of *T. pallidum* can be observed in wet mounts and is one of the characteristics which helps distinguish this organism from other spirochetes. The coiled appearance of *T. pallidum* is retained despite active motility. Forward and backward movements as well as rotation about the long axis can be observed. *T. pallidum* exhibits little flexibility and does not move rapidly from place to place. Dark-field examination for detection of *T. pallidum* has been carried out for many years and is a well-accepted method, but it has the following drawbacks: (1) *T. pallidum* can be confused with nonpathogenic spirochetes such as *T. microdentium* in the mouth and *T. genitalis* in the genital area; (2) the wet-mount slides must be examined immediately while the treponemes are still motile; (3) in order to obtain reliable results, the examination must be made by someone who has had considerable experience in differentiating *T. pallidum* from other spirochetes on the basis of structure and kind of motility.

11-5 Direct fluorescent-antibody technique This technique can be used for detection of *T. pallidum* in suspected syphilitic lesions. When results obtained with the dark-field method described above and the direct FA technique were compared, there was good correlation between the two tests. For the direct FA technique, serous fluid from the lesion to be examined is placed on a slide, allowed to dry, and fixed. A drop of antiserum containing specific antibody conjugated with fluorescein isothiocyanate, a fluorescent dye, is added to the dried and fixed smear of chancre fluid. After a suitable incubation period, the slide is washed, dried, and examined with an ultraviolet-light microscope. All ultraviolet-light microscopes have a dark-field condenser. If *T. pallidum* spirochetes are present on the smear, the labeled antibodies attach and are not removed by washing, so that the spirochetes show a yellowish-green fluorescence against the dark background. The tightly coiled spiral structure of the organism can be clearly visualized (Fig. 11-1). The direct FA test for *T. pallidum* in lesions is known by several abbreviations, such as FADF (fluorescent antibody dark field) and DFATP (direct fluorescent antibody *T. pallidum*). The direct FA method has several advantages over the dark-field wet

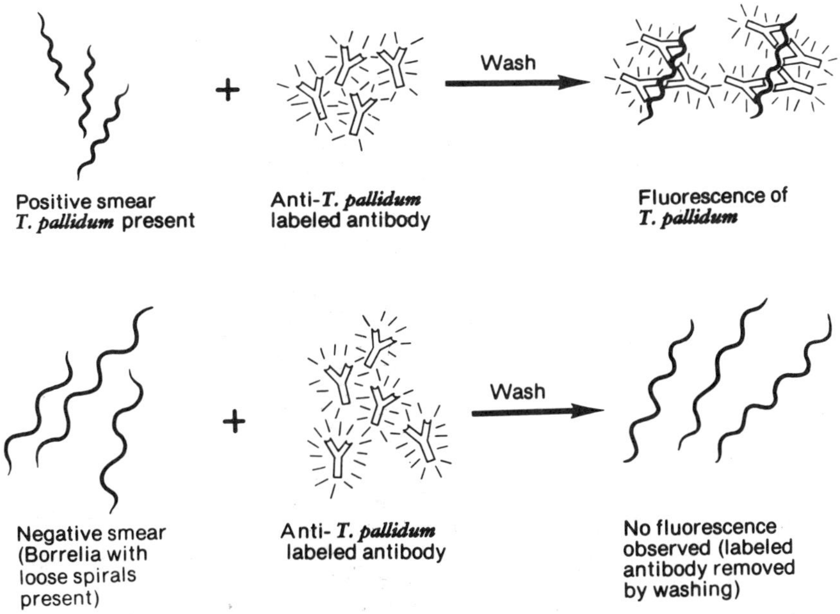

Figure 11-1 Direct fluorescent-antibody technique on exudates from suspected syphilitic lesions. Antibody is labeled with fluorescein isothiocyanate.

mount in that (1) the slide does not have to be examined immediately and (2) the slide can even be shipped to another laboratory for staining and examination. The principle and method of the direct FA technique for detection of *T. pallidum* on a slide is the same as the direct FA technique for detection of other organisms, e.g., group A streptococci (review Sec. 4-42).

11-6 The antiserum used to perform the above test is usually obtained from a patient with a high titer of antibodies to *T. pallidum.* In order to eliminate cross reactions with nonpathogenic treponemes, such as *T. microdentium*, the antiserum is absorbed with a suspension of the nonpathogenic Reiter strain. Since the Reiter strain is a nonpathogenic species of *Treponema* which can be grown in culture, a sufficient amount can be obtained to absorb out group-specific antibodies for the genus *Treponema* without absorbing species-specific antibodies for *T. pallidum.* After suitable incubation, the nonpathogenic treponemes used for absorption are removed by centrifugation. The supernatant fluid should contain antibodies specific for *T. pallidum.* The direct FA test carried out with absorbed antiserum is useful for the examination of smears from suspected syphilitic lesions in the mouth. The absorbed antiserum should not react with nonpathogenic treponemes such as *T. microdentium.*

Questions for Secs. 11-1 to 11-6

1. (*a*) Why is it difficult to see *T. pallidum* in stained smears using the light microscope? (*b*) Why is it difficult to obtain specific antigen for serologic tests?

2. (*a*) Do all cases of untreated syphilis progress to the tertiary stage? (*b*) What is meant by latent syphilis?

3. When a primary chancre suggestive of syphilitic infection appears, what general procedure usually allows the earliest possible diagnosis of syphilis? Why?

4. (*a*) What two methods are used for the detection of *T. pallidum* in lesions? (*b*) What are the advantages and disadvantages of these two methods?

Answers

1. (*a*) Although *T. pallidum* is stainable, it is very narrow and therefore difficult to observe with the light microscope. (*b*) *T. pallidum* has never been cultured in the laboratory in a way to obtain a sufficient quantity for antigen. (Sec. 11-1.)

2. (*a*) No. (*b*) A patient with latent syphilis shows no clinical evidence of syphilis at the time but does have a reactive serologic test on blood serum. (Sec. 11-2.)

3. The examination of the chancre fluid for spirochetes characteristic of *T. pallidum* usually allows the earliest possible diagnosis of syphilis because in primary syphilis the chancre may appear before the blood serum gives a positive serologic test for syphilis. (Sec. 11-3.)

4. (*a*) The two methods are the dark-field examination of wet mounts and the direct FA technique. (*b*) For the dark-field examination no special equipment or reagents are needed except a microscope with a dark-field condenser. The technique does require a person with a great deal of experience in recognizing the organism, and even so, it is difficult to differentiate between *T. microdentium* and *T. pallidum* by this method when the lesion is in the mouth. The direct FA test requires a special ultraviolet-light microscope and special reagents but has the advantage that slides can be shipped to a laboratory equipped to carry out this test. Also this serologic technique allows differentiation between *T. pallidum* and morphologically similar oral treponemes if antiserum is used which has been absorbed with nonpathogenic species of *Treponema.* A culture of the Reiter strain is usually employed for absorption. (Secs. 11-4 to 11-6.)

Serologic Tests for Reagins Using Cardiolipin as "Antigen"

11-7 Principle of tests for reagins of syphilis Serologic tests for syphilis (STS) at first employed nonspecific nontreponemal cardiolipin "antigens." The first test for syphilis, the Wassermann test, was developed in 1906. This test and the many others which followed up to 1949 were all carried out with nontreponemal "antigens." As pointed out previously, infection of a human host with *T. palli-*

dum brings about the formation of antibodies of two basic types; one type has its specificity directed to antigens of the microorganism; the specificity of the other type is to a lipid component of mammalian tissue, now known as cardiolipin. Antibodies of the second type, called *reagins*, are not specific for *T. pallidum*; they are induced following the interaction of *T. pallidum* with tissue. Cardiolipin, extracted from beef heart with alcohol, is employed as "antigen" in nontreponemal serologic tests for syphilis. Cardiolipin fits the definition of a hapten but not of an antigen. Purified cardiolipin is diphosphatidylglycerol. See Fig. 11-2 for the chemical structure of cardiolipin.

11-8 A brief historical description of the development of tests for syphilis employing nontreponemal antigens will help explain the choice of beef-heart-extracted cardiolipin for "antigen" and the origin of the term reagin. Since *T. pallidum* had not been grown in culture, Wassermann used as antigen in 1906 an extract of syphilitic fetal liver. Noting that spirochetes were very numerous in the liver of stillborn syphilitic infants, he thought that an extract of this tissue would contain antigens of the spirochetes. His extract of infected liver tissue seemed to work satisfactorily as antigen. A few years later, it was found that an extract of normal liver tissue reacts in the same manner. Furthermore, it was shown that a number of animal organs contain the active principle, which was determined to be lipoidal. Beef heart was chosen as the source of antigen because the Forssman antigen, which is widely distributed in nature and is responsible for many cross reactions, is not present in the tissues of cattle. It is important to choose a tissue devoid of Forssman antigen since many normal individuals have heterophile antibodies to it (for a review of the Forssman antigen, see Sec. 4-2).

11-9 The term reagin was used instead of antibody because it was difficult then for anyone to believe that the host would produce antibodies to his own tissue. Although it is generally accepted that syphilis reagin is an autoantibody, the real nature of the antibody has not been studied extensively and is not well understood. It has been shown that syphilis reagin may be IgG and IgM. It is not IgE. Since the term reagin has been used also with IgE antibody in atopy, some physicians refer to syphilis reagin as Wassermann antibody in order to avoid confusion. How antibody is formed to homologous lipid hapten is still a matter of conjecture. It has been postulated that tissue destruction by *T. pallidum* causes the lipid hapten to be exposed so that the body reacts to this exposed hapten (in combination with protein) as though it were foreign (or a neoantigen) and produces antibody to it. Another mechanism postulated for the production of autoantibody is that *T. pallidum* growing in vivo reacts with cardiolipin in such a way that *T. pallidum* acts as a foreign protein carrier for bound cardiolipin, which acts as an immunogenic determinant. Another theory states that mammalian tissue and *T. pallidum* have a common antigen and a cross reaction occurs. The common-antigen theory is not widely accepted. The observation that antibodies to cardiolipin are also produced in other diseases where considerable tissue damage occurs lends support to the theory that reagins of syphilis are produced as autoantibodies. Reagins produced in syphilis do not seem to play any role in pathogenesis of the disease and disappear as the patient responds to treatment.

11-10 Several times in the preceding pages reference has been made to positive test results as reactive and to negative test results as nonreactive. The use of new terminology for reporting results of serologic tests for syphilis was recommended in the 1953 report of the National Advisory Serology Council to the Surgeon General of the U.S. Public Health Service. The new system provided uniformity of

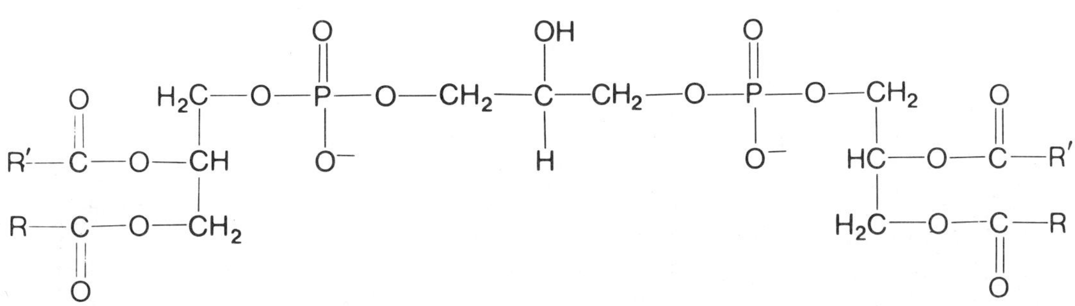

Figure 11-2 Chemical structure of cardiolipin (diphosphatidylglycerol).

reporting and avoided diagnostic connotations. In accordance with these recommendations, the terms *reactive*, *weakly reactive*, and *nonreactive* were substituted for the terms positive, weakly positive or doubtful, and negative in reporting test results by laboratories in the United States.
11-11 Although serologic tests for syphilis employing cardiolipin are not specific, they are still valuable provided physicians are aware of the limitations of these tests (Secs. 11-15 and 11-16). Some of the reasons serologic tests employing cardiolipin are still widely used are the following:

Reliability: when supported by clinical findings and history of syphilis, reactive tests have a high degree of reliability.

Cost and ease of performance: the extract of beef heart (cardiolipin) used to perform these tests is easy to obtain and relatively inexpensive, in contrast to *T. pallidum* antigen. The test procedures can be carried out easily and rapidly.

Screening tests: because of the low cost and ease of performance, tests for reagins are valuable as screening tests.

Evaluation of therapy: the reagin titer of quantitative tests drops noticeably as the patient responds to therapy (Sec. 11-27)

Aid in diagnosis of suspected congenital syphilis: the reagin titer of quantitative tests rises if the child is infected but drops if the reagins were acquired by transplacental passage (Sec. 11-30).

Flocculation Tests for Reagins

11-12 The nontreponemal antigen tests are basically of two types, complement-fixation tests and flocculation tests. The Wassermann test, the first complement-fixation test for syphilis, was later modified by several investigators. The Kolmer test was one of the most successful modifications; now, however, complement-fixation tests for syphilis are seldom done (for the procedure of the complement-fixation test, review Sec. 4-38). Complement-fixation tests for reagins are more difficult to perform and have been replaced almost entirely by flocculation tests. Lecithin and cholesterol are added to cardiolipin to increase its reactivity. In the VDRL test (developed by the Veneral Disease Research Laboratory), the clear solution of cardiolipin with lecithin and cholesterol is mixed just before use with buffered saline to form a colloidal suspension. The cardiolipin collects around insoluble cholesterol to form a micelle. Lecithin increases the sensitivity of the reaction. When this "antigen" preparation is mixed with serum free of reagin, the particles (micelles) remain dispersed, but when antibody is present, aggregation of the particles occurs. This type of aggregation usually is called flocculation.
11-13 The first flocculation test for syphilis was developed in 1933 and was known as the *Kahn test.* Over the years many flocculation tests were developed to test for reagins of syphilis, including the Hinton, Kline, Mazzini, VDRL, USR (unheated serum reagin), and RPR (rapid plasma reagin). The basic mechanisms of these flocculation tests are the same. They require as reagents besides the patient's serum only cardiolipin and saline. These tests were developed in an attempt to increase sensitivity and specificity. The sensitivity of the test refers to the abiltiy to react in the presence of syphilis; specificity refers to the property of not reacting in the absence of syphilis. Sensitivity and specificity are often delicately balanced. Some extremely sensitive tests sacrifice specificity. Probably the VDRL and RPR are used more frequently now than other flocculation tests. They are reliable and easy to perform. The RPR test is a passive agglutination test. In this test, cardiolipin is adsorbed on charcoal particles so that the test can be carried out on white cards and agglutination easily observed macroscopically.
11-14 When syphilis of the central nervous system is suspected, spinal fluid should be collected and tested for antibodies. Reagins in the blood do not pass the blood-brain barrier to reach the spinal fluid. A reactive test for reagins carried out on spinal fluid indicates that tissue of the central nervous

system is infected with *T. pallidum.* The flocculation tests used with spinal fluid are essentially the same as those used for blood serum. Only slight modifications are required.

Biologic False Positive Reactions

11-15 When results obtained with nontreponemal antigen tests such as the VDRL or RPR are reactive on the serum of a patient with no history or clinical evidence of syphilis, the physician should consider the possibility that the patient has a biologic false positive (BFP) reaction and does not have syphilis. The patient's serum should be rechecked by a test employing treponemal antigen. Patients exhibiting BFP reactions are often found to have associated infections or neoplastic or autoimmune diseases. Table 11-1 summarizes some of the conditions in which BFP reactions have been reported. They may be of a temporary or chronic nature; chronic cases are much more perplexing. There are fewer BFP reactions observed today with tests employing nontreponemal antigens than were observed a number of years ago. BFP reactions are less frequent since cardiolipin was purified in 1942 by Pangborn. For example, when the sera of patients with malaria were tested against purified cardiolipin, the number of BFP reactions approached zero; tested against crude lipoidal antigen, the number of BFP reactions approached 100 percent.

False Negative Serologic Reactions

11-16 False negative reactions may occur in patients in the very early stages of primary infection. Fuimara et al. (1956) reported that during the first week of primary syphilis, reagins can be detected in the serum of 25 percent of patients; second week, 50 percent; third week, 75 percent; and by the fourth week all patients with syphilis have a positive test. Most physicians are aware of the possibility of a negative or nonreactive test for syphilis during the early stages of syphilitic infection so that a

Table 11-1 Nonsyphilitic Conditions in Which BFP Reactions for Reagins Have Been Reported

Bacterial infections	Chancroid Leprosy Mycoplasma pneumonia Pneumococcal pneumonia Rat-bite fever Scarlet fever Subacute bacterial endocarditis Tuberculosis (advanced)
Spirochetal diseases	Relapsing fever Leptospirosis
Rickettsial infections	Typhus
Chlamydial infection	Lymphogranuloma venereum Trypanosomiasis
Viral infections	Chickenpox Infectious hepatitis Infectious mononucleosis Measles
Protozoan diseases	Malaria
Autoimmune diseases	Lupus erythematosus Periarteritis nodosa Rheumatoid arthritis Rheumatic fever
Neoplasia	
Heroin addiction	
Following immunizations	DTP Vaccinia

negative or nonreactive test at this stage usually does not present a serious problem. It is important for physicians to be aware that in secondary or tertiary syphilis, serologic tests for reagins may be nonreactive. In many cases it has been shown that the nonreactive results obtained were due to a prozone reaction. Most of the tests used today to detect reagins are flocculation tests, which are subject to prozone reactions. These reactions occur when there is a large excess of antibody in relation to antigen. A patient's serum with a very high titer of reagins could be responsible for a prozone reaction. Prozone reactions can be detected by dilution of the serum (review Sec. 4-7).

11-17 It has been estimated that prozone reactions occur in 1 to 2 percent of sera from patients with secondary syphilis. The sera of patients with tertiary syphilis tested for reagins give a much higher percentage of negative reactions: about 10 percent of patients with late benign syphilis; 20 percent with cardiovascular symptoms; and 33 percent with clinical tabes dorsalis or involvement of the central nervous system. These percentages cited vary from test to test, but it should be emphasized and reemphasized that a large percentage of patients with tertiary syphilis will show a negative or nonreactive test for reagins. Many of these nonreactive tests in tertiary syphilis have been found to be due to a prozone reaction and become reactive or positive when the serum is diluted. Spangler and associates (1964) studied a number of such cases, one of which is summarized here.

Case of syphilis involving the central nervous system A 38-year-old woman with a negative blood test for syphilis had a history of right-sided focal seizures of 8 months' duration. Her behavior in general was observed to be both childish and irascible. She was referred to a psychiatrist and received electric shock therapy. After 3 months she was discharged but given maintenance shock therapy at a local hospital for the next 3 weeks. An encephalogram was done and she was referred to the neurological service of the hospital with a diagnosis of possible brain tumor. Additional tests were made, including a *T. pallidum* immobilization (TPI) test, which was positive. A quantitative serologic test for reagins was positive in the following dilutions:

Undil	1:2	1:4	1:8	1:16	1:32	1:64	1:128
–	–	+	+	+	+	+	–

In all, three routine serologic tests for reagins were made and were nonreactive before the quantitative reagin test was performed and also the specific test with treponemal antigen. The patient was placed on penicillin therapy and made a remarkable recovery. Serologic tests employing specific treponemal antigens are much more reliable for diagnosis of tertiary syphilis than tests employing cardiolipin extracted from beef heart. Table 11-2 shows the comparative sensitivity of nontreponemal and treponemal tests in tertiary syphilis.

11-18 The 1969 U.S. Public Health Service Manual for Syphilis states that weakly reactive or "rough" nonreactive results obtained in the VDRL test may be due to prozone reactions. The manual further states, "that it is therefore recommended that all serums producing weakly reactive or 'rough' nonreactive results in the qualitative test be retested by using the quantitative procedure before a report of the VDRL slide test is submitted." Garner and Grantham (1968) reported that of 519 "rough" VDRL serum specimens, 189 were reactive in the *T. pallidum* immobilization (TPI) test. Their results emphasize the importance of recognizing a false negative reaction.

Questions for Secs. 11-7 to 11-18

5. (*a*) Are reagins antibodies? (*b*) Are the reagins observed in syphilitic infection the same as the IgE reagins observed in atopy? (*c*) What other name has been given to syphilis reagins? (*d*) With which of the following antigens or haptens do syphilis reagins react, cardiolipin extracted from beef heart or *T. pallidum*? (*e*) Why was beef heart chosen as the source for cardiolipin? (*f*) Does the term Wassermann antibody refer just to reagin detected in the Wassermann test or to all syphilis reagins (regardless of the name of the test) provided cardiolipin is employed?

6. Give two theories to explain the production of reagins.

7. Why are the terms reactive and nonreactive preferred to positive and negative for recording the results of serologic tests for syphilis?

8. Why are tests for reagins still considered valuable tests in the diagnosis of syphilis?

9. A patient has a reactive VDRL test but no history or clinical evidence of syphilis. Could the physician confirm that this was not a BFP reaction by doing an RPR test? Explain your answer.

10. A pregnant woman is found to have a reactive VDRL test. She has no history or clinical evidence of syphilis. Should the physician wait and try to find out if she has a BFP reaction before treating her? Explain your answer.

11. What does a reactive test on spinal fluid indicate?

12. What are some of the conditions responsible for BFP reactions?

13. A doctor sees a patient with symptoms that are suggestive of tertiary syphilis. A VDRL test is negative. The test is repeated and is still negative. Should the physician decide on the basis of two negative tests for reagins that the patient does not have syphilis and look for another diagnosis? Explain your answer.

14. Explain how an excess of antibody interferes with flocculation in the VDRL test and is responsible for the prozone reaction.

Answers

5. (*a*) Yes. (*b*) No. (*c*) Wassermann antibody. (*d*) Cardiolipin. (*e*) It does not contain Forssman antigen. Nonsyphilitic serum may contain antibodies to Forssman antigen, which is widely distributed in nature. (*f*) All. (Secs. 11-7 to 11-9.)

6. Reagins may be produced to a normal tissue component because of autoimmunization or because tissue and *T. pallidum* possess a common antigen. There is more support for the theory of autoimmunization. (Sec. 11-9.)

7. The terms reactive and nonreactive standardize the way of reporting and emphasize that test results alone should not be used by the physician to make a diagnosis of syphilis. (Sec. 11-10.)

8. There are several reasons, e.g., the tests for reagins are inexpensive and simple to perform, they usually give reliable results if interpretation of test results is made in the light of clinical findings, and the titer of reagins drops during treatment, which aids in evaluation of therapy. (Sec. 11-11.)

9. No. The VDRL and RPR tests are based on the same principle and employ similar antigens which are nonspecific. The physician should send the patient's serum to a laboratory for a test with the specific treponemal antigen. (Secs. 11-13 and 11-15.)

10. No. As soon as the physician has evidence that a pregnant woman has syphilis, she should be treated to protect the baby. However, the physician should collect another sample of blood to send to a laboratory for a specific serologic test with treponemal antigen. (Secs. 11-2 and 11-15.)

11. Infection with *T. pallidum* has reached the central nervous system. (Sec. 11-14.)

12. Persons with infectious diseases may show BFP reactions but especially patients with autoimmune diseases such as lupus erythematosus. Patients with various other conditions such as heroin addiction may show BFP reactions. (Sec. 11-15.)

13. No. If there is evidence of tertiary syphilis, two nonreactive VDRL tests are not sufficient reason for the doctor to change the diagnosis. It is known that tests for reagins are often nonreactive in tertiary syphilis. The physician should request a quantitative VDRL test in order to rule out a prozone reaction and also have a test run with specific treponemal antigen because such tests are usually reactive in tertiary syphilis. (Secs. 11-16 and 11-17.)

14. In the prozone reaction there are a very large number of antibody molecules in relation to antigen combining sites. These sites are rapidly saturated by antibodies. Antigen and antibodies are not present in proportions which allow lattice formation or in this case flocculation. Steric hindrance may be partially responsible. (Sec. 11-17.)

Serologic Tests for Syphilis with the Specific Causative Agent, as Antigen

11-19 The first test for syphilis using the specific causative organism was the *T. pallidum* immobilization test (TPI), described in 1949 by Nelson and Mayer. This was a major breakthrough for a number of reasons: it showed that the host produces immobilizing antibodies to *T. pallidum*, and it provided a means for recognizing BFP reactors. The TPI test was difficult to carry out because it required motile treponemes and complement besides the patient's serum. If specific antibody was present, the actively moving treponemes were immobilized. For the TPI and other specific tests for syphilis, *T. pallidum* is propagated in the rabbit testicle, separated from testicular tissue, and used as antigen. The TPI test is seldom used now except as a reference test. It is useful when diagnostic problems arise.

Fluorescent *Treponema* Antibody-Absorption Test (FTA-ABS)

11-20 The FTA-ABS test, an indirect fluorescent-antibody test, is now used extensively in the diagnosis of syphilis. The patient's serum is absorbed with the Reiter strain to remove antibodies to nonpathogenic treponemes. This absorbed serum is added to a smear of *T. pallidum* on a slide, a suitable time is allowed for incubation, and the slide is washed to remove antibodies not attached to *T. pallidum.* To this is added serum containing antibodies to human globulin labeled with fluorescein isothiocyanate. The preparation is incubated again and washed to remove the antibodies which failed to attach to the human globulin. The slide is dried and examined by the ultraviolet-light microscope for fluorescence. Fluorescence of *T. pallidum* indicates that the patient did have antibodies to the specific organism. Reactions in this test are diagrammed in Fig. 11-3.

11-21 The FTA-ABS test can be carried out more easily than the TPI test and has the advantage that live organisms are not required. The antigen can be stored at 6 to 10°C or processed by lyophilization. Smears fixed in acetone or methanol and dried can be stored at −20°C for a long time. At first when the FTA test was used, the patient's serum was diluted in order to dilute out group-specific cross-reacting antibodies to nonpathogenic treponemes such as *T. microdentium* in the mouth, but this method proved too insensitive. The test is made more sensitive by absorbing out antibodies to nonpathogenic species of treponemes rather than diluting these antibodies out. The procedure for the

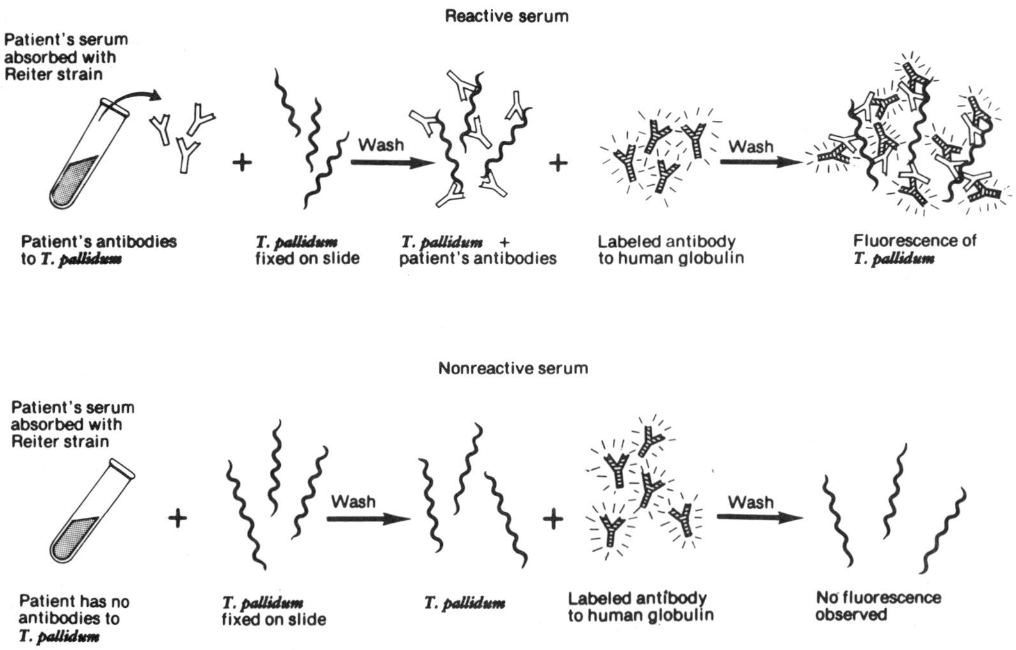

Figure 11-3 The FTA-ABS test for syphilis on patients' sera employing the indirect fluorescent-antibody technique.

FTA-ABS test is standardized now, and commercial reagents are available from several manufacturers.

11-22 The FTA-ABS test is one of the best tests available for differentiating between patients with BFP reactions and those with syphilis. This test should be used also for patients with tertiary syphilis. Table 11-2 shows the comparative sensitivity of nontreponemal and FTA and TPI treponemal tests in untreated syphilis. The FTA-ABS test was the most sensitive for detection of primary syphilis. Duncan, Knox, and Wende, (1974) report that the FTA-ABS test was performed on 77 consecutive patients with dark-field positive primary syphilis and that the FTA-ABS test was positive in 70 (91 percent) of these patients. The FTA-ABS test does not distinguish between syphilis and other treponematoses such as yaws and pinta and is not useful in measuring the effectiveness of therapy.

11-23 In a study by Mackey and associates (1969) on the specificity of the FTA-ABS test, among 827 persons tested there were 5 with a reactive FTA-ABS test but a nonreactive TPI test accompanied by no clinical evidence or history of syphilis. Three of these had diseases in which abnormal globulins are frequently found. All were more than 50 years old. Whether these five cases represented old syphilis or false positive reactions with the FTA-ABS test was not known. It was emphasized that an absolute diagnosis of syphilis cannot be made on the basis of a serologic test alone and that the management of patients with a questionable diagnosis of syphilis must depend on the total evaluation of each individual case. There also have been reports that FTA-ABS test results on some patients with lupus erythematosus may show spirochetes with an atypical beaded appearance. At present the patient's serum to be examined by the FTA-ABS test is absorbed with Reiter protein in an attempt to remove antibodies for nonpathogenic treponemes. The specificity of the FTA-ABS test might possibly be improved if antigens from still other nonpathogenic treponemes could be used for absorption of serum before carrying out the test.

T. pallidum Hemagglutination Test

11-24 The *T. pallidum* hemagglutination test (TPHA) is an indirect, or passive, hemagglutination test in which *T. pallidum* is adsorbed on the surface of red blood cells (review the technique of passive hemagglutination in Secs. 4-16 and 4-17). Although the passive hemagglutination technique was investigated many years ago for detection of specific antibodies to *T. pallidum*, only recently have the procedure and reagents been standardized for performance of this test in hospital laboratories. The test has the following advantages: (1) it is simple to perform; (2) the reagents are available commercially; (3) no special equipment such as an ultraviolet-light microscope is required. The Nichols strain of *T. pallidum* propagated in the rabbit testicle is used for antigen. This is the same strain of *T. pallidum* which is used for the FTA-ABS test. Sheep red blood cells tanned and preserved by treatment with formaldehyde serve as carriers for *T. pallidum.* The patient's serum is absorbed with a mixture of cultured nonpathogenic treponemes (Reiter strain), sheep and beef red blood cells, and normal testicular tissue. The absorption mixture is designed to remove antibodies which could give

Table 11-2 Comparative Sensitivity of Treponemal and Cardiolipin Tests in Untreated Syphilis at Different Stages of Infection

Stage of syphilitic infection	Sera expected to give reactive test results, %*			
	FTA-ABS (*T. pallidum*)	*T. pallidum* immobilization test (TPI)	VDRL slide (cardiolipin)	Kolmer CF† (cardiolipin)
Primary	86	53	76	65
Secondary	100	98	100	100
Latent, early	99	94	95	95
Late	96	89	72	65
Tertiary	97	93	70	60

*These values are approximate; †CF = complement fixation. Data from Syphilis: A Synopsis, *U.S. Public Health Serv. Publ.* 1660, 1968.

false positive results. The absorption mixture would remove antibodies to nonpathogenic treponemes which cross-react with *T. pallidum*, antibodies to the carrier red blood cells, or antibodies to the tissue in which *T. pallidum* is propagated. To carry out the hemagglutination test, the patient's absorbed serum is mixed with sheep red blood cells on which *T. pallidum* has been adsorbed. In addition, the absorbed serum is mixed with control normal sheep red blood cells. Hemagglutination is read by allowing the red blood cells to settle out and observing the pattern of settling on the bottom of the tubes or wells in a microtiter plate. Agglutinated cells form a mat of cells on the bottom of the tubes. This result is interpreted as a reactive serum. Cells which do not agglutinate form a compact button, and this reaction is interpreted as nonreactive.

11-25 The sensitivity of the TPHA test compares favorably with that of the FTA-ABS test except that the TPHA test is less sensitive than the FTA-ABS test in early primary syphilis but slightly more sensitive than the VDRL test. In the tertiary stage, the sensitivity of the TPHA test is as high as that of the FTA-ABS test. With regard to specificity, there are reports in the literature that the TPHA test failed to recognize certain BFP reactions. One advantage of the TPHA test over the FTA-ABS test is that intact treponemes are not required. In the future it may be possible to sensitize erythrocytes with an antigen specific for *T. pallidum* alone in order to achieve a completely specific serologic test.

Enzyme-Linked Immunosorbent Assay with *T. pallidum* Antigen

11-26 The enzyme-linked immunosorbent assay (ELISA) technique, using an ultrasonicate of *T. pallidum* as antigen, is now being evaluated as a serological test for syphilis. The ELISA technique adapted for serodiagnosis of syphilis appears simple and reliable with its sensitivity in all stages of syphilis equal to that of the FTA-ABS test, even in early primary syphilis. ELISA also appears to be highly specific and to be able to distinguish BFP reactions. Like the TPHA test, the ELISA technique has the advantage of not requiring intact *T. pallidum.* The ELISA technique is relatively new; it is now being used experimentally for the diagnosis of many diseases besides syphilis. The general procedure for this test was described in Sec. 4-57. ELISA adapted for syphilis was described by Veldkamp and Vissir (1975). ELISA and the other specific treponemal tests described above can be carried out using micro techniques. This conserves *T. pallidum* antigen, which is propagated by infection of rabbit testicular tissue. The use of *T. pallidum* antigen in micro volumes helps to compensate for our inability to culture it.

Questions for Secs. 11-19 to 11-26

15. (*a*) What was the first specific serologic test for syphilis? (*b*) How was it carried out? (*c*) What is the source of *T. pallidum* for the TPI and the FTA-ABS tests?

16. (*a*) Is intact living *T. pallidum* required for the FTA-ABS test? (*b*) What is the mechanism of the FTA-ABS test?

17. (*a*) Does the serum of persons with yaws and pinta show a reactive FTA-ABS test? Explain your answer. (*b*) Why has it been difficult to study the antigenic composition of *T. pallidum*?

18. (*a*) Does the TPHA test require intact *T. pallidum*? (*b*) What is the mechanism of this test? (*c*) How do the results obtained with this test compare with those obtained with FTA-ABS test?

19. With what substance(s) is antibody labeled for (*a*) the FTA-ABS and (*b*) the ELISA test?

Answers

15. (*a*) *T. pallidum* immobilization (TPI) test. (*b*) By mixing the patient's serum with complement and motile *T. pallidum* and after incubation observing microscopically for immobilization. (*c*) Infected rabbit testicle. (Sec. 11-19.)

16. (*a*) Intact but not living *T. pallidum* is required. (*b*) The FTA-ABS test is based on the indirect FA test. The patient's serum is absorbed to remove antibodies to nonpathogenic treponemes and then added to a smear of *T. pallidum* fixed on a slide. If antibodies to *T. pallidum* are present in the patient's serum, they combine with antigen and are not removed by washing; next they are demonstrated by reaction with fluorescein-labeled antihuman globulin. (Secs. 11-20 and 11-21.)

17. (*a*) Yes. The causative agents of yaws and pinta, *T. pertenue* and *T. carateum*, respectively, are very similar antigenically to *T. pallidum*. (*b*) It is difficult to obtain a pure preparation of *T. pallidum* for study since it must be separated from rabbit testicular tissue. (Secs. 11-19 and 11-22.)

18. (*a*) *T. pallidum* but not intact. (*b*) Passive hemagglutination. (*c*) Less sensitive than FTA-ABS in early primary syphilis. (Secs. 11-24 and 11-25.)

19. (*a*) Fluorescein isothiocyanate. (*b*) Enzyme (alkaline phosphatase). (Secs. 11-20 and 11-26.)

Quantitative Serologic Tests for Reagins of Syphilis to Evaluate Effectiveness of Treatment

11-27 Since reagins disappear from the serum as the patient is freed from infection with *T. pallidum*, quantitative reagin tests employing cardiolipin afford a means of evaluating the effectiveness of treatment. Because antibodies to *T. pallidum* persist longer, tests for these antibodies, e.g., the FTA-ABS, TPHA, and other tests for specific antibodies with the exception of IgM (see Sec. 11-31), are not useful for evaluation of treatment. Adequate treatment of syphilis is shown by a decline in titer of reagins. On the other hand, a rising titer may indicate a recent infection, reinfection in an adequately treated patient, relapse in an adequately treated patient, or an acute false positive reaction.

11-28 Whenever a reactive VDRL test is observed in a diagnostic laboratory, a quantitative test is also carried out and the highest dilution which gives a reactive test is reported to the physician. This gives valuable information for use in following the patient's response to treatment. After treatment of primary syphilis, titers become nonreactive in 6 to 12 months; for secondary syphilis, in 12 to 18 months. The serum of some cases of tertiary syphilis remain reactive in low titer regardless of the amount of treatment. The reason for this is not understood. Table 11-3 shows a typical serologic response of a patient with secondary syphilis to treatment. The effectiveness of treatment is followed at intervals by the VDRL test. In the same report from which the data in Table 11-3 were taken, a patient with primary syphilis was found to have a reactive VDRL test on a 1:2 dilution of serum at the time therapy was started. Approximately 4 months later the serum became nonreactive.

Significance of IgM Antibodies to *T. pallidum* in Serum from Newborn Infants

11-29 Antibodies of the IgM class are the first kind of antibodies produced in response to infection (review Sec. 3-5). IgM antibodies are produced in utero if infection is acquired from the mother before birth. The presence of IgM antibodies to *T. pallidum* in the blood serum from a newborn infant is evidence that the child was infected in utero and has congenital syphilis. IgG but not IgM antibodies

Table 11-3 Response of a Patient with Secondary Syphilis to Therapy

	VDRL slide test	
Days after therapy	Qualitative	Quantitative
0	Reactive	1:64*
34	Reactive	1:32
65	Reactive	1:16
91	Reactive	1:4
118	Reactive	1:4
180	Weakly reactive	Undiluted
245	Nonreactive	
299	Nonreactive	

*Highest dilution of patient's serum to show flocculation. Data from Syphilis: A Synopsis, *U.S. Public Health Serv. Publ.* 1660, 1968.

may be transferred from mother to the fetus transplacentally. IgM antibodies to *T. pallidum* in an infant's serum can be detected by a modified FTA-ABS procedure. The modification varies from the standard FTA-ABS test in that specific antihuman IgM labeled with fluorescein isothiocyanate is used instead of labeled anti-human globulin, which reacts with all classes of immunoglobulins. The test for IgM antibodies is known as the FTA-ABS (IgM) test. It was hoped that this test would allow the physician to take a baby's blood at birth, send it to the laboratory, and a few days later receive a report on whether or not the child was infected in utero. Then an infected child could be treated immediately. The FTA-ABS test for IgM is still in the experimental stages, but results at the present time are disappointing in that nonreactive results are not reliable. In cases of congenital syphilis, only reactive FTA-ABS (IgM) tests are useful to the physician. Some of the false negative FTA-ABS (IgM) tests in congenital syphilis may be associated with the fact that the main antibody response to *T. pallidum* is IgG. IgM is formed first and then a switch occurs, so that IgM is present in much smaller amounts than IgG. Also some babies with late-onset type of congenital infection may not develop IgM antibodies to *T. pallidum* until several weeks after birth.

11-30 Adequate treatment of a syphilitic pregnant woman before the fifth month of pregnancy should prevent congenital syphilis; however, a child born of a syphilitic mother without evidence of infection should be carefully followed for several months. For many years quantitative reagin tests such as the VDRL have been used to differentiate between an infected child and a child which received antibodies by way of the placenta from the mother. The main antibody response to cardiolipin is reported to be the production of IgM reagins, but IgG reagins which pass the placenta are also formed. If a child whose serum was reactive at birth is followed by quantitative tests for reagins, a falling titer indicates catabolic loss of passively transferred reagins; a rising titer indicates active infection requiring treatment. The same is true for antibodies to *T. pallidum*, which are mainly IgG. *T. pallidum* antibodies passively transferred from mother to fetus do not persist but are catabolized; a rising titer in the child's serum indicates infection. Both types of quantitative tests, those for reagins and those for antibodies to *T. pallidum*, have the disadvantage of taking several weeks to determine whether the antibody titer is falling or rising. During this time, the physician could lose contact with mother and child.

The Effect of Treatment on IgM Antibodies to *T. pallidum*

11-31 It has been observed that during treatment the titer of IgM antibodies to *T. pallidum* drops more rapidly than the titer of specific IgG antibodies. This is true for both children and adults. It appears that within a few months following adequate treatment for syphilis, patients stop producing IgM antibodies to *T. pallidum* but continue to produce specific IgG for several years. The drop in specific IgM antibodies during treatment is not as rapid as the drop in reagins (review Sec. 11-27). The The FTA-ABS (IgM) test is not performed routinely but offers valuable information when it is carried out properly.

Summary of Serologic Tests for Syphilis

11-32 Serologic tests for syphilis are summarized in Table 11-4.

Questions for Secs. 11-27 to 11-32

20. Which antibodies disappear much earlier from the serum of a syphilitic patient during therapy, (*a*) reagins which react with cardiolipin or (*b*) antibodies to *T. pallidum*?

21. What is the difference between a qualitative and a quantitative VDRL test?

22. What is the significance of IgM antibodies to *T. pallidum* in the serum of a newborn child?

23. What is the significance of a rising titer of reagins or of antibodies to *T. pallidum* in the serum of a child following birth whose mother had syphilis during pregnancy?

24. What is the significance of a decreasing titer of reagins or of antibodies to *T. pallidum* in the serum of a child following birth whose mother had syphilis during pregnancy?

Table 11-4 Expected Serologic Test Results in Different Stages of Syphilis, Untreated and Following Treatment

Stage of syphilitic infection or treatment	Chancre fluid, Direct FA	Serum				
		VDRL or RPR	TPHA	FTA-ABS	FTA-ABS IgG	FTA-ABS IgM
Primary, early	R	NR	NR	R	R	R
Late	R	R	R	R	R	R
Treated	Not done	NR	R†	R†	R†	NR
Secondary	R	R	R	R	R	R
Treated	Not done	NR	R†	R†	R†	NR
Tertiary	Not done	R or NR	R	R	R	R
Treated	Not done	NR?	R†	R†	R†	NR?
Congenital	R (if lesions)	R	R	R	R	R
Treated	Not done	NR	R†	R†	R†	NR

*R = reactive; NR = nonreactive.

†After several years these tests may become nonreactive.

25. If only IgG antibodies to *T. pallidum* are detected in the serum of a newborn child born of a syphilitic mother, should the physician still follow the antibody titer after birth? Explain your answer.

26. Is there a difference in the rate of disappearance of IgG and IgM antibodies to *T. pallidum* following treatment? Explain your answer.

Answers

20. (*a*) Reagins. (Sec. 11-27.)

21. The qualitative VDRL test for reagins tells only whether or not reagins are present, while the quantitative test gives the amount or titer of reagins. Since it takes several months for a VDRL test to become completely nonreactive during treatment, the quantitative test tells the physician whether the titer of reagins is dropping. (Sec. 11-28.)

22. Since IgM antibodies to *T. pallidum* do not pass the placenta, their presence in the serum of a newborn infant indicates infection in utero. (Sec. 11-29.)

23. Syphilis reagins have been found in both IgG and IgM immunoglobulins; IgG reagins cross the placenta, so that an infant's blood at birth may contain reagins if the mother had syphilis. A titer of reagins in the infant's serum that continues to rise after birth indicates that the infant was infected in utero. The same is true for specific antibodies to *T. pallidum.* (Sec. 11-30.)

24. If the titer of syphilis reagins in the serum of an infant decreases after birth (without treatment), this indicates that the child is not infected and the reagins were acquired transplacentally from the mother. The same is true for antibodies to *T. pallidum.* (Sec. 11-30.)

25. Yes. A nonreactive FTA-ABS (IgM) test here is unreliable. In order to be sure that the infant was not infected in utero, the physician should continue to observe the infant and check the infant's serum for reagins and antibodies to *T. pallidum* and ascertain that the titer of these antibodies has dropped and not increased. (Sec. 11-30.)

26. Yes. Following treatment for syphilis, the body usually stops making IgM antibodies to *T. pallidum* but continues for some time to make IgG antibodies. (Sec. 11-31.)

REFERENCES

Briody, B. A., and R. E. Gillis (1974): "Microbiology and Infectious Disease," McGraw-Hill, New York.

Cannefax, G. R., L. C. Norins, and E. J. Gillespie (1967): Immunology of Syphilis, *Annu. Rev. Med.*, **18**:471-482.

Duncan, W. C., J. M. Knox, and R. D. Wende (1974): The FTA-ABS Test in Dark-field-positive Primary Syphilis, *JAMA*, **228**:859-860.

Fitzgerald, J. J., J. N. Miller, and J. A. Sykes (1975): *Treponema pallidum* (Nichols Strain) in Tissue Culture: Cellular Attachment, Entry, and Survival, *Infect. Immunol.*, **11**:1133-1140.

———, B. Appel, W. Hill, and H. Mescon (1956): Syphilis and Its Management: Present-Day Problem, *New Engl. J. Med.*, **254**:1127-1130.

Fuimara, N. J. (1963): Biologic False Positive Reaction for Syphilis: Massachusetts, 1954-1961, *New Engl. J. Med.*, **268**:402-405.

Garner, M. F., and N. M. Grantham (1968). The VDRL Test: Significance of "Rough" Results, *Br. J. Vener. Dis.*, **44**:131-133.

———, J. L. Blackhouse, G. Daskalopoulos, and J. L. Walsh (1973): *Treponema pallidum Haemagglutination* (TPHA) Test in Biological False Positive and Leprosy Sera, *J. Clin. Pathol.*, **26**:258-260.

Johnston, N. A. (1972): Neonatal Congenital Syphilis: Diagnosis by the Absorbed Fluorescent Treponemal Antibody (IgM) Test, *Br. J. Vener. Dis.*, **48**:464-469.

Jue, R., J. Puffer, R. M. Wood, G. Schochet, W. H. Smartt, and W. A. Ketterer (1967): Comparison of Fluorescent and Conventional Darkfield Methods for the Detection of *Treponema pallidum* in Syphilitic Lesions, *Am. J. Clin. Pathol.*, **47**:809-811.

Julian, A. J., L. C. Logan, and L. C. Norins (1969): Early Syphilis: Immunoglobulins Reactive in Immunofluorescence and Other Serologic Tests, *J. Immunol.*, **102**:1250-1259.

Kaufman, R. E., D. C. Olansky, and P. J. Wiesner (1974): The FTA-ABS (IgM) Test for Neonatal Congenital Syphilis: A Critical Review, *J. Am. Vener. Dis. Ass.*, **1**:79-84.

———, S. Weiss, J. D. Moore, V. Falcone, and P. J. Wiesner (1974): Biological False-positive Serological Tests for Syphilis among Drug Addicts, *Br. J. Vener. Dis.*, **50**:350-353.

Kellogg, D. S. (1970): The Detection of *Treponema pallidum* by a Rapid, Direct Fluorescent Antibody Darkfield (DFATP) Procedure, *Health Lab. Sci.*, **7**:34-41

Kraus, S. J., J. R. Haserick, and M. A. Lantz (1970): Fluorescent Treponemal-Antibody-Absorption Test Reactions in Lupus Erythematosus: Atypical Beading Pattern and Probable False-positive Reactions, *New Engl. J. Med.*, **282**:1287-1290.

Leskiski, J., J. Krach, and E. Kadziewicz (1974): Specificity, Sensitivity and Diagnostic Value of the TPHA Test, *Br. J. Vener. Dis.*, **50**:334-339.

Mackey, D. M., E. V. Price, J. M. Knox, and A. T. Scotti (1969): Specificity of the FTA-ABS Test for Syphilis, *JAMA*, **207**:1683-1685.

Moore, J. E., and C. F. Mohr (1952): Biologically False Positive Serologic Tests for Syphilis: Type, Incidence and Cause, *JAMA*, **150**:467-473.

Nelson, R. A., Jr., and M. M. Mayer (1949): Immobilization of *Treponema pallidum in Vitro* by Antibody Produced in Syphilitic Infection, *J. Exp. Med.*, **89**:369-393.

Nicholas, L., and H. Beerman (1965): Present Day Serodiagnosis of Syphilis: A Review of some of the Recent Literature, *Am. J. Med. Sci.*, **249**:466-483.

O'Neill, P. (1976): A New Look at the Serology of Treponemal Disease, *Br. J. Vener. Dis.*, **52**:296-299.

———and C. S. Nicol (1972): IgM Class Antitreponemal Antibody in Treated and Untreated Syphilis, *Br. J. Vener. Dis.*, **48**:460-463.

Pangborn, M. C. (1942): Isolation and Purification of a Serologically Active Phospholipid from Beef Heart, *J. Biol. Chem.*, **143**:247-256.

Pusch, A. L. (1974): Serodiagnostic Tests for Syphilis and Other Diseases, pp. 1216-1238 in I. Davidson and J. B. Henry (eds.), "Todd-Sanford Clinical Diagnosis by Laboratory Methods," 15th ed., Saunders, Philadelphia.

Schroeter, A. L., J. B. Lucas, E. V. Price, and V. H. Falcone (1972): Treatment for Early Syphilis and Reactivity of Serologic Tests, *JAMA*, **221**:471-476.

Spangler, A. S., J. H. Jackson, N. J. Fuimara, and T. A. Warthin (1964): Syphilis with a Negative Blood Test Reaction, *JAMA*, **189**:87-90.

Sparling, P. F. (1971): Diagnosis and Treatment of Syphilis, *New Engl. J. Med.*, **284**:642-653.

Shore, R. N. (1974): Hemagglutination Tests and Related Advances in Serodiagnosis of Syphilis, *Arch. Dermatol.*, **109**:854-857.

U. S. Department of Health, Education, and Welfare, Public Health Service, Communicable Disease

Center, Venereal Disease Branch (1969): Manual of Tests for Syphilis, *Pub.* 411.
Veldkamp, J., and A. M. Vissir (1975): Application of the Enzyme-linked Immunosorbent Assay (ELISA) in the Serodiagnosis of Syphilis, *Br. J. Vener. Dis.*, **51**:227-231.
Wilkinson, A. E., and P. Rodin (1976): IgM-FTA Test in Syphilis in Adults: Its Relation to Clinical Findings, *Br. J. Vener. Dis.*, **52**:219-223.
Wood, R. M. (1976): Tests for Syphilis, pp. 341-351 in N. R. Rose and H. Friedman (eds.), "Manual of Clinical Immunology," American Society for Microbiology, Washington, D.C.
Wright, D. J. M., M. H. Lessof, A. S. Grumble, D. Doniach, J. L. Turk, and R. D. Catterall (1970): New Antibody in Early Syphilis, *Lancet*, **1970**(1):740-744.

Review Questions

Review each case cited; select the appropriate substance(s) used for immunization from the list of vaccines and globulins (normal and immune) and other choices and record in the first column. In the second column state whether the type of immunization is active (Ac), passive (Pa), both (Ac and Pa), or no answer (NA).

A. Sabin vaccine
B. Salk vaccine
C. Tetanus toxoid
D. Tetanus antitoxin
E. Specific bacterial vaccine
F. Normal adult globulin
G. Diphtheria toxoid
H. Diptheria antitoxin
I. Rabies duck-embryo vaccine (DEV)
J. Rabies antiserum
K. Influenza whole-virus vaccine
L. Influenza split-virus vaccine
M. Vaccinia
N. BCG vaccine
O. BCG seldom used in the United States for immunization
P. Should not be given
Q. Material not listed
R. No vaccine available

1. Routine immunization of child against poliomyelitis with attenuated virus ____ ____
2. Booster tetanus injection of previously immunized child ____ ____
3. Treatment of child diagnosed as having diphtheria ____ ____
4. Immunization of adult with deep lacerations from accident; no known immunization for tetanus ____ ____
5. Adult bitten on leg by rabid dog ____ ____
6. Adult bitten on face by rabid dog ____ ____
7. Treatment of child with agammaglobulinemia ____ ____
8. Immunization of adult for influenza ____ ____
9. Immunization of child for influenza ____ ____
10. Patient requests immunization for gonorrhea and syphilis ____ ____
11. Pregnant women requests immunization for German measles (rubella) ____ ____
12. Routine immunization of healthy child for whooping cough ____ ____
13. For purpose of travel, immunization of nonpregnant healthy woman for smallpox ____ ____
14. For purpose of travel, immunization of child with immunodeficiency disorder for smallpox ____ ____
15. Parent inquires about immunization of child for tuberculosis ____ ____

Answers

1. A; Ac
2. C; Ac
3. H; Pa
4. C and D; Ac and Pa
5. I; Ac
6. I and J; Ac and Pa
7. F; Pa
8. K; Ac
9. L; Ac,
10. R; NA
11. P; NA
12. E; Ac
13. M; Ac
14. P; NA
15. O; NA

Select the best answer (one) from the list of cells below. An answer may be used more than once.

A. B lymphocytes	B. T lymphocytes	C. Null cells
D. Plasma cells	E. Lymphoblasts	F. Macrophages
G. Monocytes	H. Neutrophils	I. Basophils
J. Eosinophils	K. Mast cells	L. Memory cells
M. Kupffer cells	N. Histiocytes	O. Osteoclasts

_____ **16.** Main cells of reticuloendothelial system
_____ **17.** Blood leukocytes which are precursor cells of macrophages
_____ **18.** Antibody-producing cells
_____ **19.** Cells shown to have immunoglobulin receptors for antigen recognition
_____ **20.** Lymphocytes transformed after stimulation by antigens or mitogens to undergo clonal expansion
_____ **21.** Cells concerned with production of cell-mediated immunity or delayed-type hypersensitivity
_____ **22.** Lymphocytes of both B and T cell origin which are responsible for the anamnestic response
_____ **23.** Cells which act as helper cells in antibody production to certain antigens
_____ **24.** Cells which act as suppressor cells to regulate the immune response
_____ **25.** Blood leukocytes which bind IgE and after reaction with antigen undergo degranulation with release of vasoactive amines
_____ **26.** Tissue cells which contain numerous intracytoplasmic granules and are associated with atopy and anaphylaxis
_____ **27.** Cells which release lymphokines after activation and reexposure to specific antigen
_____ **28.** Lymphocytes without identifying surface markers for either B or T cells
_____ **29.** Cells which form rosettes with sheep red blood cells
_____ **30.** Lymphocytes which characteristically have Fc receptors for IgG

Answers

16. F	**17.** G	**18.** D	**19.** A	**20.** E
21. B	**22.** L	**23.** B	**24.** B	**25.** I
26. K	**27.** B	**28.** C	**29.** B	**30.** A

Select the best answer from the list of immunoglobulins, immunoglobulin allotypes, fragments, etc. An anwer may be used more than once.

A. IgG	B. IgM	C. IgA
D. IgD	E. IgE	F. Fab
G. $F(ab')_2$	H. Fc	I. Heavy chains
J. Light chains	K. Variable region	L. Constant region
M. Km	N. Gm	O. Am

_____ **31.** Immunoglobulin found in secretions; contains a secretory component
_____ **32.** Region of immunoglobulin molecule responsible for idiotypy or antigen specificity
_____ **33.** Divalent fragment obtained by pepsin digestion; causes precipitation but cannot fix complement
_____ **34.** Fragment obtained by papain digestion; it is monovalent and inhibits precipitation of antigen by specific antibodies
_____ **35.** Only immunoglobulin known to be capable of transplacental passage
_____ **36.** Antibody with longest half-life; responsible for effectiveness of passive immunization of children with agammaglobulinemia
_____ **37.** Antibody formed first during primary active immunization
_____ **38.** Composition of Bence Jones proteins found in urine of patients with multiple myeloma

_____ 39. Part of immunoglobulin molecule associated with complement fixation, transplacental passage, and attachment to mast cells
_____ 40. Immunoglobulin produced when infection occurs in utero
_____ 41. Immunoglobulin which is homocytotropic in human beings
_____ 42. Monovalent immunoglobulin fragment which contains part or all of both heavy and light chains
_____ 43. Part of immunoglobulin molecule responsible for specificity of immunoglobulin class
_____ 44. Immunoglobulin found in macroglobulinemia during abnormal proliferation of malignant plasma-cell clone
_____ 45. Immunoglobulin present as receptor on B lymphocytes of newborn but appearing to have little, if any, recognized antibody activity
_____ 46. Antibody detected by Jerne plaque technique (direct method)
_____ 47. Immunoglobulin with structure of pentamer and with J chain, which secretory IgA also has
_____ 48. Part of immunoglobulin molecule composed of either kappa or lambda chains
_____ 49. Immunoglobulin present in highest concentration in normal human serum
_____ 50. Immunoglobulin present in lowest concentration in normal human serum
_____ 51. Allotypic marker present on the heavy chain of IgG
_____ 52. Allotypic marker present on immunoglobulins with kappa chains
_____ 53. Allotypic marker present on the heavy chains of IgA_2
_____ 54. Allotype formerly known as InV
_____ 55. Region of molecule in which hinge is found

Answers

31. C	32. K	33. G	34. F	35. A
36. A	37. B	38. J	39. H	40. B
41. E	42. F	43. I	44. B	45. D
46. B	47. B	48. J	49. A	50. E
51. N	52. M	53. O	54. M	55. L

For each set of reagents used in the cases described below employing diagnostic serologic tests, select the most approximate name for the test from the list. An answer may be used only once.

A. Agglutination
B. Passive hemagglutination
C. Hemagglutination inhibition
D. Coombs test (direct)
E. Precipitation
F. Agar-gel diffusion Elek test
G. Complement-fixation test
H. Neutralization
I. Direct fluorescent-antibody test
J. Indirect fluorescent-antibody test
K. Quellung reaction
L. ASO titration

_____ 56. Red blood cells (tanned) with thyroglobulin adsorbed on surface + serum of patient suspected of having autoimmune disease
_____ 57. Suspension of *Brucella abortus* + serum of patient with symptoms of brucellosis
_____ 58. Tissue-culture cells + poliomyelitis virus type 1 + serum of child believed to have poliomyelitis
_____ 59. Rubella virus (4 HA units) + serum of pregnant woman thought to have been exposed to German measles (rubella) + 1-day-old chicken rbc
_____ 60. Suspension of *Rickettsia rickettsii* + serum of patient suspected of having Rocky Mountain spotted fever + fresh guinea pig serum; after incubation, addition of sheep rbc + antibody to sheep rbc
_____ 61. Culture of *Corynebacterium diphtheriae* isolated from a school teacher suspected of being a carrier of an exotoxin-producing strain + petri dish of nutrient agar medium containing

a sterile filter-paper strip saturated with diphtheria antitoxin (culture streaked on agar across antitoxin strip at right angles to it)

_____ 62. Washed red blood cells from newborn infant with symptoms of erythroblastosis fetalis (mother Rh-negative) + anti-human globulin

_____ 63. Culture of beta-hemolytic streptococci from inflamed throat of patient + antiserum to group A *Streptococcus pyogenes* containing antibodies labeled with fluorescein isothiocyanate

_____ 64. Spirochetes of *Treponema pallidum* fixed on slide + serum of patient suspected of having syphilis; after incubation and washing of slide, addition of anti-human globulin labeled with fluorescein isothiocyanate

_____ 65. Antiserum to C-reactive protein + serum of patient with symptoms of rheumatic fever (C-reactive protein is not an antibody but an abnormal protein detectable in sera of patients with acute inflammatory diseases)

_____ 66. *Hemophilus influenzae* from spinal fluid + antiserum containing antibodies to type b polysaccharide capsule

_____ 67. Serum of child who earlier had throat infection with beta-hemolytic streptococci + commercial streptolysin (hemolysin); after incubation, addition of rabbit rbc

Answers

56. B	57. A	58. H	59. C
60. G	61. F	62. D	63. I
64. J	65. E	66. K	67. L

For each case select the most appropriate diagnostic method to be used from the list below. An answer may be used only once.

A. Immediate allergic skin test
B. Delayed allergic skin test
C. Immunoelectrophoresis
D. Radial immunodiffusion
E. Reversed passive hemagglutination
F. Radioimmunoassay
G. Schick test
H. Response of lymphocytes to PHA
I. Mixed lymphocyte reaction (MLR)
J. Cytotoxicity (dye-exclusion) test

_____ 68. A surgeon would like to determine that the blood to be used in an operation does not contain hepatitis B virus. What is the most sensitive method for this purpose?

_____ 69. Another surgeon wants to determine that the blood to be used does not contain hepatitis B virus, but the hospital does not have the equipment for the most sensitive test (like that for Question 68). What is another very sensitive method that does not require expensive equipment to perform?

_____ 70. A surgeon would like to determine that a patient is not sensitive to horse protein because it is planned to inject him with antilymphocyte globulin (from horse) before transplantation. What test is usually employed?

_____ 71. An intern would like to know whether or not she has been exposed to tuberculosis. What is the method of the test she would use?

_____ 72. Because of an outbreak of four cases of diphtheria in the state a school physician would like to know whether or not the pupils (all of whom have been immunized against diphtheria) are resistant. What test was developed to screen for susceptibility to diphtheria?

_____ 73. A child has recurrent bacterial infections. A physician would like to determine whether the child has agammaglobulinemia. What method can be used?

_____ 74. What method can be used to determine the amount of C3 complement component in a patient's serum?

_____ 75. What test can be made on the cells of a patient who appears to be lacking in cell-mediated immunity?

_____ 116. Complement
(1) Is a heat-stable protein found in guinea pig serum
(2) Is made up of four components
(3) Is increased by immunization
(4) Is fixed by IgG or IgM and the specific antigen

_____ 117. The Rh antigen
(1) Is present on red blood cells but not on tissue cells
(2) May cause erythroblastosis fetalis if the mother is Rh-negative and the fetus is Rh-positive
(3) May cause a transfusion reaction if Rh-positive blood is given to an Rh-negative patient
(4) May cause rejection of an allograft if the donor is Rh-positive and the recipient is Rh-negative

_____ 118. Atopy may be caused by inhalation of the following allergens:
(1) Pollens of plants
(2) Mites in house dust
(3) Animal danders
(4) Mold spores

_____ 119. The following contribute to the Arthus reaction:
(1) Precipitins and specific antigen
(2) Complement
(3) Polymorphonuclear leukocytes
(4) Endotoxin

_____ 120. Donors with blood group O:
(1) Have natural alloantibodies to A and B blood-group antigens in their sera
(2) Have neither A nor B antigens on their red blood cells
(3) Have H antigen on their red blood cells
(4) Can act as universal blood donors in an emergency because their red blood cells would not be agglutinated by either anti-A or anti-B antibodies if present in serum of the recipient.

Answers

111. A	112. A	113. C	114. E	115. A
116. D	117. A	118. E	119. A	120. E

Answer the question by selecting A, B, C, D, or E according to the scheme below:

A. If 1, 2, and 3 are correct
B. If 1 and 3 are correct
C. If 2 and 4 are correct
D. If only 4 is correct
E. If all are correct

_____ 121. Lymphokines are
(1) Soluble proteins produced by sensitized or activated T lymphocytes after reaction with specific antigen
(2) Macrophage, neutrophil, or eosinophil chemotactic factors
(3) Macrophage-activating factor or migration-inhibition factor (MIF)
(4) Involved in cell-mediated immunity and delayed-type hypersensitivity reactions

_____ 122. With regard to delayed-type hypersensitivity (DTH) or cell-mediated immunity (CMI)
(1) The Koch phenomenon was one of the first, if not the first, example of DTH or CMI to tuberculosis
(2) A positive tuberculin skin reaction is an example of DTH
(3) BCG vaccine containing an attenuated strain of *M. bovis* causes an immunized person

to develop a positive tuberculin skin reaction
(4) Both Freund's adjuvant (complete) and BCG vaccine stimulate the cells of the reticuloendothelial system

_____**123.** With regard to anergy
(1) Patients with advanced cases of tuberculosis often become anergic
(2) Patients with advanced cases of fungus diseases such as blastomycosis often become anergic
(3) Patients with advanced cases of cancer often become anergic
(4) Anergy may be reversed by antibiotic therapy in case of infection or by surgery, adjuvant immunotherapy, or chemotherapy in the case of cancer

_____**124.** With regard to activation of T lymphocytes
(1) T lymphocytes can be activated by contact with the specific or corresponding antigen
(2) The events following activation of T lymphocytes may be favorable to the host or harmful, depending on the particular situation
(3) T lymphocytes are activated by mitogens such as phytohemagglutinin (PHA)
(4) In vitro, more T lymphocytes are activated by contact with a mitogen than by contact with a specific antigen

_____**125.** With regard to rejection of grafts
(1) The first-set rejection is caused mainly by delayed-type hypersensitivity reactions
(2) The white graft is caused mainly by delayed-type hypersensitivity reactions
(3) Autografts and syngrafts are not rejected
(4) Allografts were formerly called heterografts and are rejected

_____**126.** With regard to tissue typing for transplantation
(1) HLA antigens on lymphocytes are used for tissue typing
(2) Typing sera are obtained from multiparous women
(3) The HLA antigen at the D locus is one of the most important to match to prevent rejection
(4) Preformed cytotoxic antibodies in serum of recipient to donor cells do not cause graft rejection

_____**127.** With regard to autoimmune diseases
(1) Host response to self tissue is believed to cause injury
(2) Incidence increases with age
(3) Some autoimmune diseases are associated with genetic factors which determine HLA antigens
(4) Autoimmune diseases may be antibody-mediated or cell-mediated

_____**128.** Rheumatoid factor
(1) Is an IgM molecule but may also be IgG
(2) Reacts with altered Fc region of homologous IgG
(3) Is elevated in sera of patients with rheumatoid arthritis
(4) Can be detected by agglutination of latex particles coated with IgG when mixed with serum of a patient with rheumatoid arthritis

_____**129.** Contact dermatitis
(1) Requires covalent bonding between small molecules and skin protein
(2) Occurs in the condition known as poison ivy
(3) Occurs when DNCB (dinitrochlorobenzene) is applied to human or guinea pig skin
(4) Sensitivity can be passively transferred with serum of the patient

_____**130.** The following tests use heterophile antibodies:
(1) Weil-Felix test for rickettsial infections
(2) Widal test for typhoid fever
(3) Paul-Bunnell test for infectious mononucleosis
(4) Elek test for toxigenic strains of diphtheria

Answers

121. E	122. E	123. E	124. E	125. B
126. A	127. E	128. E	129. A	130. B

Answer the question by selecting A, B, C, D or E according to the scheme below:

A. If 1, 2, and 3 are correct
B. If 1 and 3 are correct
C. If 2 and 4 are correct
D. If only 4 is correct
E. If all are correct

_____ 131. Macrophages
(1) Are phagocytic cells and are important in host resistance
(2) Interact with antigen, helper T cells, and B cells for induction of antibody formation to T-cell-dependent antigens
(3) Usually act in a nonspecific manner but can be specifically "armed" with antibodies or with substances (possibly T-cell receptors) released by interaction of T cells with antigen
(4) In tissue are usually observed in close association with lymphoid cells during an immunologic reaction

_____ 132. With regard to antibody formation
(1) T-cell-independent antigens or immunogens are large polymers such as pneumococcal polysaccharide with many copies of the same determinant group per molecule
(2) T-cell-independent immunogens appear to induce mainly IgM antibodies
(3) T-cell-dependent immunogens induce formation of antibodies to both IgM and IgG, which appears after IgM
(4) T-cell receptors combine with the carrier and B-cell receptors with the hapten when helper T cells and B cells interact to induce antibody

_____ 133. Monoclonal proteins
(1) Are produced by a malignant plasma-cell clone
(2) May be either IgG, IgM, IgA, or IgE
(3) Are found in multiple myeloma
(4) Are heterogenous proteins

_____ 134. In Waldenström's macroglobulinemia
(1) Immunoglobulins produced have been called pathological immunoglobulins, paraproteins, and M proteins
(2) Immunoglobulins produced in excessive amounts by a single clone have the same specificity (variable region is the same)
(3) Production of IgG is depressed
(4) Excessive production of immunoglobulin (one class) can be observed in immunoelectrophoresis

_____ 135. T-cell immunodeficiency of a child can be reconstituted or helped by
(1) Thymus transplant
(2) Adoptive immunization
(3) Transfer factor
(4) Answers (1) to (3) may all cause a graft-versus-host reaction

_____ 136. Specific immunological tolerance can be induced experimentally by
(1) Immunosuppressive drug
(2) Removal of spleen
(3) Antilymphocyte serum to T cells in general
(4) Injection of an antigen

_____ 137. The following cells or immune complexes are removed from blood by macrophages:
(1) Rh-positive red blood cells which have reacted with anti-Rh antibodies
(2) Red blood cells which have reacted with autoantibodies
(3) Platelets which have reacted with antibodies
(4) Large immune complexes formed with IgM

_____ 138. Children with only B-cell deficiency have
(1) Hypogammaglobulinemia
(2) Depletion of paracortical region of lymph nodes
(3) Normal resistance to viral infections
(4) Normal resistance to bacterial infections

_____ 139. In congenital syphilis or in child born of a syphilitic mother
(1) IgG reagins pass the placenta
(2) Reagins in the child's serum increase in titer if the child is infected
(3) Reagins in the child's serum decrease in titer if the child is not infected
(4) Detection in the newborn of IgM antibodies to *T. pallidum* by a modified FTA test indicates fetal infection

_____ 140. The serum of a patient with a biologic false positive reaction for syphilis
(1) Is positive with tests for reagins with cardiolipin
(2) Is negative with tests with the specific *T. pallidum* antigen
(3) Is negative with the TPI and FTA-ABS tests for syphilis
(4) May be positive with both VDRL and RPR tests

Answers

131. E	132. E	133. A	134. E	135. A
136. D	137. E	138. B	139. E	140. E

Answer by selecting A, B, C, D, or E according to the scheme below:

A. If 1, 2, and 3 are correct
B. If 1 and 3 are correct
C. If 2 and 4 are correct
D. If only 4 is correct
E. If all are correct

_____ 141. Complement is required for
(1) Opsonic adherence of Rh-positive cells with attached anti-Rh antibodies
(2) Immune C3b adherence
(3) Antibody-dependent cytolysis by K cells
(4) Specific lysis of group A or group B red blood cells by their respective antibodies

_____ 142. Anti-Rh_0 (D) antibodies as a cause of erythroblastosis fetalis have the following properties:
(1) They are IgG and are divalent
(2) They do not fix complement, possibly because of the sparse distribution of Rh antigen on the red-blood-cell surface
(3) They do not agglutinate specific Rh_0 (D-positive) red blood cells when the cells are suspended in saline
(4) They do agglutinate Rh_0 (D-positive) red blood cells when the zeta potential is reduced following suspension in albumin, a colloidal medium, or by treatment with enzyme

_____ 143. With regard to the Schick test for susceptibility to diphtheria
(1) The test is carried out with diphtheria toxoid and is read in 96 h
(2) The test is based on neutralization of toxin by antitoxin
(3) If an erythematous reaction followed by a brown desquamation of the skin occurs at the injection site of test material, the patient had neutralizing antibody

(4) A negative test indicates that a reaction between skin-test antigen and neutralizing antitoxin occurred and the patient is resistant

_____**144.** Specific antiglobulin reagent has many uses, such as the following:
(1) Agglutination of Rh-positive cells with IgG attached (suspended in saline) by spanning the zeta potential
(2) Agglutination of red blood cells with autoantibodies attached
(3) In blood matching to detect a very small amount of antibody on the blood cells
(4) In the indirect fluorescent-antibody technique

_____**145.** B lymphocytes have the following characteristics
(1) They have Ig surface receptors for antigen recognition
(2) They have Fc receptors for IgG
(3) They form EA or Fc rosettes
(4) They have receptors for complement component C3

_____**146.** With regard to systemic lupus erythematosus
(1) Patients often have a biologic false positive reaction for syphilis
(2) May have a positive test for rheumatoid factor
(3) Characteristically have antinuclear antibodies
(4) Have glomerulonephritis with the same smooth pattern of immunofluoresence along the basement membrane as that seen with Goodpasture's syndrome

_____**147.** Evidence at the present time indicates that cancer cells are destroyed by
(1) Sensitized T lymphocytes
(2) Armed macrophages
(3) K cells responsible for antibody-dependent cytolysis
(4) A phenomenon known as immunological enhancement

_____**148.** With regard to killer cells
(1) T lymphocytes which react directly with target cells by virtue of target-cell receptors are sometimes called killer cells
(2) Cells which are responsible for antibody-dependent cytolysis (ADC) are called killer or K cells
(3) Killer cells may cause destruction of cancer cells in patients with cancer or normal tissue cells following transplantation
(4) Killer cells require complement for their action

_____**149.** K cells have the following properties
(1) They do not have receptors for target cells
(2) Their Fc receptors react with antibodies on target cells
(3) They take part in a reaction often referred to as antibody-dependent cytolysis (ADC) or antibody-dependent cell-mediated cytotoxicity (ADCC)
(4) They are small mononuclear cells in peripheral blood and spleen, but their exact identity is not clear

_____**150.** Oncofetal antigens such as CEA
(1) Often are not found in the serum of a patient during the early stages of cancer
(2) May be found in very small amounts in the sera of persons without cancer
(3) Are usually found in the serum of a patient in large amounts after metastasis occurs
(4) Have limited diagnostic value at present

Answers

141. C	**142.** E	**143.** C	**144.** E	**145.** E
146. A	**147.** A	**148.** A	**149.** E	**150.** E

Index